THE BODY DIVIDED

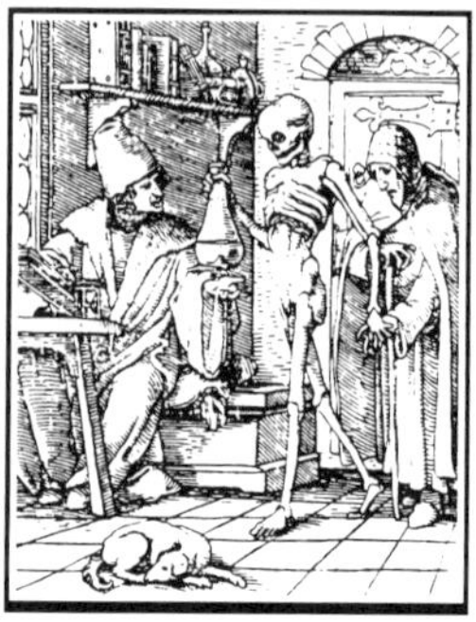

The History of Medicine in Context

Series Editors: Andrew Cunningham and Ole Peter Grell

Department of History and Philosophy of Science
University of Cambridge

Department of History
Open University

Titles in this series include

Medicine, Government and Public Health in Philip II's Spain
Shared Interests, Competing Authorities
Michele L. Clouse

Nursing before Nightingale, 1815–1899
Carol Helmstadter and Judith Godden

Secrets and Knowledge in Medicine and Science, 1500–1800
Edited by Elaine Leong and Alisha Rankin

Henri de Rothschild, 1872–1947
Medicine and Theater
Harry W. Paul

The Anatomist Anatomis'd
An Experimental Discipline in Enlightenment Europe
Andrew Cunningham

Centres of Medical Excellence?
Medical Travel and Education in Europe, 1500–1789
Edited by Ole Peter Grell, Andrew Cunningham and Jon Arrizabalaga

The Body Divided

Human Beings and Human 'Material' in Modern Medical History

Edited by
SARAH FERBER
University of Wollongong, Australia
and
SALLY WILDE
University of Queensland, Australia

ASHGATE

Published by
Ashgate Publishing Limited
Wey Court East
Union Road
Farnham
Surrey, GU9 7PT
England

Ashgate Publishing Company
Suite 420
101 Cherry Street
Burlington
VT 05401-4405
USA

www.ashgate.com

British Library Cataloguing in Publication Data
The body divided : Human Beings and Human 'Material' in Modern Medical History. -- (The history of medicine in context)
1. Human experimentation in medicine--Australia--History--19th century.
2. Human experimentation in medicine--Australia--History--20th century.
3. Human experimentation in medicine--Great Britain--History--19th century.
4. Human experimentation in medicine--Great Britain--History--20th century.
5. Human dissection--Australia--History--19th century. 6. Human dissection--Australia--History--20th century. 7. Human body--Social aspects--Australia--History.
8. Human body--Social aspects--Great Britain--History.
I. Series II. Ferber, Sarah, 1957- III. Wilde, Sally, 1949-
306.4'61'09-dc22

ISBN-13: 9780754668343

Library of Congress Cataloging-in-Publication Data
Ferber, Sarah, 1957-
The body divided : human beings and human 'material' in modern medical history / Sarah Ferber and Sally Wilde.
p. cm.
Includes bibliographical references and index.
ISBN 978-0-7546-6834-3 (hbk) -- ISBN 978-0-7546-9481-6 (ebk)
1. Human dissection. 2. Human anatomy. 3. Medical sciences--History. 4. Medicine--Philosophy. I. Wilde, Sally, 1949- II. Title.
QM33.4.F47 2011
611.009--dc23

2011026574

ISBN 9780754668343 (hbk)
ISBN 9780754694816 (ebk)

MIX
Paper from responsible sources
FSC® C013056
FSC www.fsc.org

Printed and bound in Great Britain by
TJ International Ltd, Padstow, Cornwall.

Contents

List of Figures

List of Contributors

Leo Brown is currently the Bequest Programme Manager at the School of Biomedical Sciences, University of Queensland. In this role he coordinates all aspects of the whole body donation process. He has been involved in this programme for many years and has heard many stories from potential donors. Leo is also the chairman of the Thanksgiving Service Organizing Committee for body donors, which is conducted in May every year. Leo regularly accepts invitations as guest speaker at service club meetings and professional conferences, as well as radio and print media interviews. Outside of the university, Leo is President of the Qld Branch of the Australian Army Water Transport Association and has been appointed as the Honorary Colonel of Army Cadets in South Queensland. He is also actively involved in Toc H, a community organization providing support and assistance to those in need.

Sarah Ferber is Associate Professor of History at the University of Wollongong. She has published widely in early modern French history, as well as researching and teaching on modern medical ethics history. Her book *Bioethics in Historical Perspective* (forthcoming) was funded by a Discovery Grant from the Australian Research Council. She is Chair of the Human Research Ethics Committee (Health and Medical) at the University of Wollongong.

Ross L. Jones is Australian Research Council Postdoctoral Fellow, Department of History, University of Sydney. He completed his PhD in the Education Faculty at Monash University in 2001. He also has a Masters in Educational Studies from Monash and a BA (Hons) and Dip Ed from the University of Melbourne. He has taught the history of medicine and biology at the University of Melbourne. He has published in the areas of the history of anatomy, eugenics and education, including *Humanity's Mirror: 150 Years of Anatomy in Melbourne* (Haddington Press, 2007).

Helen MacDonald is an Australian Research Council Future Fellow at the University of Melbourne. She researches the histories of organ transplantation, human dissection and post-mortem examinations. Helen is the author of *Possessing the Dead: The Artful Science of Anatomy* (2010) and *Human Remains: Dissection and its Histories* (2006), which won the Victorian Premier's Literary Award (History category) and was shortlisted for the Ernest Scott History Prize. She is a member of the Advisory Board of The Writing Centre for Scholars and Researchers at the University of Melbourne.

Dolly MacKinnon is Senior Lecturer in the School of History, Philosophy, Religion and Classics at the University of Queensland. She co-edited *'Madness' in Australia: Histories, Heritage and the Asylum* (2003), and also *Exhibiting Madness in Museums: Remembering Psychiatry through Collections and Display* (2011), both with Catharine Coleborne. Her other cultural history publications include 'Music, Madness, and the Body: Symptom and Cure', *History of Psychiatry* (2006), and '"Amusements are Provided": Asylum Entertainment and Recreation in Australia and New Zealand *c.*1860–*c.*1945', in G. Mooney and J. Reinarz (eds), *Permeable Walls: Historical Perspectives on Hospital and Asylum Visiting* (2009).

Nicola J. Marks is Lecturer in Science and Technology Studies at the University of Wollongong. She is the Australian Committee representative for the Asia-Pacific Science and Technology Studies Network. She holds degrees in Natural Sciences and Genetics respectively from Cambridge University and the University of Edinburgh, and a PhD on the social aspects of science also from the University of Edinburgh. Her doctoral and post-doctoral research focused on public engagement in stem cell research. She recently published 'Defining Stem Cells? Scientists and Their Classifications of Nature' (2010) in a special issue of *The Sociological Review* on 'Nature after the Genome'.

Susan K. Martin is Associate Professor in English and Associate Dean of Research for the Faculty of Humanities and Social Science, at La Trobe University, Melbourne. She teaches Australian studies and Victorian literature, and publishes on nineteenth- and twentieth-century Australian literature and culture. Her work has appeared in various books, including *The Oxford Literary History of Australia* and *Imagining Australia: Literature and Culture In The New New World*. She has published in journals including *Australian Literary Studies*, *Studies in The History of Gardens and Designed Landscapes* and *Southern Review*. Her interest in death and bodies is reflected in her work on Garden Cemeteries, which includes the article 'Monuments in the Garden: The Garden Cemetery in Australia' in *Postcolonial Studies* (2004). Her books include *Reading the Garden: The Settlement of Australia*, with Katie Holmes and Kylie Mirmohamadi (Melbourne University Press, 2008) and *Sensational Melbourne: Reading, Sensation Fiction and Lady Audley's Secret in the Victorian Metropolis*, with Kylie Mirmohamadi (Australian Scholarly Publishing, 2011).

Jo Robertson has a PhD in Literature from the University of Queensland. She is a former Research Officer to the ILA Global Project on the History of Leprosy, Wellcome Unit for the History of Medicine, Oxford University, and is currently attached to the Institut d'Histoire de la Médecine et de la Santé, Centre Médicale Universitaire (CMU), Geneva. She is currently working on a monograph on the recent history of leprosy (1948–2005), which places anti-leprosy work within the context of the politics of international health.

Elizabeth Stephens is an ARC Research Fellow and Deputy Director of the Centre for the History of European Discourses at the University of Queensland. She is the author of *Queer Writing: Homoeroticism in Jean Genet's Fiction* (Palgrave Macmillan, 2009) and *Anatomy as Spectacle: Public Exhibitions of the Body From 1700 to the Present* (Liverpool University Press, 2011).

Paul Turnbull is Professor of History at the University of Queensland. He has written extensively on the theft and repatriation of Indigenous Australian bodily remains and cultural property. His recent publications include the co-edited volume *The Long Way Home: The Meaning and Values of Repatriation* (Oxford: Berghahn, 2010). Paul is also known internationally for his work on presenting history and cultural heritage in networked digital media, notably on South Seas, a major online information resource devoted to exploring the history of cross-cultural encounters during James Cook's momentous first Pacific voyage (1769–1771).

Sally Wilde completed her MPhil in economic history in the 1970s, at the University of Nottingham, and her PhD in the history of medicine more than 20 years later, at the University of Melbourne. In the interim, she worked for the Labour Party in England for far too long, before migrating to Australia, teaching economic history at Monash University, and writing 10 books on various aspects of Australia's social, economic and medical history. Sally held an ARC postdoctoral research fellowship at the University of Queensland (2007–2009), and is currently an Honorary Research Fellow there. She is researching the history of relationships between doctors and patients, especially in surgery.

Acknowledgements

The editors wish to acknowledge the Faculty of Arts, University of Queensland, for its support of a seminar based around the work of Helen MacDonald. We also thank Helen MacDonald for her early editorial work on this project. Thanks are also due to Kerry Ross for her assistance at the indexing and proof stages.

The Body Divided in Time and Place: An Introductory Essay*

Sarah Ferber and Sally Wilde

In 1988, early in the history of human *in vitro* fertilization (IVF), a bioethics commentator suggested that the bodies of brain-dead women could, with hormonal assistance, provide suitable incubation for implanted embryos, to bring them to term. Dr Paul Gerber, a medical law academic, argued 'I can't see anything wrong with it, and at least the dead would be doing some good', adding that such a development would represent 'a magnificent use of a corpse'. The front page newspaper article which reported his claim, added: 'A specialist in reproductive physiology … said that a neomort would probably be able to sustain a pregnancy. "I can't see any reason why the pregnancy shouldn't go ahead normally, as long as the female incubator is receiving the appropriate nutrients and care", said the specialist, who preferred to remain unnamed'.[1] In response, the inaugural chair of the world's first IVF regulatory committee, lawyer Professor Louis Waller, responded: 'If these women are dead, then bury them decently. That's what we do with dead people in our society'.[2] The matter was apparently not publicly discussed again. Yet notwithstanding Professor Waller's assertion that there exists an underlying social consensus about what might constitute a limit case in medical ethics, the article itself shows no such consensus, thus his statement needs to be read more for rhetorical force than factuality.

Who constitutes the 'we' of this imagined consensual social world? How do 'we' know where to draw the line? And on whose authority are these lines drawn? These are some of the questions which underscore the research presented in this book. As new ideas about medical education and new technologies have come into being, particularly since the mid-nineteenth century, the idea of what 'we' do in 'our' culture has been subject to continuous negotiation and change. The 1988 report in many ways resembles those medical debates which were staked out in the mid-nineteenth century: a wish for secrecy under the light of media scrutiny;

* The editors wish to thank Dolly MacKinnon and Kerry Ross for their help in the preparation of this chapter.

1 Calvin Miller, 'The Brain-Dead Could Be Surrogates, Say Scientists', *The Herald* (Melbourne), 24 June 1988, p. 1.

2 Waller chaired the Standing Review and Advisory Committee on Infertility, created under the Victorian Infertility (Medical Procedures) Act, 1984.

intense medico-legal debate; and the problems of a donor culture. This book is about some of the ways in which, over the last two centuries, humans have made use of other people's bodies in and through medicine and how these changes have brought into play questions about social consensus, individual identity, the nature of the sacred, and the role of language and the imagination.

The Disciplinary Context

This book presents the work of researchers trained in science, social science, literature and history, reflecting the multidisciplinary mood of modern 'medicine studies' and of recent bioethics itself. The book advances an investigative agenda similar to that of the new journal *Medicine Studies*, the editor of which, Norbert W. Paul, states: 'By exploring the shifts of knowledge production in medicine we may be able to see the driving forces behind the ongoing development of medicine and the associated transformation of its social functions in a new light'.[3] More is required of scholars in medicine studies than to provide a mantra of condemnation or a reiteration of constructivist ideas which assume an unchanging power base of medicine, and which anticipate or even incapacitate the personal views of medicine's global clientele. The medical–social matrix is increasingly complex. Couples undergoing IVF, for example, are encouraged to bond with embryos still under the microscope. This kind of interaction represents a fundamental reconstitution of human intimacy – it both responds to and creates a new form of desire – and is indicative of developments which cannot be contained within a traditional 'medical dominance' analysis.

Recent research in the social history of medicine has also pressed the case for greater dialogue between historical research and modern bioethics.[4] Social history of medicine and bioethics were until relatively recently seen as largely unconnected, a consequence in part of the dominance of philosophy in major bioethics fora. Informed by intellectual history, Alastair V. Campbell has made

---

3 1/1 (2009): 3–10, p. 3. In 2010 the journal devoted a special issue (2/1) to anatomical history, from early European studies up to the present-day medical school classroom.

4 Alastair V. Campbell's 2009 *The Body in Bioethics* (London) moves the debate into the realm of history of ideas in order to advocate a reorientation of bioethics discourse away from what he sees as the influence of Cartesian dualism. For a definition of 'cultural bioethics', see D. Callahan, 'Bioethics', in S.G. Post (ed.), *Encyclopedia of Bioethics*, 3rd edn (Farmington Hills, MI, 2004): pp. 278–87. For the work of social and cultural historians in the bioethics field, see: R.S. Cowan, *Heredity and Hope: The Case for Genetic Screening* (Cambridge, MA, 2008); R. Falk, D.B. Paul and G. Allen (eds), *Eugenic Thought and Practice: A Reappraisal*, Special Double Issue, *Science in Context*, 11/3–4 (2005); Diane B. Paul, *The Politics of Heredity: Essays on Eugenics, Biomedicine, and the Nature-Nurture Debate* (Albany, 1998); and for the same view coming back from philosophy: P. Borry, P. Schotsmans and K. Dierickx, 'The Birth of the Empirical Turn in Bioethics', *Bioethics*, 19/1 (2005): pp. 49–71.

a case in *The Body in Bioethics* for the integrity of the body and the ideal of its coming 'together at last'.[5] Yet the notion of the integrity of the body, in some sense sacralized by being 'undivided', is not necessarily the nub of the debate: many people in the past and in the present have seen the dispersal of the body as at least ennobling if not indeed itself sacred. This applies not only to many medical scientists, who hold as 'sacred' the secular notion of healing, but to donors of many kinds. (And indeed, as Bruno Latour has argued, with typically engaging extremism, 'the apparent unity of our body … is only the superficial impression left by the routine of life'.)[6] This goes to questions of where identity resides: does it reside in a human gamete? Does it reside in a genetically distinctive cell line? Does it reside in the retention of all of the body being in one place? The divided body is not so much a matter for the resolution of philosophical and conceptual disintegration: rather, what holds the human body together is the social discourses which surround it, the discourses which legitimate both claims for its singularity and integrity and the moral exigencies of its division.

But can or should empirical and interpretative works stake any kind of moral, implicitly normative, claim? Inevitably, elements of analysis as basic as subject choice or word choice reflect tacit normative assumptions. These are clearly evident in this book, yet the job of the scholar is always to listen for differences, for departures from even their own original scripts, and there is also much evidence of this listening here, too. The archive in written form, or in interview, becomes the place where metaphorical and literal voices can be heard for nuance, for individuality, for uncertainty. Identifying these contours of sensibility and of debate are the central enterprise of this book. In this way, soundings in the archive can resonate ethically as well as factually, not to provide answers to a clinical or policy question, but to deepen understanding of the ways in which questions are asked, and the reasons some questions are asked while others remained either unasked or unanswered.

Chapter Outline

The time frame of the book traverses three centuries, making it possible to reflect on similarities and differences between former and present practices. In particular, the long view makes it possible to consider how the bodies of individual human beings and groups – ranked by others either high or low on the economic or evolutionary scale – have in different times and places mediated social relations, gaining or losing value in the light of medical or public curiosity.[7] The book begins

[5] Campbell, *Body in Bioethics*, pp. 119–25.

[6] 'Body, Cyborgs and the Politics of Incarnation', in Sean T. Sweeney and Ian Hodder (eds), *The Body* (The Darwin College Lectures) (Cambridge, 2002), pp. 127–41 on p. 127.

[7] The spaces for social mediation provided by new biotechnology are the subject of N.L. Sunderland, 'Biotechnology as Media: A Critical Study of the Movement of Meanings

with several chapters on the history of anatomical science, which in its modern form was closely aligned to the spread of professionalization of medical training in rapidly expanding university systems, to the project of race science, and in the emerging mental sciences in England and its colonies.[8] The first five chapters show the different ways in which middle-class colonial doctors and medical students conducted post-mortems on those who died in asylums, dissected the bodies of those who died in prisons or charitable hospitals, and collected the bones of Australian Aboriginal people. These acts were all, broadly speaking, performed for defensible reasons and within the law of the time, in the interests of current scientific enquiry or for the purposes of medical education. But they were also in the main acts performed without the consent of those whose bodies were appropriated for the benefit of others and their morality was contested in many cases at the time, as well as drawing opprobrium in hindsight. They were performed, in some cases more, in some cases less, hidden from public view, because the actors believed that public knowledge of what they were doing would risk outrage. As Frederic Wood Jones, Professor of Anatomy at the University of Melbourne in 1933 (cited by Ross L. Jones in this collection) was aware, there was a deep cultural investment attendant on the pursuit of his specialism:

> The subject of dissection of the human body cannot be approached without some understanding of the prejudice which inevitably clings to it. We must admit that there is, interwoven in the whole story, the idea of the sanctity of the human body, the dislike for its mutilation and the demand that it should find sepulchre intact.[9]

Wood Jones acknowledged these widespread public sensibilities in the face of a widely held view in his own profession that human corpses were useful and even necessary things for the purposes of study and healing. This view became mediated through law, in a climate of acute social division. As Helen MacDonald argues in the opening chapter, the British Anatomy Act of 1832 turned the 'institutionalized poor into useful things' seeing 'a body buried [as] a body wasted'. During the process of dissection, bodies ceased to be recognizable as such. Disassembled parts and 'waste' seldom left a 'body' to be decently interred, as required by the Anatomy Act. Instead, the remains of multiple bodies, operating theatre waste and even parts of animals were at various times placed in coffins. As MacDonald notes, anatomy inspectors sought to both obtain bodies 'as quietly as possible' and supervise the inconspicuous removal of remains, in an attempt to avoid public scrutiny and opposition to the practical workings of the Anatomy Act. In this, they were not always successful, and there was considerable opposition to the treatment of the corpses of those who died in workhouses, hospitals and prisons.

Associated with Contemporary Biotechnology', Thesis for the Doctor of Philosophy, Queensland University of Technology, 2003.

[8] J.H. Cassedy, *Medicine in America: A Short History* (Baltimore, MD, 1991).

[9] Cited in Chapter 2, this volume, p. 48.

In Chapter 2, Ross L. Jones picks up these themes in a study of the relationship between students of a major colonial medical school at Melbourne and the bodies that they dissected, in the era of both democratization and eugenics. As he points out, by the mid-nineteenth century, medical schools had developed a dependence on an abundant supply of human corpses, but this 'new thirst for cadavers for dissection took place concurrently with the growth of the modern democratic polity'. However, the nineteenth-century spread of democracy did not extend to inhabitants of charitable institutions or people with no fixed abode and neither did it imply any widespread belief in equality. At Melbourne, Jones has found that Professor of Anatomy, Richard Berry, was also an active eugenicist for most of the first quarter of the twentieth century and his belief that slum dwellers were inherently biologically inferior underpinned the use of the corpses of the institutionalized poor by his students.

Susan K. Martin argues further in Chapter 3 that colonial Victoria's Anatomy Act of 1862, like the British act of 1832 on which it was modelled, was essentially a punishment for being poor. This was in contrast to the earlier dissection of the bodies of hanged murderers, which was seen as an additional punishment for the crime of murder. As Martin shows, for this to be possible within an increasingly democratic system, the poor body had first to be construed as 'other' by key groups within the middle classes, and subsequently as a useable commodity available to the state. Doctors and medical students came to understand non-white and non-middle class bodies in different ways to their own bodies and those of their friends and family. However, Martin also highlights some of the complexities of the relationships between bodies and their dissectors in her tale of Christopher Harrison, a convicted murderer who tried to give his brain to the University of Melbourne. The recent work of Tatjana Buklijas for Vienna shows that Harrison can be seen to belong to an emerging trend of individuals' voluntary provision to science of the body after death.[10] In Harrison's case, however, the government sheriff contended that the convict's brain was not his to give. After his execution in 1864, it belonged to the government.[11] If Harrison's poignant offer was rebuffed, a mood of democratization at Melbourne's Benevolent Asylum made it possible for those whose bodies were at risk of dissection after death to sometimes avoid that fate. The inmates of the asylum petitioned their committee of management in the 1860s and for some years the committee refused to hand over any bodies to the medical school.

Notwithstanding pressure from the medical profession, relatively few bodies of those who died in colonial Victoria's asylums ended up at the medical school for dissection, but many were subject to the prior claims of the asylums' medical staff.[12] Struggles over handling rights of the bodies of asylum inmates are explored

[10] Tatjana Buklijas, 'Public Anatomies in *Fin-de-Siècle* Vienna', *Medicine Studies*, 2/1 (2010): pp. 71–92.

[11] Chapter 3, this volume, p. 53.

[12] Cressida Fforde, *Collecting the Dead: Archaeology and the Reburial Issue* (London, 2004); Elizabeth Hurren, 'A Pauper Dead-House: The Expansion of the Cambridge

in Dolly MacKinnon's study of the surviving archives from an archipelago of asylums that grew up in the gold-rush colony of mid-to-late nineteenth-century Victoria. Some post-mortems were performed because of an asylum doctor's interest in the pathology of madness, while in some cases post-mortem took place as a result of a statutory requirement, to investigate allegations of staff brutality or mistreatment. As MacKinnon notes, 'Asylum doctors knew their patients inside and out', but the appropriation of such bodies did not go uncontested and letters survive from family members pleading to be notified of deaths so that they could collect the body themselves for burial.[13] Medical authorities in government posts also sought access to the dead from mental asylums: in one case from 1900 the body of the asylum patient became a contested scientific object, its 'ownership' by medical men with official appointments the subject of public debate.

Paul Turnbull (Chapter 5) examines the post-mortem treatment of Aboriginal bodies towards the turn of the twentieth century. It is clear from his evidence that the degree to which Aboriginal bodies were constructed as 'other' was particularly extreme. He argues that the correspondence of Adelaide surgeon Edward Charles Stirling 'throws into question the adequacy of recent revisionist claims that frontier violence was never a systematic phenomenon'.[14] On the contrary, settler reactions to Aboriginal people were profoundly affected by their ideas about race and evolutionary genealogy. Aboriginal bodies and body parts were seen as appropriate objects for collection and study and Stirling was particularly enthusiastic in collecting skulls and leg bones, because he saw resemblances between the shape of the crania and tibias of Aboriginal people and those of Palaeolithic specimens from Europe.

In Chapter 6, Jo Robertson addresses the history of the treatment of people with Hansen's disease (leprosy), the condition most often associated with a loss of bodily integrity. Her study shows some of the ways in which leprosy-affected people in Japan, the Philippines and Norway 'have had to struggle for sovereignty over their own bodies, in the face of assumptions that they were research material or a resource of some kind'.[15] However, the behaviour of doctors was by no means

---

Anatomical Teaching School under the late-Victorian Poor Law, 1870–1914', *Medical History*, 48/1 (2004): pp. 69–94; Ross L. Jones, *Humanity's Mirror: 150 Years of Anatomy in Melbourne* (South Yarra, Victoria, 2007); Helen MacDonald, 'In the Interests of Science: Gathering Corpses from Lunatic Asylums', in Catharine Coleborne and Dolly MacKinnon (eds), *Exhibiting Madness in Museums: Remembering Psychiatry through Collections and Display* (New York, 2010): pp. 139–60; Helen MacDonald, *Human Remains: Episodes in Human Dissection* (Carlton South, 2005) and also as *Human Remains: Dissection and its Histories* (New Haven, 2006); Helen MacDonald, *Possessing the Dead: The Artful Science of Anatomy* (Carlton South, 2010).

[13] Chapter 4, this volume, p. 98.

[14] Chapter 5, this volume, p.111.

[15] Chapter 6, this volume, p. 133. The book's subtitle seeks to draw attention to contrasting perceptions: the term 'human material' has been used widely and unproblematically, without inverted commas, in the modern history of anatomy. See, for example: Thomas H. Gillingwater, 'The Importance of Exposure to Human Material in

uncontested and Robertson describes how the Norwegian doctor, Gerhard Hansen, the man who first identified the *Mycobacterium leprae*, was taken to court in 1880 and removed from his hospital post following a complaint from a patient about her use in one of his experiments. By the mid-twentieth century, it was no longer acceptable to simply expropriate the bodies of the poor or the stigmatized for medically determined uses, a change accelerated by the revelations surrounding the excesses of Nazi 'science' during the Second World War. Robertson charts the shift in what was considered appropriate behaviour in her study of changing attitudes to people affected by leprosy, and much of her evidence comes from a 2005 Japanese committee, which investigated the impact of attempts to restrict child-bearing in Japanese leprosy sanatoria from 1907 to 1996. In contrast to the behaviour of doctors described in the first five chapters, the doctors described by Robertson as treating those affected by leprosy on the Philippines island of Culion or in Japan in the early twentieth century do not seem to have felt any particular need to hide what they were doing in their attempts to restrict the rights to sexual activity and/or child bearing of those people segregated in their sanatoria.

In the late twentieth century probably the most distinctive shift occurred in uses for human body parts, when the body became not only a source of education or new scientific knowledge, but a direct source of healing. In Chapter 7, Sally Wilde discusses some of the issues raised by the regular replacement of an ever-increasing range of components of the body. In keeping with the spread of liberal ideas on equality in the early twenty-first century, it is hard to find anywhere in the world where the body parts of the poor are openly expropriated for transplantation. Rather, there is now widespread argument that the poor can be paid for their body parts and that the body should be straightforwardly commodified in this way, with organs bought and sold in an international market. However, this avoids the question of whether the project of the self, the twenty-first century concept of renewable bodies, entitles the rich and well educated to use parts of other people's bodies. It is as if many twenty-first-century advocates of the sale of body parts agree with nineteenth-century supporters of the various anatomy acts, that a body buried is a body wasted. Globalization of medical commodities has in important ways reinforced some of the lines of dominance of colonialism, but has also been accommodated by a new emphasis on the imagined autonomous liberal individual, removed from the cultural contexts which lead them to seek to sell their body parts.[16]

Nicola J. Marks' chapter builds on the recent work of literary and history of science scholars who have investigated the power of the 'biological imaginary', not just in science fiction, but in the constitution of scientific discourse itself, showing

---

Anatomical Education: A Philosophical Perspective', *Anatomical Sciences Education*, 1/6 (2008): pp. 264–6.

[16] 'Rent-a-Womb Trend is a Form of Neo-colonialism', interview with Catherine Waldby. Available at: http://digital.dnaindia.com/epaperpdf%5C24072010%5C23pune%20main%20edition-pg10-0.pdf (accessed 9 December 2010).

the ways in which practising scientists draw on science fiction-based cultural tropes to validate and underscore the social meaning of their work.[17] Marks considers the ways in which cloned bodies (both reproductive and therapeutic) have been *described* and *constituted* in discourses about cloning, focusing specifically on scientists' imagining of various futures for cloning. Her chapter then investigates the paradox of scientific discourse which works at the same time to discredit fears about stem cell research and cloning by associating fear with the unstable realm of fantasy. Her chapter shows for the case of cloning that fiction – including science fiction and speculative fiction, utopian and dystopian visions – has become an important way for us to express both unease and excitement about the future of science and medicine.

In Chapter 9, Elizabeth Stephens brings the story back to where the book began, to the uses of dissected bodies for educational purposes. But in line with the increasing democratization of the uses of the body in the twenty-first century, public displays of anatomy are presented as educational not for middle-class medical students, but for the broader public. As Stephens points out, this process of public display has interesting parallels with the popularity of eighteenth- and nineteenth-century displays of body parts, whether primarily designed as spectacle or as a contribution to medical science. Stephens argues that from the eighteenth to the twenty-first centuries, the combination of the medical and the spectacular in public displays of dissection serves 'to reinforce the cultural status of medicine'.[18] However, her main argument is to link such public anatomical displays to changing conceptions of the self and the invention of 'the healthy subject who is assumed to be rational about and individually responsible for, the condition of his or her body'.[19] Drawing on concepts from Foucault's work, she uses the history of such displays to track the invention of health as a process, a relationship we have with our body through self-surveillance and the self-cultivation of a healthy body.

The public acceptability of the dissections still performed by our medical students (although now as a far less prominent part of the medical curriculum) is aided by the fact that the cadavers are now gifted by public-spirited individuals, rather than stolen from the poor and stigmatized, a change highlighted by Leo Brown in his concluding chapter on the now widespread thanksgiving ceremonies for those who donate their bodies to medical teaching.

---

[17] See, for example, Catherine Waldby and Susan Squier, 'Ontogeny, Ontology, and Phylogeny: Embryonic Life and Stem Cell Technologies', *Configurations*, 11/1 (2003): 27–46; Susan Merrill Squier, *Liminal Lives: Imagining the Future at the Frontiers of Biomedicine* (Durham and London, 2004); Lily E. Kay, *Who Wrote the Book of Life? A History of the Genetic Code* (Stanford, 2000).

[18] Chapter 9, this volume, p. 235.

[19] Chapter 9, this volume, p. 235.

Chapter 1

A Body Buried is a Body Wasted: The Spoils of Human Dissection

Helen MacDonald

In January 1847, parliamentarian Thomas Dunscombe revealed in the House of Commons the latest scandal concerning the ways in which British convicts were treated on board the hulks moored in the Thames at Woolwich. Dunscombe demanded that a Select Committee investigate the medical treatment meted out to those awaiting exile to Britain's colonies aboard these makeshift prisons and what became of their corpses when they died. Prisoners' corpses were being subjected to post-mortem examinations during which, Dunscombe asserted, surgeons threw entrails into the river rather than burying the bodies intact in the marshland graves that had for decades served this purpose. The convicts on board the Woolwich hulks told Dunscombe that they feared they were being allowed to die so that their bodies could be sent to a school under the Anatomy Act of 1832. In parliament, Dunscombe demanded to know how many hulk corpses went to such destinations rather than to graves, but the government brought a halt to his disclosures. Home Secretary Sir George Grey remonstrated with Dunscombe for raising the matter, suggesting that instead he should have quietly expressed his concerns with the executive government. In this way, one call among many made during the nineteenth century for an investigation into how the Anatomy Act worked was effectively sidelined.[1]

In her history of the making of Britain's Anatomy Act, *Death, Dissection and the Destitute* (1988), Ruth Richardson demonstrated that the Act radically changed the source from which British medical schools obtained corpses for their students to dissect. Prior to 1832 murderers' bodies provided the only legal source of subjects, under an Act of Parliament that made dissection a punitive measure

[1] Hansard's Parliamentary Debates, House of Commons, 28 January 1847, cols 511–28. For the history of governments silencing debate on the Anatomy Act, see Helen MacDonald, *Possessing the Dead: The Artful Science of Anatomy* (Melbourne, 2010). On the hulks and transportation, see A.G.L. Shaw, *Convicts and the Colonies: A Study of Penal Transportation from Great Britain & Ireland to Australia & Other Parts of the British Empire* (Kilkenny, 1998), pp. 335–60; and Angeline Brasier's PhD thesis, 'Prison or Paradise: An Investigation into Conditions in the Bermudian Convict Establishment', which also discusses England's hulks (in preparation, School of Historical and Philosophical Studies, University of Melbourne).

inflicted on corpses. An Act for Better Preventing the Horrid Crime of Murder (25 Geo. 2, c. 37, 1752) had been designed with deterrence in mind by men who knew how far destroying a corpse and denying it burial strayed from customary ways of dealing with the dead. It attached a 'peculiar Mark of Infamy' to murderers' bodies and was meant to induce 'Terror' in those who heard the sentence of dissection pronounced.[2] However the gallows proved to be an uncertain source of subjects for Britain's medical schools. Few people were hanged for murder in any given year, and their corpses were sent to the Colleges of Surgeons rather than being distributed among the schools. The supply was grossly inadequate. As Sir Robert Inglis pointed out during the parliamentary debate in 1832, in the previous year a mere 11 corpses had been 'legally disposed of as subjects', while 800 students of medicine required one or more each to dissect and upon which to practise operative surgery.[3] This left most schools and students to find subjects where they could. Medical men attached to hospitals made good use of these institutions' mortuaries. They and others also purchased corpses from grave-robbers who sold the freshest bodies they obtained intact – and took what they could get for the limbs they cut from putrefying remains.[4]

The Act to Regulate Schools of Anatomy brought this risky business to an end by authorizing the men in charge of the institutions in which large numbers of poor people died – workhouses, hospitals, prisons and, later in the century, lunatic asylums – to dispose of these corpses to a medical school. This increased supply and effectively reduced the cost of a corpse, thereby putting the resurrectionists out of work. So long as the patient or inmate had not recorded a formal protest against being dissected should they die and no relative claimed the body for a private burial instead within 48 hours of the death, it could be sent to a school. Then, after six weeks, that school was to pay for the remains to be buried.

This chapter focuses on an aspect of the history of human dissection that has thus far been little explored: how the concept of waste was mobilized under the British Anatomy Act. Waste-talk featured in nineteenth-century discussions of dissection in two ways. It was deployed in the utilitarian sense favoured by those advocating increasing supplies of corpses for medical schools. To these people, any corpse that left an institution to be buried rather than dissected was a wasted thing. Second, waste featured as the detritus that was created in dissecting rooms. In highlighting what became of the devastated remains left behind following a dissection, the Anatomy Act's critics effectively mobilized opposition to the statute.

---

[2] Douglas Hay, 'Property, Authority and the Criminal Law', in D. Hay, P. Linebaugh, J. Rule, E.P. Thompson and C. Winslow (eds), *Albion's Fatal Tree: Crime and Society in Eighteenth-Century England* (London, 1975), pp. 65–117 on pp. 76–8.

[3] Hansard's Parliamentary Debates, House of Commons, 17 January 1832, col 578.

[4] Joshua Naples, Diary of a London Resurrectionist, 1811–1812, held by the Royal College of Surgeons, London.

Disposing of the Dead

The Anatomy Act's burial clause appeared clearly to set out how a corpse was to be removed to a school from the place in which the death had occurred, and subsequently interred. This clause had been a late inclusion in the Act, which was surprising given that thwarted burials of one kind or another had been instrumental in bringing the legislation into being. Initially, the Bill's promoter parliamentarian Henry Warburton had expressed the view that a burial service was only important to the living, and since under his Bill only 'unclaimed' corpses would be sent to the schools there was no need to provide for their subsequent interment. The burial clause was only included when it became clear to Warburton that some of the Bill's parliamentary critics would support the legislation if subjects for dissection were ultimately disposed of in consecrated ground.[5]

The clause was designed with an eye to notions of public decency. Every corpse was to be 'placed in a decent Coffin or Shell' for removal to a school, and following the anatomical examination it was to be 'decently interred in consecrated Ground, or in some public Burial Ground in use for Persons of that religious Persuasion to which the Person whose Body was so removed belonged'. Then, a burial certificate was to be sent to the Inspector of Anatomy.[6]

For the rest of the century, Section XIII caused the inspectors appointed under the Anatomy Act no end of trouble, for perversely it used the word 'body' to describe what would ultimately be interred. This implied that dissected remains retained a form of identity and integrity which, after six weeks in a dissecting room, was not the case. It was as if words had failed the parliamentarians or, more likely, that using a more accurate descriptor of the contents of those coffins needed to be avoided lest it raise the spectre of waste in people's minds. The end products of a dissection – the mess of fats, fluids, tissues and bones that actually remained to be disposed of – needed to be disguised and using the word 'body' accomplished that. It enabled *The Times* to assure readers that dissection did not destroy a corpse

---

5 Hansard, Vol. IX. House of Commons, Sir Robert Inglis, 17 January 1832, col 578 and unnamed member, 24 January 1832, col 826; Hansard, Vol. X, 7 February to 8 March 1832. House of Commons, Sir Robert Inglis, 27 February 1832, col 834; Hansard, Vol. XIV, 3 July to 16 August 1832. House of Lords, Earl of Harewood, 19 July 1832, col 535.

6 'An Act for Regulating Schools of Anatomy', *Statutes of the United Kingdom of Great Britain and Ireland* (London), p. 893. The Bill's initial omission of a burial clause is also surprising in light of the fact that an earlier Anatomy Bill which Henry Warburton had presented in 1829 *had* contained such a clause. Then, Warburton stated that denying 'the rites of the tomb … to any of our fellow-creatures was naturally repulsive to their feelings'. His first Bill therefore provided that 'after the purposes of dissection had been completed, the remains should be interred, according to the custom of the country' (Hansard, Vol. XX (6 February to 30 March 1829). House of Commons, Henry Warburton, 12 March 1829, col 1000).

as the 'parts may afterwards be put together and decently conveyed to the earth'.[7] In practice, little remained of a body to bury at its conclusion and this became a potent weapon for the Act's critics for the rest of the century.

Repugnance to Dissection

First, though, who was this public that was opposed to dissection and therefore feared by the Act's promoters and mobilized by its critics?

Demand for corpses during the nineteenth century outstripped the number that could be obtained under the Anatomy Act. Hardly anyone donated their own bodies or those of their relatives to be dissected, to the point that when a few people did so, theirs was considered to be an idiosyncratic choice.[8] Dissection was therefore talked about from a base understanding that 'the public' was strongly opposed to it. This public was frequently invoked as if it comprised pretty much everyone – or at least everyone whom the Act had made vulnerable to being dissected. During parliamentary debates in 1829 and 1831/1832 dissection was said to be 'extremely unpopular out of doors' (outside parliament) and offensive to 'the community'.[9] 'The great mass of the British public' argued Mr Sadler in the House of Commons 'was alive to this subject, and they contemplated with extraordinary disgust any advancement in science that was to be made at their expense'.[10] More specifically, parliamentarians believed that 'destitute' people felt 'the most unconquerable objection to the dissection of their bodies'.[11]

After the Anatomy Act had passed, the anatomy inspectors appointed under it also strongly believed that most lay people abhorred corpses being sent from institutions to schools to be dissected.[12] They therefore strove to keep any discussion of the practices that arose under the Act out of the public domain. More specifically, the inspectors worried about certain elements of the British population whose prejudices they thought were particularly strong. In Scotland, home of the infamous Burke and Hare murders that had supplied Robert Knox's anatomy school prior to the Act passing, Inspector James Somerville was particularly wary

---

7 *The Times*, 3 December 1831, p. 2. In a later edition 'as much of it will be conveyed … to the earth, as if an artery had never been laid open, or a gland displayed' (6 December 1831, p. 2).

8 See, e.g., reports of Alfred Carlile's donation (*John Bull*, 18 February 1843) and Sarah Searl's 'curious bequest' (*The Lady's Newspaper*, 14 October 1848, p. 309).

9 Earl of Malmesbury, House of Lords, 20 May 1829, col 1489 (who himself experienced 'a sort of conflict between the head and the heart on the subject'); Archbishop of Canterbury, House of Lords, 5 June 1829, col 1747.

10 11 May 1832, col 900.

11 Lord Tenterden, House of Lords, 5 June 1829, col 1749.

12 On the anatomy inspectorate see Helen MacDonald, 'Procuring Corpses: England's Anatomy Inspectorate, 1842 to 1858', *Medical History*, 53/3 (July 2009): pp. 379–96.

of the immigrant Irish population and the 'lower orders'.[13] He believed that the 'peculiar difficulties' experienced in obtaining corpses north of the border were due to the fact that the 'poorer classes' there had strong kindred ties and so did not lose sight of relatives who entered poor houses. But Somerville thought that an abhorrence against dissection also existed more widely – among 'all classes of the Community' – and had been 'heightened by the exposure of the means by which the Schools were supplied'.[14]

In this context, quiet arrangements needed to be made by those promoting the Anatomy Act, as that legislation *enabled*, rather than compelled, institutions' officials to send corpses to medical schools, and they often declined to do so. This left the inspectors needing to persuade parochial officers, which they did by discreetly contacting them to ask them to 'comply' with the Act, and trying to ensure that when they agreed, body removal was stealthily accomplished. Inspector Somerville pointed out to one Edinburgh anatomist that it would be better in 'the eyes of the public if teachers should not appear interested parties' when that city's funeratories were established.[15] During a later scandal that threatened to expose much about the working of the Anatomy Act in Scotland, an official involved warned that bodies must be obtained without arousing 'suspicions'. Arrangements must work 'quietly' lest those distributing corpses were 'stoned in the neighbourhood'.[16] Both the inspectors and anatomy teachers must work behind the scenes to increase corpse supply while avoiding 'public clamour'.[17]

The inspectors therefore approached men like parish medical officers, who could be relied upon to share their belief that a pauper's corpse that was buried rather than dissected was a wasted thing. In the words of Somerville's successor John Rutherford Alcock, burying an unclaimed corpse was 'to the pecuniary disadvantage of the Parishes and the injury of Science'.[18] Deals were struck with

---

[13] Public Records Office, National Archives [hereafter NA], Ministry of Health, Anatomy Office, Outletter Book, General (1835 to 1841) [hereafter MH 74/13], Somerville to Phillipps, 11 March 1837; Somerville to Lizars, 13 April 1837. On the Burke and Hare murders, see Lisa Rosner, *The Anatomy Murders* (Philadelphia, 2009).

[14] Somerville to Fox Maule, 27 September 1839, MH 74/13. That may have been so, though the 'lower orders' did not all think in just one way about dissection which Somerville knew. Some among them clamoured for entry to witness dissections. In 1837 Somerville found, to his horror, that members of the 'labouring classes' were in the University of Edinburgh's practical rooms participating in indecent and revolting levities there (Somerville to Fox Maule, 11 September 1837, MH 74/13; Fox Maule to Monro (23 September 1837, NA, HO 83/1, Home Office, Anatomy, Volume 1 (1832 to 1842)).

[15] Somerville to Lizars, 30 November 1840, MH 74/13. On the funeratories, see MacDonald, *Possessing the Dead*, pp. 31–3, pp. 37–42.

[16] NAS, Inspector of Anatomy for Scotland, Letterbook (1875–1882) [hereafter MH 3/6], Explanation by Mr Kennedy, March 1880.

[17] Kennedy to Wood, 26 July 1880, MH 3/6.

[18] NA, Ministry of Health, Anatomy Office, Outletter Books, Metropolitan District, 1842–1858, MH 74/15 [hereafter MH 74/15], Alcock to Howell, 11 November 1842, p. 12.

sympathetic members of parochial boards while others were kept in ignorance of the arrangements made. In 1892, Councillor Kinnaird, who sat on the South Leith Parochial Board, learned that for 50 years corpses had been secretly disposed of in this way from the local poorhouse without board members knowing of this. The Scottish anatomy inspector, James Russell, defended the practice by nicely turning the notion of a public interest which was at stake on its head. He argued that the public had 'a right to expect that such disagreeable subjects as Anatomy should be conducted in private'.[19]

Exposing the Act

Each of the men who successively served as Britain's anatomy inspectors was himself a medical man with intimate knowledge of what it meant to dissect a corpse. Yet he was required to ensure that a 'body' was later buried. The inspectors knew that if this was not done, adverse publicity would result and imperil the supply of corpses. They therefore constantly warned anatomists to be 'vigilant' in not offending parish feelings and prejudices and counselled them to send remains for burial in less than the six weeks that the Act allowed and 'in the Evening' as quietly as possible.[20] The inspectors emphasized that all '*possible* decency' was to be taken with regard to the contents of each coffin, bearing in mind that a parish official may open its lid with disastrous consequences;[21] and the funerals held for these remains should be 'superior' in quality to an ordinary pauper's burial.[22] Everything must be done in such a way as to ensure that the public was not 'influenced against' the Anatomy Act.[23]

However, one of the Act's most vociferous critics, the surgeon William Roberts, proved to be adept at rallying opinion against it by appealing to people's

[19] NAS, Letter Book, Inspector of Anatomy for Scotland, MH 3/8 (1885–1889) [hereafter MH 3/8], Russell to Cleland, 9 August 1888.

[20] For example, NA, Ministry of Health, Anatomy Office, Out letter Books, General including Scotland, 1832–1835, MH 74/12 [hereafter MH 74/12], Somerville to Teale, 25 September 1833, p. 97; Circular to Metropolitan Teachers, 14 November 1842, pp. 13–14, Bacot to Benjamin Alcock, September 1853, p. 339, MH 74/15.

[21] NA, Ministry of Health, Anatomy Office, Out letter Books, Metropolitan District, 1858–1881, MH 74/6 [hereafter MH 74/6]. Hawkins to the Teachers of Anatomy in the Metropolitan Schools, 27 September 1858, p. 36.

[22] See, e.g., Somerville to Teale, 25 September 1833, p. 97, MH 74/12. On pauper burials see e.g. Thomas Laqueur, 'Bodies, Death, and Pauper Funerals', *Representations*, 1/1 (1983): pp. 109–31 and Julie-Marie Strange, '"Only a Pauper Whom Nobody Owns": Reassessing the Pauper Grave *c.*1880–1914', *Past and Present*, 178 (February 2003): pp. 148–75.

[23] Letter to Teachers of Anatomy in the Metropolitan Schools, 27 September 1858, p. 36, MH 74/6.

sensibilities with regard to the fact that only poor persons' corpses were vulnerable to being sent to a medical school and how their remains were being disposed of. Roberts published placards and papers, wrote letters to newspapers, held meetings in public houses and forced his way into workhouses to expose how the Act worked in practice. He also threatened to publish the names of those parish guardians who voted to supply workhouse inmates' bodies to the schools.[24]

Roberts charged that corpses were little more than commodities to the schools, the base material that enabled their proprietors to extract large fees from students. He claimed that soon after entering a school each body was cut into pieces and sold to the students 'at an aggregate charge of 70/- or 80/-'.[25] Corpses were also being treated in disrespectful ways. Roberts asserted that if the public knew what actually occurred in dissecting rooms no person in the middle or upper class walks of life – that is, no one with a choice in the matter – would ever consent to their own or their relatives' remains being used in this way.[26] As for the Act's burial clause, that was no more than a sham since at the conclusion of these transactions there was little left to be buried. Pieces were sold and much else was cut away and decomposed, 'wasted, or consigned to troughs, pits and night-carts'. At the end of six weeks all that was left was 'an assemblage of disconnected bones, well nigh denuded of the flesh' that weighed no more than a fourth of the original body. This, if anything, was consigned to a grave.[27] Such was the 'ordinary havoc and waste' in a dissecting room. As for the inspector's role in administering the Act, Roberts accused Inspector Somerville of taking care 'never to be where his presence was most wanted'. He charged that the idea of inspecting the contents of a coffin before it was buried 'never once entered his head'.[28]

---

[24] Copy of Letter to the Guardians of the Poor, 2 October 1858, p. 43, MH 74/6. Roberts' campaign had messy motives. He understood the need for subjects, but thought they should be obtained from prisons rather than workhouses and that fewer bodies would be required should the government buy his recipe for preserving corpses (for a fuller discussion, see Anna Stevenson, 'An Obscure Personality called William Roberts: The Later History of the Anatomy Act of 1832', BSc Thesis, History of Medicine, University of London, April 2004).

[25] MH 74/6, Copy of Letter to the Guardians of the Poor, 2 October 1858, p. 43.

[26] Cited in Stephenson, 'An Obscure Personality', p. 10.

[27] Roberts, William, *Mr Warburton's Anatomy Bill, thoughts on its mischievous tendency; with suggestions for an entirely new one, founded upon an available anti-septic process, in an appeal to medical practitioners, students of anatomy, and the public at large, on the injury to medical science and the hindrances to the decent interment of unclaimed pauper bodies now delivered up for anatomical 'examination', consequent upon the rejection of such a process* (London, 1843), pp. 9–10.

[28] Stephenson, 'An Obscure Personality', p. 28. In fact, the Act did not require him to do so. It left it up to the Secretary of State to direct how the Inspectors should 'transact their duties', and only specified that they must make quarterly returns detailing the sex, name and age of each corpse, and that it would be lawful for them to 'visit and inspect' places in which it was intended to practice anatomy, as well as receive the paperwork already discussed ('An Act to Regulate', pp. 891–4).

Somerville and his successors dreaded Roberts' dramatic revelations, for they resulted in the Anatomy Act being raised in parliament, calls for law reform, and Secretaries of State demanding explanations on matters that could not be satisfactorily explained. Nevertheless, the inspectors tried. Inspector John Bacot claimed that no more money was taken from the students than was necessary to cover the 'ordinary expenses of removal and interment'.[29] He asserted that parishes *gave* bodies to the schools and forthrightly denied that there was any 'trading in the Dead Bodies of Paupers' (though he simultaneously warned the Home Office not to enquire closely into these matters as the 'public exposure of the details of the dissecting room would be fatal … to the present, or any other mode of supplying [the schools] with subjects').[30]

These denials were untrue. Money and favours changed hands at every stage of the proceedings, as useful corpses were turned into tradeable objects. While the inspectors and others consistently claimed that anatomical examinations were undertaken for the good of science and the public, they knew that the workhouse masters and undertakers who supplied the schools expected to have their own, more personal, interests met in return for cooperating with the Act.[31] Until a change of law in 1844, officials in the Union workhouses that supported the Act openly sold corpses to the schools.[32] Some collected them with such zeal that scandals resulted, such as when a 'respectable' woman's remains were sent to St Bartholomew's hospital school. At Whitechapel, the parish beadle also received money in exchange for each unclaimed corpse that he sent to the London hospital school and went about his job so enthusiastically that illegalities followed.[33] When the Poor Law Amendment Act (1844) prohibited workhouse masters from selling corpses, payments were still made but now took a different form, being designated 'gratuities'.[34] In addition, undertakers were paid a contract price of £2/10/0d to cart each corpse to the school and subsequently dispose of it, which was much more than they received for burying parish paupers directly from the workhouse.[35] Sextons and ministers were paid for performing burials – whether or not the minister was actually present.[36] Messengers were rewarded for carrying notices to

[29] Bacot to Phillipps, 10 July 1843, p. 39, MH 74/15.

[30] Bacot to Secretary of State, May 1842, p. 240, MH 74/15.

[31] NA, Home Office, Anatomy, Appointment of Inspectors under Anatomy Act (1834, 1842–1843) HO 45/189, Alcock and Bacot to Phillipps, 3 November 1842.

[32] Somerville to Phillipps, 22 June 1833, pp. 83–4, MH 74/12.

[33] Somerville to Phillipps, 12 January 1835, p. 175, MH 74/12.

[34] The £5 penalty the Act imposed was meaningless, given that as much could be obtained for each body sold (see MH 74/12, Somerville to Phillipps, 12 January 1835, p. 175).

[35] Hawkins to Dix, 16 April 1858, p. 20, MH 74/6.

[36] It emerged during a case at the Yorkshire summer assizes that one provincial school paid 13 shillings to the local sexton, which he in turn shared with the minister of religion who should have been present at the burial of the remains but was not (*Leeds Mercury*, 25 July 1862).

the inspectorate office.[37] Dissecting room assistants, and the school porters who received corpses at the gate after dark, were paid emoluments. Many of these costs were then passed on to medical students, including in the price each paid for the dismembered parts that he obtained.[38]

Useless Corpses

The anatomy inspectors spent much of their time stamping out brush-fires with regard to the waste products leaving British dissecting rooms. Much of the problem lay in the fact that the men with whom they dealt held different conceptions of what comprised waste where a useful corpse was concerned.

Those that arrived in a school out of the winter dissecting season were of little value to teachers or students, who therefore refused to accept them after March each year.[39] This left the inspectors in a difficult situation, for workhouse inmates were most likely to die at winter's end and this was also the time when the inspectors' urgent winter requests to the workhouses were taking effect. They tried to persuade the schools to accept these worthless corpses and quietly bury them rather than let the parishes know that they were not required.[40] The schools declined to do that – burying corpses cost them money – so Inspector Alcock was reduced to asking the Home Office for permission to pay for such interments from the inspectorate purse.[41]

Of even less value than an unseasonable corpse was one which arrived at a school having already been 'mutilated' by being subjected to a post-mortem examination at the hospital, prison or other institution in which the person had died. Here, too, the inspectors were placed in a difficult situation. They had no oversight of post-mortem examinations, with which the Anatomy Act had not been concerned.[42] However to avoid the scandals that would inevitably result if these spoiled corpses were

---

37 These payments were eventually abolished in 1893 (NA, Ministry of Health, Anatomy Correspondence 1890–1904, MH 74/37, Bennett to Pemberton, 12 January 1893).

38 For students paying the undertakers' fees, see Hawkins to Dix, 16 April 1858, p. 20, MH 74/6. Workhouse inmate John Darwin's body was found to have been 'cut up into quarters', each of which had then been sold for nine shillings to students (NA, Ministry of Health, Anatomy Office, Outletter Books, Provincial Districts, 1842–1879, MH 74/10 [hereafter MH 74/10]. Cursham to Gregory, 24 May 1847, p. 51).

39 Dix to Gregg, 18 May 1858, p. 23, Gregg to Governor of Millbank Prison, 19 May 1858, p. 23, MH 74/6.

40 Hawkins to Holden, 22 March 1860, p. 93, MH 74/6.

41 Alcock to Phillipps, 9 March 1843, p. 33, MH 74/15. In addition, the inspectors pointed out to the Council of Medical Education the benefits of extending the dissecting season into the middle of April (Hawkins to President of the General Council of Medical Education, 30 April 1860, p. 99, MH 74/6).

42 On post-mortem examinations, see MacDonald, *Possessing the Dead*, pp. 96–106.

discovered en route to a school or were returned to a parish having been rejected, they instructed undertakers to examine each body prior to taking it to a school and assess its suitability for dissection. They were to reject a corpse from which 'all the parts are taken out' or which was putrefying as it would be of no possible use.[43]

Like autopsied corpses, those of foetuses and stillborn infants also lay outside the inspectors' purview, being non-persons in law. Until 1838, such deaths required no registration and the remains could be treated as waste material.[44] However, the inspectors worried when they learned of schools obtaining infants' remains, not least because these could be those of victims of infanticide – evidence of which would be destroyed by the dissection.[45] The inspectors asked the schools not to receive such bodies. When these requests were ignored, they sought burial certificates for them 'to prevent the possibility of any enquiry hereafter being made'.[46] When they learned that the schools were disposing of infants' corpses as rubbish by placing them in a single coffin along with dissected adult remains they expressed their dismay.[47]

Then there was the problem of the waste that medical students created in dissecting rooms. Much has been written of the high jinks with corpses and body parts in which nineteenth-century students indulged.[48] Such behaviour brought the schools unwelcome attention, making people suspect that corpses were generally treated in offensive ways during dissections. Sketches and photographs sometimes captured this behaviour, which John Harley Warner and James Edmondson have recently argued illustrated a rite of passage through which medical students passed. The images also include words that the students' inscribed on their dissecting tables and blackboards – reinforcing the view that these corpses would have gone to waste had they not been dissected: 'Such the vultures love' appears above one corpse; 'She lived for others but died for us' beneath another.[49]

---

43 Bacot to Harwell, 18 January 1855, pp. 354–5, MH 74/15.

44 However as Nicky Hart has argued, the distinction between stillborn infants, and those who died soon after birth, could be a slippery one, as a parent could be reluctant to register a death and arrange a burial for several reasons. Both processes could be avoided by construing the death as a stillbirth (Nicky Hart, 'Beyond Infant Mortality: Gender and Stillbirth in Reproductive Mortality before the Twentieth Century', *Population Studies*, 52/2 (1998): pp. 215–29, on pp. 220–21).

45 Somerville to Fox Maule, 16 December 1840, p. 344, MH 74/13.

46 Those enquiries might be made by a coroner, if a death was referred to him, or by a mother who discovered that her infant's body had been sent to a school without her knowledge (Gregg to Roper, 20 December 1871, p. 429, MH 74/10).

47 Bacot to Barnett, 15 November 1850, p. 325, MH 74/15.

48 See, for example, Ross L. Jones, *Humanity's Mirror: 150 Years of Anatomy in Melbourne* (South Yarra, 2007); Keir Waddington, 'Mayhem and Medical Students: Image, Conduct, and Control in the Victorian and Edwardian London Teaching Hospital', *Social History of Medicine*, 15/1 (2002): pp. 45–64.

49 John Harley Warner and James M. Edmonson, *Dissection: Photographs of a Rite of Passage in American Medicine 1880–1930* (New York, 2009).

Valuable Parts

The Anatomy Act had not contemplated that parts would be removed from corpses and retained as specimens or be preserved as preparations for the individual use of students, for teachers with a particular research interest, and for museum collections – private, hospital and public. Yet this commonly occurred, with parts being retained. Concern about this practice had been expressed during the anatomy debates. It struck some commentators with particular revulsion, including influential surgeon George Guthrie. He spoke of 'the horror' a relative would feel on learning that 'various parts of the person he most esteemed and loved [were] exposed in bottles, for the contemplation of the learned and the gaze of the curious'.[50] People also worried about how the detritus left behind after specimens were taken might be disposed of. Fears were expressed that it would be cast away as 'mere filth' – or be fed to animals, thrown into a lime hole, be taken away by students to be used as grisly souvenirs.[51]

Those with experience in dissecting rooms revealed that few corpses would subsequently be buried, 'either whole or in detail'. Any person who claimed otherwise, George Guthrie argued, either wilfully deceived others or himself.[52] As Jonathan Reinarz has argued, nineteenth-century medical students learned as much of their anatomy in museums as they did in books and dissecting rooms.[53] Any interesting part that was disposed of through burial, rather than being salvaged, therefore came to be viewed as something that had been 'lost' to a museum, in which it would have been preserved for students' further use – or displayed, exchanged, discarded, the usual things – and lost, too, to individual students who acquired specimens and preparations for their own personal use.[54]

---

[50] George Guthrie, *A letter to the Right Honorable the Secretary of State for the Home Department containing remarks on the report of the Select Committee of the House of Commons on anatomy, and pointing out the means by which the science may be cultivated with advantage and safety to the public* (London, 1829), on p. 9.

[51] 'Medicus', *An exposure of the present system of obtaining bodies for dissection and a more consistent plan suggested* (London, 1829), on p. 9; The souvenirs 'Medicus' had in mind were those of which he had personal knowledge: students converting skulls into a sugar-basin or a drinking-cup (*An exposure*, p. 9).

[52] Guthrie, *A letter*, p. 14.

[53] Jonathan Reinarz, 'The Age of Museum Medicine: The Rise and Fall of the Medical Museum at Birmingham's School of Medicine', *Social History of Medicine*, 18/3 (2005): pp. 419–37. On anatomy museums see also Samuel Alberti, 'The Museum Affect: Visiting Collections of Anatomy and Natural History', in A. Fyfe and B. Lightman (eds), *Science in the Marketplace: Nineteenth-Century Sites and Experiences* (Chicago, 2007), pp. 371–403; Sam Alberti, 'Wax Bodies: Art and Anatomy in Victorian Medical Museums', *Museum History Journal*, 2 (2009): pp. 7–36; Simon Chaplin, 'Nature Dissected, or Dissection Naturalized? The Case of John Hunter's Museum', *Museum and Society*, 6/2 (2008): pp. 135–51.

[54] The phrase 'lost to the museum' is that of Edinburgh-trained Professor J.T. Wilson (University of Sydney Archives, Department of Anatomy, Letter Book G63-1, 1890–1894,

Lists circulated of the many parts each well-trained man required for his own use. John Flint South recommended that a student's preparations should consist of one set of separate bones, one skeleton, one upper and one lower extremity, one head and neck (injected to show the blood-vessels), a wet specimen side-view of one male and one female pelvis, preparations of particular parts, and in addition, one small subject to show the distribution of the nerves.[55]

Only when the retention of this material threatened to become, in Inspector James Somerville's words, 'notorious', did the inspectors seek to bring it to a halt with reference to the Anatomy Act's burial clause. This occurred in 1838 when Somerville found that the janitor who worked in the practical anatomy rooms at Edinburgh University was selling dried bones.[56] And when police in Edinburgh reported to a later inspector what they thought must clearly be a contravention of the Anatomy Act – a wooden box emitting a peculiar smell had been found on the platform of Waverley railway station and was discovered to contain a human arm, leg, foot, two skullcaps and two clean thigh bones – Inspector Russell advised them to return the bones to 'the owner', a medical student, but to bury the other 'anatomical specimens'.[57]

Waste Disposal

But what of the material left behind once valuable specimens like these had been extracted from a corpse: those solid parts that were not considered worthy of being turned into specimens, the fluids, fat and soft tissue that stuck to a man's clothes and caused his fingers to become covered in rough patches of discoloured skin as he learned his craft from long immersion in morbid tissue rather than the 'unsoiling pages of a quarto'?[58] Where did the wreckage of a body go?

Waste, as David Halperin notes, is inevitable; it is how we deal with it that matters.[59] On this, anatomy inspectorate, hospital and museum records are usually

---

Wilson to Stuart, 20 June 1890, p. 23). For a discussion on the cultural biography of museum objects, in particular body parts, see Samuel Alberti, 'Objects and the Museum', *Isis*, 96 (2005): pp. 559–71.

55 John Flint South, *The Dissector's Manual, New Edition with Additions and Alterations* (London, 1825) on pp. xix–xx.

56 Somerville to Monro, 14 September 1838, p. 213, MH 74/13. For porters' duties including cleaning and scraping bones, see 'Joint statement by Dr Knox's principal assistants', cited in William Roughead (ed.), *Burke and Hare* (London, 1948), on p. 396.

57 NAS, Letter Book, Inspector of Anatomy for Scotland, MH 3/7 (1881–1885) [hereafter MH 3/7], Henderson to Russell, 8 April 1884; MH 3/7, Russell to Henderson, 9 April 1884.

58 South, *The Dissector's Manual*, p.viii.

59 David Halperin, cited in Gay Hawkins and Stephen Muecke (eds), 'Introduction', *Culture and Waste: The Creation and Destruction of Value* (Maryland, 2003), p. xv.

resolutely silent. Some teachers were genuinely puzzled about how to dispose of the offals and 'fragments' left behind after a dissection.[60] London's Inspector of Nuisances asked Anatomy Inspector Charles Hawkins whether 'the portions of muscular and other tissues' could not be taken away by undertakers and decently buried as the dissection progressed, '*before the whole body* is done with', for as things stood, saturating them with carbonic acid only substituted 'one stink for another', both to the disgust of the neighbours of his anatomy school.[61]

Waste only became the subject of writing when it was part of a larger scandal, something for which someone needed to account. After the Burke and Hare murders were discovered in Edinburgh in 1828, anatomist Robert Knox's students exposed his porter as being a man employed to dispose of the 'offals of the dissecting room'.[62] During an Irish scandal, a coffin was found to contain 'nothing in the form of a human body' but merely 'a bundle of some disgusting matter', in this case the intestines and some clothing.[63] When an undertaker was not paid his due in an Australian colonial hospital mortuary he took his revenge by informing the public that his work required him to use a shovel to scrape up bodily remnants and tip them into a coffin.[64] And photographs taken in American dissecting rooms sometimes captured the factotums who worked in these, mop or bucket in hand, cleaning up after young men dissected.

Quite a deal of bodily material was clearly escaping the Anatomy Act's burial clause. Nor were that clause's other elements being followed, those that specified that remains must be placed in a 'decent Coffin or Shell' for transport both to a school, and later from the school to a grave.

Where coffins and shells were concerned, those in which parish paupers' remains were buried were poor enough, so cheaply made that nails split the wood, gaps and holes exposed the corpse, leakages occurred.[65] But when bodies were

---

60 NA, Ministry of Health, Anatomy Office, General Correspondence and Papers, 1834–1890, MH 74/36, Windle to Birkett, 3 February 1890, pp. 2–3.

61 Saunders to Hawkins, 16 December 1876, p. 370, MH 74/6.

62 'Joint statement', cited in Roughhead, *Burke and Hare*, p. 396.

63 *Freeman's Journal and Daily Commercial Advertiser*, 1 April 1878. Ina Scherder is currently investigating the history of the Anatomy Act in Ireland (pers. comm.).

64 MacDonald, *Possessing the Dead*, p. 162.

65 Undertakers tendered to obtain parish contracts. Pauper shells and coffins were made of soft woods such as elm (see Julie-Marie Strange, *Death, Grief and Poverty in Britain, 1870–1914* (Cambridge, 2005), pp. 148–9). Nor were paupers' corpses secure once they were under the ground. As Julie-Marie Strange notes, wasteland rather than the 'best ground' was likely to be chosen for paupers' remains; and when the demand for burial sites outstripped available land, public graves were re-opened, the coffins 'broken up and trampled down' and the anonymous remnants of the corpses they contained exposed before being deposited elsewhere (Strange, 'Only a Pauper', pp. 159–60). Thomas Laqueur has argued that the pauper funeral was but 'the final ignominy' for the destitute, one that degraded them as 'social outcasts' beyond life ('Bodies, Death', p. 122).

being sent to a school rather than directly to a grave, some anatomy teachers even construed this parsimonious choice of container to be a wasteful outlay. In Surrey, corpses were sometimes removed from the St Mary Newington workhouse to the Guy's Hospital school trussed up in bags.[66] Until 1866 in Galway, workhouse paupers' corpses were also bagged up – then tossed over the workhouse wall at night into the waiting hands of representatives of the Queen's College medical school.[67] One Sheffield school which had been discovered sending remains for burial in a box rather than a coffin, justified the practice by claiming to have chosen this container to prevent public feelings against dissection being aroused (besides which, this school's proprietor pragmatically explained, as the corpse had been dismembered and the body otherwise much 'reduced in volume', no more than a *small* box was required).[68] The remains sent out of this school became part of a broader scandal which resulted in the local sexton and parish minister being charged with offences under the Burial Act: the sexton had been tipping uncoffined corpses into a pit that he grandiloquently named 'the catacombs'; the minister had been editing the burial register and signing the burial certificates required by the Anatomy Act for remains over which he had performed no service, and which had not been buried.[69]

Sometimes remains never entered a burial ground. *The Times* reported that a partial female skeleton had been found on the Vauxhall Bridge Road in circumstances that implicated the King's College school.[70] When a school of medicine in Surgeon Square, Edinburgh, closed in 1898, portions of a subject continued to dwell there in a tank for two years before a new occupant discovered them. Isabel Veuters wrote to Inspector Russell to alert him to their presence, but Russell responded that according to the certificates in his possession all of the bodies from that school had been buried. He had no papers relating to the 'material still in the tank', and no responsibility to bury them, but informed Miss Veuters that to avoid a scandal he would have a licensed anatomy teacher remove them.[71]

To the anatomy inspectors' horror, they also learned that corpses, extremities and otherwise mutilated remains were being packed into containers to travel around the country in public conveyances where they might be discovered at any moment 'in their transit to & fro'.[72] Inspector Somerville warned one Bath doctor that the 'discovery by the Public of the disgusting practice' he used in removing 'portions of a body from one town to another' would rekindle

66 MacDonald, *Possessing the Dead*, p. 86.

67 *Freeman's Journal and Daily Commercial Advertiser*, 3 April 1878.

68 Waddington to Home Office, 3 July 1862, pp. 312–13, MH 74/15.

69 *Leeds Mercury*, 24 June 1862.

70 Bacot to Partridge, 5 May 1847, p. 215, MH 74/15.

71 NAS, Inspector of Anatomy for Scotland letter book, MH 3/11 (1899–1905), Veuters to Russell, 9 December 1900 and Russell to Veuters, 10 September 1900.

72 Cursham to Sands Cox, 10 January 1851, p. 96, MH 74/10.

prejudices against dissection.[73] Sending corpses by train was always risky for the contents of each 'package' could be discovered and a great 'hubbub' would be raised.[74]

In addition, the inspectors learned that coffins were leaving medical schools containing more than the debris of the body that was specified on the burial certificate. Different people's remains were being mixed together in single coffins, together with non-human rubbish. One teacher who did this received a stern letter from Inspector John Bacot and promised that in future he would take care to render dissected parts 'as decent & proper as the necessities of the circumstances will allow'.[75] Bacot sent a circular to warn all of the metropolitan teachers against subjects being sent for burial so carelessly and 'so mixed with extraneous matter' as to cause outrage should this be discovered.[76] In another case, a teacher at St Thomas's hospital school wrote to complain about his own institution. The hospital was using the dissecting-room coffins as a means of disposing of hospital waste – amputated limbs from the operating theatre, 'odds and sods' from the museum.[77] Schools also sent coffins for burial that contained no body parts at all and forwarded fraudulent burial certificates to the inspector's office.[78] Worst of all, human and non-human animal remains were being disposed of together in single coffins. A certain Mr Philpot, speaking at a meeting of the Paddington Board of Guardians in December 1869, reported one such case 'in which various members of the body of a "subject" were found to be missing, and the bones of a dead donkey were used to fill up the coffin'. To Philpot's particular horror, the Christian burial service was then read over these remains.[79]

A further problem arose when remains that were sent for interment were disposed of in unconsecrated ground. The fact that a minister of religion signed a burial certificate did not mean that he had actually been present at the event.[80] Knowing the outrage that this would cause should it become public knowledge,

---

73 Somerville to Manlo, 13 August 1835, pp. 186–7, MH 74/12.

74 Cursham to Humphrey, 15 April 1861, p. 292, MH 74/10. For the later, routine use of the railway system to send bodies to Cambridge, see Elizabeth Hurren, 'A Pauper Dead-House: The Expansion of the Cambridge Anatomical Teaching School under the Late-Victorian Poor Law, 1870–1914', *Medical History*, 48/1 (2004): pp. 69–94.

75 Woods to Bacot, 15 November 1852, pp. 325–6, MH 74/15.

76 Circular to Metropolitan Teachers, 2 October 1853, p. 340, MH 74/15.

77 Copy of letter from Reid to Hawkins, November 1879, p. 425, MH 74/6.

78 Hawkins to Liddell, 25 November 1874, p. 337, MH 74/6.

79 *Daily News*, 2 December 1869.

80 Hawkins to Dix, 13 April 1858, p. 19, MH 74/6; Hawkins to Burridge, 31 December 1873, pp. 305–6, MH 74/10, Gregg to Stephens, 4 October 1855, MH 74/6, p. 184. This was also part of a broader problem at the time. By the 1840s the disreputable state of London's burial grounds was common knowledge and the subject of investigation (Catharine Arnold, *Necropolis: London and its Dead* (London, 2006) pp. 95–119). The city burial grounds were closed in 1852.

the inspectors tried to stop it.[81] But market forces were at work then, as they are now, and waste travelled to the cheapest dumping ground. In 1835, this was revealed when a farmer sent a man in a wagon to remove night soil from an East London hospital. Upon arriving, the wagoner found that the soil contained more body parts than excrement. Threatened by hospital officials, he shovelled the 'soil' into his wagon and took it away to deposit in the farmer's field. Onlookers there saw exposed to view 'legs, thighs, arms, in fact fragments of every part of the human body; also several heads, some bald, others with hair on, and their teeth remaining', as well as the body of a child which was in near perfect condition. The farmer ordered that a deep pit be dug for most of these remains, but he had the child's body buried 'in the normal way'.[82]

Conclusion

That learning anatomy required corpses was something which few people taking part in debating the matter during the nineteenth century disputed. Substitutes, in the form of wax models and books, could not replace them. The problem lay in deciding specifically whose bodies should be devoted to this unpopular purpose. The 1832 Anatomy Act legalized the contentious choice to turn the institutionalized poor into useful things. It set in place a regime under which it became possible for those with the power to dispose of corpses, to view any that went to the grave rather than to a dissecting table as being things wasted to science. In this context, over the course of the century Britain's anatomy inspectors sought to obtain bodies for medical students as quietly as possible to prevent exposure of the system which the Act had put in place. They feared that if the public learned that human remains were frequently treated as if they were no more than waste material that could be used and disposed of in cavalier ways, the hard-fought Anatomy Act would be revisited and perhaps even repealed.

Bibliography

Manuscript Sources

Edinburgh City Archives, Town Council Minutes.

National Archives of Scotland, Inspector of Anatomy for Scotland, Letterbook (1875–1882), MH 3/6.

National Archives of Scotland, Inspector of Anatomy for Scotland, Letterbook (1881–1885), MH 3/7.

81 Hawkins to Dix, 13 April 1858, p. 19, MH 74/6.

82 *Bell's Life in London and Sporting Chronicle*, 20 September 1835.

National Archives of Scotland, Inspector of Anatomy for Scotland, Letterbook (1885–1889), MH 3/8.
National Archives of Scotland, Inspector of Anatomy for Scotland, Letterbook (1899–1905), MH 3/11.
National Archives, Home Office, Anatomy, Appointment of Inspectors under Anatomy Act (1834, 1842–1843), HO 45/189.
National Archives, Home Office, Anatomy, Volume 1 (1832 to 1842), HO 83/1.
National Archives, Ministry of Health, Anatomy Office, Out letter Books, General including Scotland (1832–1835), MH 74/12.
National Archives, Ministry of Health, Anatomy Office, General Correspondence and Papers (1834–1890), MH 74/36.
National Archives, Ministry of Health, Anatomy Office, Outletter Book, General (1835 to 1841), MH 74/13.
National Archives, Anatomy Office, Outletter Books, Metropolitan District (1842–1858), MH 74/15.
National Archives, Ministry of Health, Anatomy Office, Outletter Books, Provincial Districts (1842–1879), MH 74/10.
National Archives, Ministry of Health, Anatomy Office, Outletter Books, Metropolitan District (1858–1881), MH 74/6.
National Archives, Ministry of Health, Anatomy Correspondence (1890–1904), MH 74/37.
University of Sydney Archives, Department of Anatomy, Letter Book G63-1 (1890–1894).

Printed Primary Sources

Bell's Life in London and Sporting Chronicle.
Daily News.
Freeman's Journal and Daily Commercial Advertiser.
John Bull.
The Lady's Newspaper.
Leeds Mercury.
The Times.
'An Act for Regulating Schools of Anatomy', *Statutes of the United Kingdom of Great Britain and Ireland* (London).
Guthrie, George, *A letter to the Right Honorable the Secretary of State for the Home Department containing remarks on the report of the Select Committee of the House of Commons on anatomy, and pointing out the means by which the science may be cultivated with advantage and safety to the public* (London, 1829), on p. 9.
'Medicus', *An exposure of the present system of obtaining bodies for dissection and a more consistent plan suggested* (London, 1829), on p. 9.
Naples, Joshua, Diary of a London Resurrectionist, 1811–1812, held by the Royal College of Surgeons, London.

Parliamentary Papers, United Kingdom, Hansard's Parliamentary Debates, Volumes IX, X, XIV, XX.

Roberts, William, *Mr Warburton's Anatomy Bill, thoughts on its mischievous tendency; with suggestions for an entirely new one, founded upon an available anti-septic process, in an appeal to medical practitioners, students of anatomy, and the public at large, on the injury to medical science and the hindrances to the decent interment of unclaimed pauper bodies now delivered up for anatomical 'examination,' consequent upon the rejection of such a process* (London, 1843).

South, John Flint, *The Dissector's Manual*, New Edition with Additions and Alterations (London, 1825).

Theses

Brasier, Angeline, 'Prison or Paradise: An Investigation into Conditions in the Bermudian Convict Establishment', PhD Thesis, School of Historical and Philosophical Studies, University of Melbourne, in preparation.

Stevenson, Anna, 'An Obscure Personality called William Roberts: The Later History of the Anatomy Act of 1832', BSc Thesis, History of Medicine, University of London, 2004.

Secondary Sources

Alberti, Samuel, 'Objects and the Museum', *Isis*, 96 (2005): pp. 559–71.

Alberti, Samuel, 'The Museum Affect: Visiting Collections of Anatomy and Natural History', in A. Fyfe and B. Lightman (eds), *Science in the Marketplace: Nineteenth-Century Sites and Experiences* (Chicago: University of Chicago Press, 2007), pp. 371–403.

Alberti, Samuel, 'Wax Bodies: Art and Anatomy in Victorian Medical Museums', *Museum History Journal*, 2 (2009): pp. 7–36.

Arnold, Catharine, *Necropolis: London and its Dead* (London: Simon & Schuster, 2006).

Chaplin, Simon, 'Nature Dissected, or Dissection Naturalized? The Case of John Hunter's Museum', *Museum and Society*, 6/2 (2008): pp. 135–51.

Hart, Nicky, 'Beyond Infant Mortality: Gender and Stillbirth in Reproductive Mortality before the Twentieth Century', *Population Studies*, 52/2 (1998): pp. 215–29.

Hawkins, Gay and Muecke, Stephen (eds), 'Introduction', *Culture and Waste: The Creation and Destruction of Value* (Lanham: Rowman & Littlefield, 2003), pp. ix–xvii.

Hay, Douglas, 'Property, Authority and the Criminal Law', in D. Hay, P. Linebaugh, J. Rule, E.P. Thompson and C. Winslow (eds), *Albion's Fatal Tree: Crime and Society in Eighteenth-Century England* (London: Pantheon, 1975), pp. 17–64.

Hurren, Elizabeth, 'A Pauper Dead-House: The Expansion of the Cambridge Anatomical Teaching School under the Late-Victorian Poor Law, 1870–1914', *Medical History*, 48/1 (2004): pp. 69–94.

Jones, Ross L., *Humanity's Mirror: 150 Years of Anatomy in Melbourne* (South Yarra: Haddington Press, 2007).

Laqueur, Thomas, 'Bodies, Death, and Pauper Funerals', *Representations*, 1/1 (1983): pp. 109–31.

Lawrence, Susan, 'Anatomy and Address: Creating Medical Gentlemen in Eighteenth-Century London', in V. Nutton and R. Porter (eds), *The History of Medical Education in Britain* (Amsterdam: Rodopi, 1995), pp. 199–228.

MacDonald, Helen, 'Procuring Corpses: England's Anatomy Inspectorate, 1842 to 1858', *Medical History*, 53/3 (2009): pp. 379–96.

MacDonald, Helen, *Possessing the Dead: The Artful Science of Anatomy* (Melbourne: Melbourne University Press, 2010).

Reinarz, Jonathan, 'The Age of Museum Medicine: The Rise and Fall of the Medical Museum at Birmingham's School of Medicine', *Social History of Medicine*, 18/3 (2005): pp. 419–37.

Rosner, Lisa, *The Anatomy Murders* (Philadelphia: University of Pennsylvania Press, 2009).

Roughead, William (ed.), *Burke and Hare* (London: Willliam Hodge & Coy Ltd, 1948).

Shaw, A.G.L., *Convicts and the Colonies: A Study of Penal Transportation from Great Britain & Ireland to Australia & Other Parts of the British Empire* (Kilkenny: Irish Historical Press, 1998).

Strange, Julie-Marie, '"Only a Pauper Whom Nobody Owns": Reassessing the Pauper Grave c.1880–1914', *Past and Present*, 178 (February 2003): pp. 148–75.

Strange, Julie-Marie, *Death, Grief and Poverty in Britain, 1870–1914* (Cambridge: Cambridge University Press, 2005).

Waddington, Keir, 'Mayhem and Medical Students: Image, Conduct, and Control in the Victorian and Edwardian London Teaching Hospital', *Social History of Medicine*, 15/1 (2002): pp. 45–64.

Warner, John Harley and Edmonson, James M., *Dissection: Photographs of a Rite of Passage in American Medicine 1880–1930* (New York: Blast Books, 2009).

Chapter 2
Cadavers and the Social Dimension of Dissection*

Ross L. Jones

In the late nineteenth century, Western medical schools developed an acute dependence on an abundant and secure supply of human cadavers, which were essential for the purpose of teaching students the new understanding of the localization of diseases in organs and tissues. As this new thirst for cadavers for dissection arose concurrently with the growth of the modern democratic polity, the question of how to source the essential bodies for the processes of medical research and education created a significant dilemma – one that has dogged medical policy planners from the nineteenth century until the present. This chapter provides a case study which examines the problem relating to the supply of cadavers in Melbourne, Australia, as well as the responses and proffered solutions to it of the medical establishment.[1]

---

* I wish to thank Tatjana Buklijas, Richard Selleck, Helen MacDonald, Cecily Hunter, John Waugh and Susan Kenny for their assistance in writing this chapter.

1 For a recent overview of anatomical education in the United States see John Harley Warner and Lawrence J. Rizzolo, 'Anatomical Instruction and Training for Professionalism from the 19th to the 20th Centuries', *Clinical Anatomy*, 19/5 (2006): pp. 403–14. The major study of anatomy for the nineteenth century in the United States (particularly in relation to cadavers) is Michael Sappol, *A Traffic of Dead Bodies: Anatomy and Embodied Social Identity in Nineteenth-Century America* (Princeton, 2002); F.W. Hafferty, *Into the Valley: Death and the Socialization of Medical Students* (Yale, 1991) For the nineteenth century in the UK see Ruth Richardson, *Death, Dissection and the Destitute* (Harmondsworth, 1988), Elizabeth T. Hurren, 'A Pauper Dead-House: The Expansion of the Cambridge Anatomical Teaching School under the Late-Victorian Poor Law, 1870–1914', *Medical History*, 48/1 (2004): pp. 69–94; and 'Whose Body is it Anyway? Trading the Dead Poor, Coroner's Disputes, and the Business of Anatomy at Oxford University, 1885–1929', *Bulletin of the History of Medicine*, 82/4 (Winter 2008): pp. 775–818; and Helen MacDonald, 'Procuring Corpses: England's Anatomy Inspectorate, 1842 to 1858', *Medical History*, 53/3 (2009): pp. 379–96. For Vienna see Tatjana Buklijas, 'Cultures of Death and Politics of Corpse Supply: Anatomy in Vienna, 1848–1914', *Bulletin of the History of Medicine*, 82/3 (2008): pp. 570–607. For Australasia, see D. Gareth Jones, 'Bequests, Cadavers and Dissections: Sketches from New Zealand History', *New Zealand Medical Journal*, 104 (1991): pp. 210–12, and Helen MacDonald, 'A Scandalous Act: Regulating Anatomy in a British Settler Colony', *Social History of Medicine*, 20/1 (2007): pp. 39–56, '"Humanity's Discards": The New South

The study of anatomy through the dissection of the human body has justifiably been portrayed as a powerful way in which social and political ideas are embodied and transmitted. Adrian Desmond has shown that dissection was a tool for radicalism in early nineteenth-century Britain, at a time when medical schools provided a way 'into the anatomical underworld, where Lamarck's and Geoffroy's doctrines mingled with anti-Church-and-state propaganda'.[2] Michael Sappol has revealed anatomy to have been a complex vehicle for social and ideological expression, most significantly an important way in which the emerging middle class in the United States became self-aware through 'the incorporation of the anatomical body into the curriculum of bourgeois self-making'.[3] The growth of allopathic medicine and the subsequent medicalization of Western societies including Australia saw the creation of a class of powerful, anatomically trained medical practitioners with an insatiable need for human corpses.

With the development of the social and political institutions that accompanied large-scale urban growth in Melbourne during the second half of the nineteenth century, the university-trained medical profession was well placed to take a leading role in the city, for the study of anatomy was an important badge of respectability and power. The University of Melbourne Medical School had been founded in 1862 (paid for, like other public institutions in this new metropolis, by the wealth created by gold), and was the first medical school in the southern hemisphere. Important distinguishing characteristics of this colonial society affected the way in which the increased demand for cadavers for this new and fast growing school was met.

Melbourne's Underclass

Following the discovery of gold in the British colony of Victoria in the early 1850s, the transformation of its capital city was rapid and dramatic. Melbourne grew from a village to a large metropolis in a decade, with all the social dislocation that such an upheaval necessarily caused.[4] In 1851 Melbourne's

---

Wales Anatomy Act 1881', *Mortality*, 12/4 (2007): pp. 365–82, and 'The Anatomy Inspector and the Government Corpse', *History Australia*, 6/2 (2009): 40.1–40.17. The literature on the much-examined later phenomenon of medicalization of certain Western societies is unusually bereft of studies of the important role played in its development by cadavers and human material. See Adele Clarke et al., 'Biomedicalization: Technoscientific Transformations of Health, Illness, and U.S. Biomedicine', *American Sociology Review*, 68/2 (April 2003): p. 163.

2 Adrian Desmond, *The Politics of Evolution: Morphology, Medicine, and Reform in Radical London* (Chicago, 1989), p. 21.

3 Sappol, *A Traffic of Dead Bodies*, p. 238.

4 See Paul de Serville, *Pounds and Pedigrees: The Upper Class in Victoria 1850–80*, (Melbourne, 1991) and Andrew Brown-May, *Melbourne Street Life: The Itinerary of Our Days* (Melbourne, 1998), especially pp. 121–2.

population was 23,000: fortune-seekers flooded into the colony, doubling that number in 1852 and within 40 years there were one million people, many of whom found no riches. As the 1886 Annual Report of the Melbourne Benevolent Asylum committee noted:

> In such a city as Melbourne, the growth of which has been so rapid, it could hardly be expected, even under the most auspicious circumstances, that all should be possessed of a competency. Such a thing would indeed be exceptional, and altogether contrary to the accepted notion that indigence more or less is to be found in every large centre of population. Whether or not the sudden maturity of our metropolis may not, so to speak, have fostered an abnormal social condition is a question for historians to determine; but one thing seems certain, and that is, that we are not without a goodly number of those who are in an absolute state of want, and unable to procure even the common necessities of life.[5]

Another consequence of this great inrush of people to Victoria was the creation of a large class of itinerant and semi-itinerant males.[6] The preponderance of men in this class is reflected in the high proportion of male inmates in the town's Benevolent Asylum in North Melbourne; and also perhaps in the high number of male cadavers that entered the Medical School's dissecting room in the early twentieth century (see Figure 2.1).[7] The first arrival noted in the surviving School archives was James Halferty, aged 53, who had been found ill at the Fitzroy Cricket Club in Brunswick Street, making it likely that Halferty was itinerant. He died on 24 October 1898 in the Melbourne Hospital of heart failure caused by arteriosclerosis and his corpse was received in the Anatomy Department at 8 p.m. the following night.[8]

---

5 *The Thirty-Seventh Annual report of the Committee of Management of the Melbourne Benevolent Asylum and list of subscriptions and donations for the year 1886* (Melbourne, 1887), p.4.

6 Ross L. Jones, 'The Rogers-Templeton and Pearson Royal Commissions: Contemporary Views of the 1872 Education Act', *History of Education Review*, 27/2 (1998): pp. 50–66.

7 For example in 1869, 369 men and 155 women were resident in the Asylum (*Argus*, 30 July 1869, p. 5); see also R.A. Cage, *Poverty Abounding, Charity Aplenty: The Charity Network in Colonial Victoria* (Sydney, 1992); Mary Kehoe, *The Melbourne Benevolent Asylum: Hotham's Premier Building: The Annals of Hotham*, vol. 1 (North Melbourne, 1998).

8 Cadaver Archives, Department of Anatomy and Cell Biology, University of Melbourne. Each of the records was signed by a medical officer at the hospital and by the Professor of Anatomy or his agent at the University. Addresses were only given for 13 of the first group of 55 bodies recorded in the surviving records (those of 1902) indicating that the information concerning place of abode was not always available.

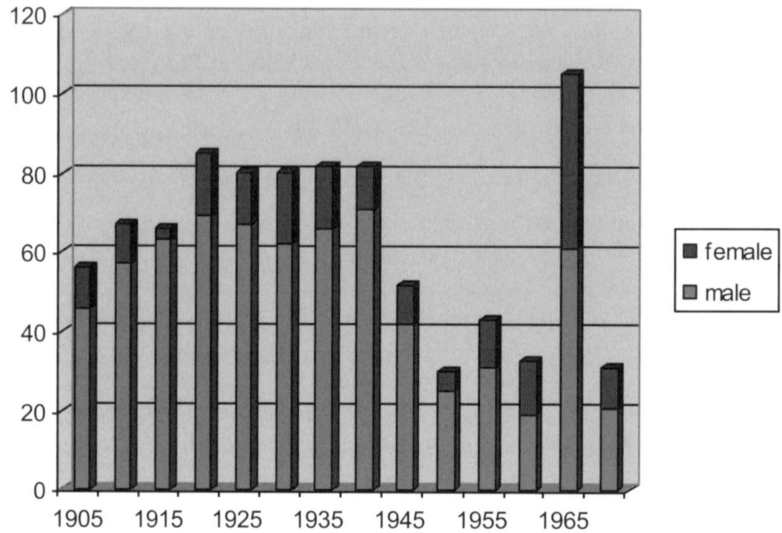

Figure 2.1 Gender of cadavers received into the Department of Anatomy, University of Melbourne, 1905–1965[9]

Whilst great rewards were possible in the mutable social structure of a new and exotic location, fate could be fickle and fortunes dramatically change for any particular individual. This occurred in Australia in the 1890s financial crash, during which Halferty died. In Victoria, from the earliest days of the gold rush through to the end of the century, class boundaries were elastic – even fluid – and anxiety characterized the efforts of groups seeking to establish respectability and influence. As Andrew Brown-May has written, 'whilst a teacher sold refreshments on a street corner, diggers lucky enough to have hit the jackpot ostentatiously paraded the streets on orgiastic sprees, eating pound notes between slices of bread, drinking champagne by the bucketful'.[10]

Medical students were aware of the need to establish respectability in the shifting sands of *fin-de-siècle* Melbourne society. They jealously guarded their hard-won gains. As one wrote in the medical student magazine *Speculum* in May 1887:

---

[9] A note on the graphs: there are tens of thousands of records in the Department of Anatomy archives and an exhaustive study would take years and considerable resources to complete. For the purposes of this chapter I have sampled cadavers received in one of every five years and categorized them as belonging to one of four groups: those from institutions; hospitals but with a home address; hospitals with no known address; and those who have only a home address – a category which commences with the donations that started trickling in at the beginning of the 1950s. I will discuss body donation in a later article.

[10] Brown-May, *Melbourne Street Life*, p. 121. For an extended discussion of the fluidity of class structure in Melbourne at this time see de Serville, *Pounds and Pedigrees*.

> In this age of cheap jewellery – and especially in a country like this, which has been populated by money-getters – it is only to be expected that there would be many willing to undertake the labour of a course, say of medicine or law for the sake of kudos, and the social standing, which are among the prerequisites of the professional man.[11]

In 1905, *Speculum* hailed the arrival from Britain of Professor Richard Berry, who had been appointed to the newly created professorship of anatomy and would revitalize anatomical teaching at the Medical School.[12] For decades the students had complained about how anatomy was taught by Berry's predecessor Harry Brookes Allen, a physiologist by inclination. After a year of Berry's tenure the student magazine could exclaim:

> Our anatomy is now no longer dry bone,
> Since Professor Berry has come to expound it;
> For, in some strange poetical way of his own
> He has weaved graceful garlands around it.[13]

As a rigid class structure like that in Britain seemed absent from Australia, Berry was aware of his opportunity to contribute to the development of Victoria and the nascent Commonwealth of Australia. In an unpublished memoir he later wrote that there was 'no aristocracy of birth in these Dominions overseas, aristocracy of intellect takes its place. Consequently a Professor of the University of Melbourne occupied a very special place in the society of my time'.[14] A relatively fluid social structure did not, however, completely absolve failure, and it was not just the itinerant that posed a problem. Berry was greatly concerned by the presence of an underclass in Melbourne. He was amongst those (including many in Melbourne's medical and intellectual establishment) who believed that slum-dwellers were biologically – and thus irreversibly – inferior beings. Berry would go on to make a significant contribution to the English eugenic movement when he returned there from Melbourne in 1929.[15]

---

11 *Speculum*, 9 (May 1887): p. 1.

12 George Britton Halford was Professor of Anatomy, Pathology and Physiology from 1862 to 1881 when his student Harry Brookes Allen was appointed Professor of Anatomy and Pathology, leaving Halford with Physiology. Berry left in 1929.

13 *Speculum*, 67 (December 1906): 120f. For the complaints see Ross L. Jones, *Humanity's Mirror: 150 Years of Anatomy in Melbourne* (Melbourne, 2007), pp. 67–71.

14 R.J.A. Berry, Chance and Circumstance, unpublished autobiography, University of Melbourne Medical Library, 1954, p. 115.

15 Penrose Memoirs – 1964: Phenylketonuria, Lionel S. Penrose Papers, University College London Archives, quoted in Daniel Kevles, *In the Name of Eugenics* (London, 2001 [1985]), p. 159.

Melbourne's demographic pattern also changed radically in the late nineteenth century as a product of the rapid expansion of the city with the growth of middle-class suburbs ringing its centre and the flight of the wealthy from the earliest suburbs which surrounded the central business district. Once-grand terraces built in the booming 1880s soon became boarding houses as whole suburbs were abandoned by the middle classes.[16] The Medical School and the public hospitals, in which its students attended clinical subjects, were situated in the middle of these declining suburbs. To the medical student who frequently passed though Carlton, the suburb that enveloped its northern and eastern boundary, its impoverished residents seemed completely foreign. As one student wrote in *Speculum*:

> Swarms of young Carltonians may be seen and heard at all times of the day and year dancing and singing – dressed in their own peculiar, and at the same time picturesque, garb – to the strains of the soul-stirring, never-wearying hurdy-gurdy or street organ, played in masterly fashion by a swarthy 'Irishman'.[17]

The Carltonian was posited as a quaint and distant character, a:

> 'singular anomaly', the Carlton masher … who, with thumbs in breeches' pockets, a large mushroom, carefully ironed, hat, 'overhanging foliage' on his forehead, and the irresistible bell-bottomed pants … saunters along, and loiters around the sunny corners of the blue-stones, dreaming love's young dream, or of pints of ale to come, and anon squirting from beneath his teeth the juice of the succulent tobacco.[18]

Battles were fought between these larrikins and the students, just one symptom of the antagonism that existed at this time between the university and significant sections of Melbourne's citizenry.[19]

The Medical School's cadaver archives up until the 1940s show that the overwhelming majority of bodies arriving in the dissecting room for which a last

---

16 George Tibbits, 'Slums and Public Housing in Southern Fitzroy', in Cutten History Committee of the Fitzroy History Society (eds), *Fitzroy: Melbourne's First Suburb* (Melbourne, 1991): pp. 126–37, p. 134; Allan Willingham, 'The Rise and Fall of a Fitzroy Villa', in Cutten History (eds), *Fitzroy: Melbourne's First Suburb* (Melbourne, 1991), pp. 118–25.

17 *Speculum*, 25 (July 1891): pp. 78–9.

18 Ibid.

19 See Jones, *Humanity's Mirror*, p. 49. The medical students expressed similar views about Parkville, the suburb in which the University was situated and in which they often found accommodation during term time. Parkville declined after the 1890s crash. *Speculum*, 116 (June 1925): pp. 45–6

place of abode was known (other than when that was a benevolent institution or the Melbourne Hospital) lived in these inner suburbs.

The Supply of Cadavers

In 1862, a Bill to regularize dissection was brought before the Upper House of the Victorian parliament by Thomas Turner a'Beckett, in preparation for the imminent foundation of the University of Melbourne Medical School.[20] A'Beckett announced that this colonial bill 'was a transcript of the English Bill, with the necessary alterations to adapt it to the circumstances of the colony'.[21] During the second reading debate, he told the Council:

> It was a misdemeanour at common law to be in possession of a deceased person's body. Of course it would be an outrage of common decency for a man to have anything of the kind; but they all knew what crimes were formerly perpetrated in obtaining possession of dead bodies, for the purpose of anatomical investigation; and how it was found necessary ultimately to legalise what, at first sight, appeared to be a violation of their natural feelings.[22]

The editor of the *Argus* newspaper argued that the Anatomy Bill was somewhat slipshod in not specifying the sources from which corpses would be obtained. He predicted that if bodies could not be procured from public institutions 'the practice of "body-snatching" will be revived'.[23] A'Beckett's reference to grave-robbing does not appear to refer to any local scandal. Whilst body-snatching had created a sensation in the nearby island colony of Tasmania, evidence of any such scandal in Melbourne had not thus far surfaced.[24] The parliamentary debate concerning the supply of cadavers passed in Victoria as a non-event, unencumbered by the important considerations that accompanied the passage of similar legislation later in the neighbouring colony of New South Wales.[25] Perhaps this was because the Victorian Act was Australia's first.

The earliest records still held by the Anatomy Department in the Medical School begin nearly three decades later on 26 October 1898. Direct evidence for the

---

[20] 4 March 1862, *Victorian Parliamentary Debates*, Legislative Council, 1862, vol. 8, p. 706.

[21] Ibid.

[22] Ibid., p. 837.

[23] *Argus*, 7 August 1869, p. 4.

[24] For the Tasmanian scandals see Helen McDonald, *Human Remains: Dissection and its Histories* (New Haven, 2006).

[25] MacDonald, '"Humanity's Discards"'.

supply of cadavers to the School from 1863 until then is lost.[26] The first complete year to be recorded is 1902, when the School received 55 cadavers at a cost of £1 each.[27] Only 13 of these came with addresses that included a street number; 21 were supplied with the name of a suburb only, with occasionally a street name also being recorded. Seven of the bodies were those of people who had no known address. Of all the cadavers more than three-quarters had been itinerant. There were 47 male and only eight female corpses, with the address supplied for the two younger women (aged 22 and 27 years) and one older woman (aged 67) being the notorious brothel district, Little Lonsdale Street. The young women had died of phthisis and the older woman of debility. Two of the male cadavers received that year were those of men who had resided on ships docked in the port. Both had died from phthisis. Seven died of alcoholism and 18 from tuberculosis. The average age of these people at death was 55 years, almost exactly the average male life expectancy in Australia in 1902 which is interesting considering the tenuous nature of these people's life circumstances. The demography of the cadavers in this first recorded year, both in the gender imbalance and degree of impoverishment, established a pattern that lasted for decades.

Corpse Supply in the Early Twentieth Century

At first, and for much of the nineteenth century, the supply for the Medical School comprised mainly unclaimed corpses from the Melbourne Hospital, although after the amendment to the *Medical Practitioners Statute 1865* Part IV in 1876 it was possible to use unclaimed asylum bodies, the bodies of prisoners and those who died unclaimed in public institutions, although it is not known to what degree this occurred.[28] However this source was inadequate for the School's needs and so the first two anatomy professors, George Britton Halford and Harry Brookes Allen, searched for alternate sources. The problem of supply became chronic as the nineteenth century drew to a close, as the number of students in the Medical School had grown from three in 1862 to 260 in 1897.[29]

On his arrival in Melbourne to take up the chair of anatomy, Berry wrote that a shortage of cadavers had bedevilled Allen's attempts to teach it but that his

[26] Anecdotal evidence suggests that any archives for the period 1860s until 1898 were destroyed during the 1980s.

[27] Cadaver Archives.

[28] Like all such institutions, this hospital was established principally for the care of the poor. It had been modelled on the charitable structure of London's hospitals, but colonial society was neither sufficiently rich nor willing to provide charitable funds to make the hospital self-sufficient. Public funding therefore supplemented donations. The colonial, then the state, government was the principal donor. See also MacKinnon, Chapter 4 this volume.

[29] See Jones, *Humanity's Mirror*, pp. 1–2; for the chronic shortage pp. 86–91.

predecessor 'got over some of his difficulties by the ingenious method of teaching anatomy in the post-mortem room [at the Melbourne Hospital], hence the forlorn appearance of the dissecting room as I first saw it'.[30] A student poem from 1894 also places the hospital as an important early source:

> When Winter saw the typhoids end,
> Pulmonic troubles did not falter.
> Then, just as 'go-betweens', there'd come
> Some 'cardiacs' or 'fractured bases',
> Chronic kidneys, or likely some
> New fangled 'op' to fill his 'cases'.[31]

The cadaver archives show that from 1898 the major source of cadavers remained the Melbourne Hospital, however Allen was also receiving bodies from a home for the indigent, the Immigrants' Home. This had been established in 1853 in the outlying suburb of St Kilda by the Immigrants' Aid Society, to provide support for those who arrived in the colony without adequate resources. Over time, the Immigrants' Home came to provide facilities similar to those of an English workhouse, including accommodation for the homeless (though Melbourne's asylums were less stark than those in the United Kingdom).[32] In 1882 abandoned industrial school buildings in Royal Park (not far from the university) housed a growing number of indigent men. Though records for this time are missing, this may have been when the Immigrants' Home first became a source of cadavers to the School. From 1899 it provided numerous bodies, with the first record in the archive indicating the purchase of 22 individuals in that year.[33]

The Medical School also attempted to obtain corpses from the local Benevolent Asylum, but failed to do so during the nineteenth century, as Susan K. Martin illustrates in Chapter 3 of this book. However, in 1920 bodies began to arrive in the School from this institution, which in 1911 had relocated from inner-city North Melbourne to the relatively distant seaside suburb of Cheltenham. As can be seen in Figure 2.2, during the first decade of the twentieth century institutions for the homeless took over from hospitals as the major supplier of cadavers.[34]

---

30 Berry, Chance and Circumstance, p. 112.

31 *Speculum*, 30 (August 1894): p. 12, 'op' being surgical operation.

32 R. Kennedy, 'Poor Relief in Melbourne: the Benevolent Society's Contribution', *Journal of the Royal Australian Historical Society*, 60 (1974): pp. 256–66.

33 In 1900–17 bodies; 1901–10; 1902–11; 1903–09; 1909–75, Cadaver Archives. It was also known as the Victorian Homes for the Aged and Infirm after 1902 and then the Victorian Benevolent Home and Hospital for the Aged and Infirm after 1925, eventually taking the name Mount Royal. See Jean Uhl, *Mount Royal Hospital: A Social History* (Parkville, 1981).

34 The Alfred Hospital in the inner suburb of Prahran had begun to supply a small number of bodies after 1900.

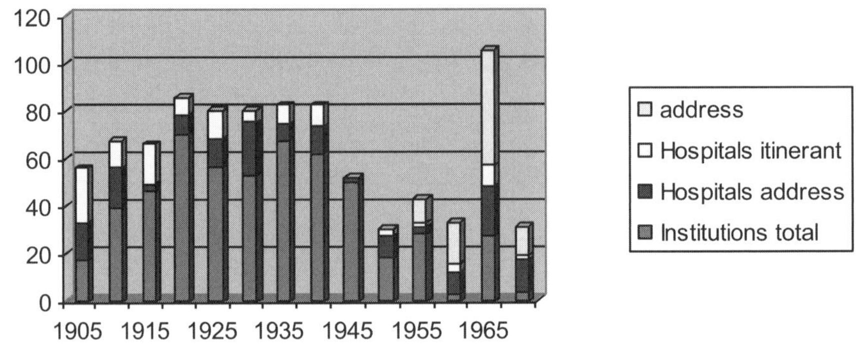

Figure 2.2 Sources of cadavers received into the Department of Anatomy, University of Melbourne, 1905–1965

Cadavers, Medical Students and Social Class

Although no studies have been made of the class background of medical students at this time, the need to pay substantial fees to study medicine and fund board and living expenses whilst studying meant that there was a clear social distinction between the students and their cadavers. The medical students recognized this. They were prickly about their perceived advantages over the common populace, to the point that *Speculum* felt impelled to argue in July 1887 that 'money is frequently a question among students, who are not *all* wealthy'.[35] A perception of biological superiority can also be found amongst the views that occasionally surfaced in *Speculum*. One report of a medical student night out at the theatre (a regular social activity of the Medical Students' Society during this period) characterized the lower-class members of the audience as scoffing at the student group as bearing a biological mark of social superiority: there was a 'general murmur of "s'help me Tommy they're all toffs, look at their faces"'. The medical student writing this article expressed his agreement with Henry Mayhew's identification of separate species within the human race, commenting to his readers: 'Please note this remark, oh! physiognomical Dr Moloney'.[36]

On the other hand, Melbourne's working-class youths were sometimes represented by the students as being particularly vigorous stock. In 1887, the university's Australian Rules football team's dismal season was reported in the following terms in *Speculum*:

---

[35] *Speculum*, 10 (July 1887): p. 10. The total cost of a medical degree at Melbourne in 1892 was £900, see *Speculum*, 28 (July 1892): pp. 25–6.

[36] *Speculum*, 2 (December 1884): 7. Henry Mayhew, *London Labour and the London Poor: A Cyclopaedia of the Conditions and Earnings of Those that will Work and Those that Cannot Work, and Those that Will Not Work* (London, 1851).

> our style of life renders it almost impossible that we should contend in strength with clubs, the players of which are mostly engaged in manual labour, and are, on an average, two stone per man heavier than we are.[37]

A grudging respect was sometimes paid to the rude physicality of the Australian working man, creating a distinction between the 'worthy' poor and the itinerant and slum-dweller.

Medical students' attitudes to the working classes exhibited all the complexity of a group establishing a profession of status in a developing society. Even in the dissecting room, *Speculum* could enquire of the Lancastrian Berry in an interview, 'You find abnormalities scarce in Australia, we believe?'.[38] Ambivalence and a degree of anxiety characterized the middle-class idea of the evolving Australian 'type'. As Warwick Anderson has written, uncertainty about identity underlay the Australian psyche from early colonial days when concerns were expressed because 'the climate was foreign, social life appeared disordered, the diseases varied, and it sometimes seemed that a new biological type might emerge from the colonial turmoil' until the 1930s, when 'the racial type was either degenerate or it was triumphant in the antipodean environment'.[39]

Little evidence remains of any extensive use of Aboriginal cadavers in the dissecting room.[40] Medical students' attitudes to the Victorian Aboriginal population seem less complex than those they expressed about working-class people. In 1891, 'Studentia' wrote in *Speculum* that '[a]nyone who visits our National Museum cannot fail to be struck with the resemblance between the specimens of the higher apes and our aboriginal brethren', although he believed that 'Poor Jacky Jacky would turn away from his hairy ancestor with about the same feelings of contempt that one of our patrician ladies would show, if her aboriginal brother claimed relationship'. Studentia concluded that '[t]aking all into consideration, there is nothing so very repulsive after all when we look back to our progenitors. It is comforting to feel that we are *evolved* from them'.[41] However, that is not to say that there was no trade in such bodies. Anatomy professors in Melbourne

---

37 *Speculum*, 9 (May 1887): p. 22.

38 *Speculum*, 76 (December 1909): p. 152.

39 Warwick Anderson, *The Cultivation of Whiteness: Science, Health and Racial Destiny in Australia* (Melbourne, 2002), p. 11; p. 2. For more on this anxiety see Geoffrey Serle, *From Deserts the Prophets Come – The Creative Spirit in Australia 1788–1972* (Melbourne, 1973), p. 55; de Serville, *Pounds and Pedigrees*, p. 140, pp. 147–8, p. 187; Jones, *Humanity's Mirror*, pp. 44–5; Geoffrey Sherington, '"A Better Class of Boy" The Big Brother Movement, Youth Migration and Citizenship of Empire', *Australian Historical Studies*, 33/120 (October 2002): pp. 267–85.

40 For one troubling exception, see *Speculum*, 40 (May 1898): 27, 'In the Dissecting Room—Very junior man gazing on a blackfellow: "See! This body is putrifying: it is all black"'.

41 *Speculum*, 23 (February 1891): p. 161, p. 162.

provided Aboriginal remains to their academic mentors in the United Kingdom. From the arrival of George Halford in 1863 until the departure of Richard Berry in 1929, Melbourne was well recognized as a centre for the study of physical anthropology. Summing up the work of Halford, Berry and others in an oration in 1934, Tasmanian surgeon and historian, William Edward Lodewyk Crowther questioned 'Is there any other school of medicine that can show such a tradition of anthropological work, and is it too much to say that the influence of George Britton Halford was responsible for its inception?'.[42] Whilst botanists and zoologists puzzled over Australia's exotic flora and fauna, Halford and Berry were more interested in the land's inhabitants, both Indigenous and those recently arrived. Collections of skeletal remains stored in the Anatomy Department, and their controversial history, are testament to the importance of physical anthropology as a discipline championed by the University of Melbourne's anatomists.[43] In his address at Jubilee celebrations in 1914, Professor Allen listed as one of a select few of the Medical School's most important research successes Berry's 'Atlas of Tasmania crania, the Atlas of Australian Aboriginal crania and other important works' of physical anthropology.[44] It is possible that Aboriginal cadavers were too valuable as academic exchange gifts to end up in the dissecting room.[45] Later, however, Frederic Wood Jones, Professor of Anatomy from 1929 to 1938, was an early supporter of Aboriginal rights.[46]

What seems certain is that the burly football players who gave the medical students such a rough time were not normally represented amongst the cadavers, for while they came from the poorer classes they did not come from those groups that had failed to benefit from the rapid growth of Melbourne during its first decades. Another important distinction between the medical students and those who would become their anatomical subjects was the different degree of engagement each had in the democratic political process that developed in Victoria and Australia, where after a flirtation from 1857 with a system of almost full male suffrage, the 1863 *Electoral Act* had instituted a qualified system of adult male suffrage in Victoria. The vote was not extended to women there until 1908. Following the creation of the Australian nation in 1901, full suffrage for most men and women was enacted

---

42 W.E.L.H. Crowther, '"1803–1876. The Passing of the Tasmanian Race", The Halford Oration', *Medical Journal of Australia* (3 February 1934): p. 148.

43 See D.J. Mulvaney, 'Reflections on the Murray Black Collection', *Australian Natural History*, 23/1 (1989): pp. 66–73; Paul Turnbull, 'Rare Work for the Professors: The Entanglement of Aboriginal Remains in Phrenological Knowledge in Early Colonial Australia', in Jeanette Hoorn and Barbara Creed (eds), *Body Trade: Cannibalism, Captivity and Colonialism in the Pacific* (Melbourne, 2001).

44 H.B. Allen, *University of Melbourne, Medical School Jubilee 1914* (Carlton, 1914), p. 53. R.J.A. Berry and A.W.D. Robertson, *Dioptrographic Tracings in Four Normae of Fifty-two Tasmanian Crania* (Melbourne, 1909).

45 See MacDonald, *Human Remains*.

46 See Jones, *Humanity's Mirror*, pp. 157–9.

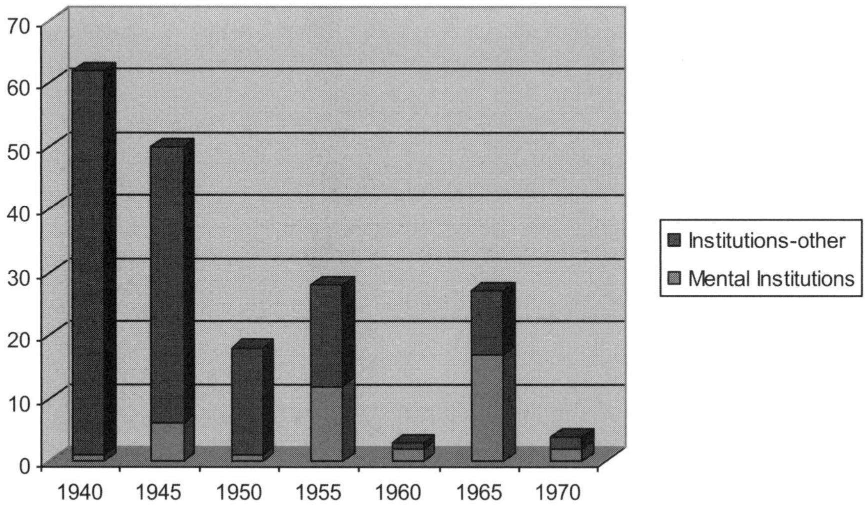

Figure 2.3 Cadavers from institutions received into the Department of Anatomy, University of Melbourne, 1940–1970

for Federal elections in 1902, however participation required registration and many eligible voters did not register until the 1920s. The itinerant were disqualified by being unable to provide a place of abode.[47] It is a reasonable conclusion therefore that the great majority of the cadavers dissected in the Anatomy Department between 1863 and the 1920s were not part of the political process as they had no known address or were from slums.[48] And those who moved into the benevolent institutions were a different case again, having been specifically disenfranchized by the 1863 *Electoral Act*. Any person who was 'receiving relief as an inmate of any eleemosynary or charitable institution' could not vote.[49] This ban was further entrenched in the State constitution in the *Constitution Act Amendment Act 1890*, only being discarded in 1975 in the *Constitution Act*.[50]

---

47 Compulsory registration for State elections did not come until 1923; one year after the measure was introduced for Federal elections. Greg Taylor, *The Constitution of Victoria* (Melbourne, 2006), p. 386.

48 It is possible that some voted in Federal elections after 1902, but registration was not compulsory for two decades, and the cadavers came from the class that traditionally failed to register in large numbers. Also, of all eligible voters registered to vote, as few as 50 per cent, and never more than 70 per cent, actually voted in Federal elections in the first two decades of the century. Gavin Souter, *Acts of Parliament: A Narrative History of the Senate and House of Representatives Commonwealth of Australia* (Melbourne, 1988), p. 35, p. 192. For 1903 see Commonwealth of Australia, *Parliamentary Papers*, 1904, vol. 2, pt 1, p. 397.

49 Barbara Kerr, *The State Franchise in Victoria, 1842–2005* (Melbourne, 2005), p. 22.

50 Kerr, *The State Franchise*, p. 11; *Victorian Parliamentary Debates*, 1910, vol. 124, pp. 416–20.

Finally, a third institutional source of bodies appeared, as can be seen in Figure 2.3, following the Second World War when mental institutions supplemented the supply of corpses from benevolent homes. In addition, as Figure 2.2 illustrates, body donations – which tentatively began in the 1950s – became increasingly important throughout the 1960s.[51] Elizabeth Hurren has pointed out that changes in the sources and numbers of cadavers for Cambridge University were dependent on the variations in official arrangements for the poor.[52] Such seems to also be the case in Melbourne, despite the differences in the arrangements.

In summary, a great gulf existed between the medical students and their subjects in terms of status, respectability, wealth and engagement in the formal political process from the 1860s until the 1960s. These were the people whose dissected bodies enabled the Medical School's students to establish professional and social superiority vis-à-vis others in the medical marketplace, which university-trained medical practitioners came to dominate in the late nineteenth century. Anatomy was central to the perceived superiority of the university-trained. It, and dissection, needed to thrive to sustain this success. In 1897 the Medical Students' Society, discussing the study of 'all-important Anatomy' pointed out that 'if our men are to retain the high name that they have heretofore borne as skilled anatomists', there needed to be a much more regular supply of cadavers for dissection.[53]

Medical Students' Attitudes to the Cadavers

In August 1889 *Speculum* published a dramatic scene by an anonymous author titled 'A Night in the Dissecting Room'. Many such pieces of doggerel appeared in the magazine's pages from the 1880s until the 1920s.[54] In this one, a student wakes up to find him or herself locked in the dissecting room for the night. The spirits of the dancing cadavers stumble on the intruder:

> 1st spirit—
> Me you left a week together
> Half dissected on the table
> In the piercing winter weather,
> Now respond if you are able.
> (Tortures him) …
> 2nd spirit—

[51] From 1951 until 1983 under direction from the Chief Secretary, the Department of Mental Hygiene supplied bodies from its institutions to the university for the purpose of dissection. See Public Record Office of Victoria series VPRS 7688 'Record of Subjects sent to School of Anatomy, University of Melbourne'.

[52] Hurren, 'A Pauper Dead-House'.

[53] *Speculum*, 39 (November 1897): p. 74.

[54] See Jones, *Humanity's Mirror*, ch. 4 for numerous examples.

And, for once about me joking,
(I was far too stout to please you),
In my side your finger poking,
By the snout I now will seize you …
3rd spirit—
And, for words and deeds atoning,
None from us can now protect him.
Musical will sound his moaning,
Hasten, spirits, and dissect him.
(proceed to dissect).[55]

Cadavers were not universally respected by students in the Medical School's dissecting room. That such would be the case had been suspected by those at the Benevolent Asylum who had rejected the School's nineteenth-century requests for corpses, when both the Professor and Victoria's Inspector of Anatomy had denied that cadavers would be misused. However when Richard Berry arrived to take up the chair of anatomy 43 years later, he found the dissecting theatre bore the mark of 'meat fights' by students.[56]

In 1890, when Berry's predecessor Professor Allen had been absent on leave, the students had published their own handbook of dissecting room etiquette as 'during the years in which the Medical School has been in existence a number of unwritten rules have come to be tacitly observed'.[57] In the dissectors' vade mecum it was pointed out that only certain rituals and costumes were acceptable:

> It is considered somewhat old-fashioned to wear an old coat and long apron in the room now-a-days. Fourth and second-year men, especially, who have to deal with surgical cases at the hospital, seldom go to the trouble of changing their coats: demi-sleeves of some blue material slipped over their ordinary coats are all that is considered necessary.[58]

Dress was particularly important. Tongue-in-cheek, the students noted that:

> college caps look jaunty, and are therefore much affected by college meds. Mortar-boards have the advantage that their tassels mop up any superfluous moisture on the part being dissected. Pot hats are extremely comfortable and 'becoming', and have the advantage of preventing the man opposite from approaching his part.[59]

---

55 *Speculum*, 18 (August 1889): p. 47.

56 Berry, Chance and Circumstance, p. 110. For more details of the meat fights see Jones, *Humanity's Mirror*, pp. 93–5.

57 *Speculum*, 21 (June 1890): p. 66.

58 Ibid.

59 Ibid.

It was possible, according to the manual, to establish those of seniority because of the confident gait they affected. They must also confirm their superiority, when arriving, by wandering around and criticizing the juniors' work because 'it impresses unsophisticated second-year men, who may mistake the senior for a demonstrator … it is considered *infra dig* to replace coverings on a part which you have examined – a porter is kept chained up on the premises for this purpose'.[60] The prohibitions on smoking and being noisy are rules 'more honoured in the breach that the observance; besides, infringement of these minor rules gives a devil-may-care air of disregard for the authorities, which suits well the conventional idea of a medical student'.[61] As far as seeking entertainment when enduring the long hours of dissecting, the student is encouraged to:

> practice aiming chunks of semi-putrid muscle across the room at their bosom friends … at first you will probably miss … and hit some inoffensive med. Unexpectedly you may be so unfortunate as to hit an aggressive med. This chance adds an element of danger to the pastime which increases its zest. Your friend will probably retaliate, according to ancient custom, by discharging some putrescent internal organ at you, which will equally probably miss you and 'land' someone else. The fun is thus kept up *ad libitum*.[62]

Throughout the nineteenth century, adequate supervision had been a problem in the dissecting room.[63] Berry was appalled by this entrenched misbehaviour, later writing:

> Had these bodies been those of an oxen instead of humans, an old time butcher would have said it was a waste of good rump steak. A grim smile was my only comment on this curious practice which ceased henceforth.[64]

Berry's reforms prompted a plaintive response in verse in *Speculum*:

> Now the work has lost its flavour,
> (Though the odour's rather high),
> Since we beggars must behave our
> Selves not lark upon the sly …
> It was jolly in the old years
> When we had some liberty;
> Then we fought like valiant soldiers
> Shying meat right royally.

60 Ibid., p. 67.

61 Ibid.

62 Ibid, pp. 67–8.

63 Jones, *Humanity's Mirror*, pp. 92–5.

64 Berry, Chance and Circumstance, p. 110.

> Then we sometimes got a jawful,
> Or we sometimes got a fine …
> And you've gallantly attempted
> Now to keep our sport in check,
> And the meat we once emptied
> Down another fellow's neck
> Must repose at peace in dishes.[65]

For the United States, Warner and Rizzolo have described dissection as alternating between an 'affective' or 'scientific' element of medical education.[66] In the late nineteenth century the experience of the dissecting room shaped professional character and was an important bonding experience, It was essentially 'affective', a catalyst for moral transformation – as seen in the rise of the group dissecting room portrait.[67] In Melbourne at the beginning of the twentieth century, in response to the perceived threat to anatomy's primacy in the curriculum from the new biological and clinical sciences, the importance of the 'scientific' nature of dissection was also emphasized. Scientific justification was a powerful reinforcement of the status of doctors. In 1889 *Speculum* explained that:

> In these days when science demands a thorough knowledge of every branch, no obstacle should be allowed to stand in the way of any design calculated to further the good of humanity. The government also should be brought to understand that if they wish the medical men of their University to rank with those of other nations, technical knowledge in this as well as other things is required. And as this technical knowledge is only acquired by the aid of morbid anatomy, we should use every legitimate ends to further that end.[68]

The behaviour in the dissecting room, as well as the cadaver poetry written by the students, can perhaps be explained as the product of a number of factors. The demise of the notion of the sanctity of the body as the temple of the soul is a tempting but elusive matter. Church attendances in Melbourne in the late nineteenth century remained steady despite the encroachment of Darwinian materialism.[69] Whether the medical students were religious is another matter. In his lectures, J.W. Springthorpe (an early Melbourne medical student and, from 1887, lecturer

---

65 Anonymous, 'A Dissecting Room Wail', *Speculum*, 65 (May 1906): pp. 22–3.

66 Warner and Rizzolo, 'Anatomical Instruction', pp. 403–14; Hafferty, *Into the Valley*.

67 Warner and Rizzolo, 'Anatomical Instruction', p. 404. J.H Warner and James Edmonson, *Dissection: Photographs of a rite of passage in American medicine, 1880–1930* (New York, 2009); Jones, *Humanity's Mirror*, p. 83.

68 *Speculum*, 16 (January 1889): pp. 13–14, pp. 17–18.

69 J. Roe, 'Challenge and Response: Religious Life in Melbourne, 1876–86', *Journal of Religious History*, 5/2 (December 1968): pp. 149–66.

in therapeutics) understood life as the expression of a non-traditional spiritual life force but one that was driven by Darwinian conflict:

> As in ordinary warfare … the battle is won by the best selected, best trained soldiery, so in the battle of life, the issue depends primarily upon heredity and development [but] … in countless instances the inherited momentum continues to be towards weakness … [this] sacrilege must continue until the public at large are made to know and appreciate its significance … There is no escape from the struggle for existence.[70]

Certainly, the appearance of the cadaver portrait at this time suggests that a ritualization of dissection or the creation of a 'rite of passage' was an important element in the development of the medical profession.[71] Perhaps it can be explained as a necessary 'blooding' to produce the dispassionate, scientific and detached medical practitioner. Certainly such familiarity, even disrespect, for the human body was not for those outside the professional class. When it was reported in the April 1899 edition of the university magazine, *Alma Mater*, that working-class youths were visiting the morgue to view the remains of fatal accidents and suicides, a medical student wrote in high dudgeon:

> With an elementary system of compulsory education [introduced in 1872], of which it is our boast that it has rescued our youth from crass ignorance, it is rather a takedown to find that young girls, in crowds, pass through this dead house and make merry over the mutilated remains of a wretched sister. We cannot remember the slums of any large city, in any part of the civilised world, ever turned out greater streams of heartless humanity than those which surged through the morgue to glare at the head of a poor young girl, who, however giddy, had been cruelly and clumsily done to death.[72]

This was not to say that the working classes were not to learn human anatomy (or even physiology). From 1899, Frank Tate's State Education Department published the *School Paper*, a textbook for working-class children in elementary schools. Detailed lessons on anatomy and physiology made up an important part of the science curriculum for children aged from 8 to 11 years.[73] In Melbourne as elsewhere, public anatomy museums were also popular from the 1860s up until the First World War. However there was no expectation that the consumers of this educational information

[70] J.W. Springthorpe, *Therapeutics, Dietetics and Hygiene: An Australian Textbook* (Melbourne, 1914), p. 5.

[71] For the United States see Warner and Rizzolo, 'Anatomical Instruction', p. 404.

[72] *Alma Mater*, iv/1 (April 1899): 19.

[73] For example see the *School Paper*, October 1899: p. 136; September 1899: p. 124; May 1900: p. 124, p. 125.

would graduate from medical school.[74] And, as Michael Sappol has written of the teaching of anatomy in the public schools in the United States:

> Sexual radicalism was always a potential theme of popular anatomical discourse … there were troublesome questions … Should children, women, the lower classes and races be taught anatomy? Who should be allowed to dissect, to have 'unmediated' knowledge of the body? Who should be allowed to view anatomically detailed representations of the body?[75]

What such an education did accomplish was the creation of an anatomically literate class who would become patients for the newly created university-trained medical profession.[76] In July 1926, one of Australia's first psychologists, Dr Chris McRae, argued in an article in the Victorian *Education Gazette and Teacher's Aid* (the journal sent out to all schools, coincidentally using the *School Paper* as the major textbook), that those children attending schools in slum areas in Melbourne 'will never go to the university [and] … should not follow the same curriculum' as those in schools in wealthier suburbs. Rather, the education of the poorer classes 'should be vocational' as 'in the main, people live in slums because they are mentally deficient, and not vice versa'.[77] Whilst both the 'scientific' and 'affective' elements were important, in Melbourne at least, dissection also provided a strong reinforcement of class difference between the medically trained and the majority of their patients.

Conclusion

In 1908, *Speculum* published 'An Outsider's View of the Medical Curriculum'. It expressed the self-confidence of the Melbourne medical establishment of the time while spelling out a proposed medical-racial experiment:

---

[74] For the anatomy museums, see Jones, *Humanity's Mirror*, pp. 6–11, pp. 25–8.

[75] Sappol, *Traffic*, p. 268.

[76] For a discussion of the rise of the Melbourne Medical School as the dominant medical educational and accrediting institution in Victoria see Jones, *Humanity's Mirror*, ch. 3. For the US situation in regard to this see Sappol, *A Traffic of Dead Bodies*, chs 6, 8 and 9.

[77] Chris R. McRae, 'Reports of the Psychological Laboratory, Teacher's College. No. V. The Relation between Intelligence and Social Status', *Education Gazette and Teacher's Aid*, (20 July 1926): p. 242. McRae became deputy Vice-Chancellor of the University of Sydney. This view was based on research conducted by McRae in an attempt to replicate an experiment conducted by Cyril Burt in England, McRae's teacher at the University of London. McRae was a member, along with Tate and Berry, of the committee that drew up the 1926 Mental Deficiency Bill in Victoria. See Ross L. Jones, 'The Master Potter and the Rejected Pots: Eugenic Legislation in Victoria 1918–1939', *Australian Historical Studies*, 30/113 (October 1999): pp. 319–42.

> A unique feature of Australian Universities is the prominence of the medical schools, both in number of students and in public estimation. This is most notable in our own University. Nor is it to be wondered at: as a people Australians are in what Emerson calls 'the era of bodily nature', the Grecian stage when harmonious bodily activity is regarded as the first index of development … The ideal man is he who can react to the most complex situations by reason of mental self-reliance, based on organic health. The work of the medical man in a modern community is more and more recognised to be the fashioning from the haphazard materials available of a race of such men.[78]

In Melbourne at least, it seems that not all its inhabitants were considered by the medical fraternity to be suitable racial stock. The bodies of those who had effectively been removed from the polity (the poor and abandoned, further diminished by political disenfranchisement) were appropriated for the benefit of the citizens of the state. For Berry these were the racially 'unfit'.[79] Springthorpe designated them medically 'sacrilegious' and the aversion of Melbourne's citizens – the beneficiaries of the development of medicine – to being dissected remained until the late 1960s. As the fourth Professor of Anatomy at the University of Melbourne, Frederic Wood Jones, told the Medico-Legal Society of Victoria in 1933:

> The subject of the dissection of the human body cannot be approached without some understanding of the prejudice which inevitably clings to it. We must admit that, there is, interwoven in the whole story, the idea of the sanctity of the human body, the dislike for its mutilation and the demand that it should find sepulchre intact.[80]

It is difficult to come to any other than suggestive conclusions about the contribution of dissection and anatomical study in the transformation of Melbourne society in the late nineteenth and early twentieth centuries. The medical profession became an important cog in the wheels of Melbourne's upper echelons, however, and dissection was an important element in achieving that accreditation. Those who benefited from Melbourne's prosperity and growth were not found on the dissecting table.

---

[78] *Speculum*, 72 (September 1908): pp. 76–7. See also Isobel Crombie, *Body Culture: Max Dupain, Photography and Australian Culture, 1919–1939* (Melbourne, 2004).

[79] Jones, *Humanity's Mirror*, pp. 103f.

[80] F. Wood Jones, 'The Legalization of the Study of Human Anatomy', in J.V. Barry and A.E. Coates (eds), *The Proceedings of the Medico-Legal Society of Victoria During the Years 1933–1934 and 1935–1936*, vol. ii (Melbourne, 1937), pp. 135–44, p. 135.

Bibliography

Manuscript Sources

Berry, R.J.A., Chance and Circumstance, unpublished autobiography, University of Melbourne Medical Library, 1954.

Cadaver Archives, Department of Anatomy and Cell Biology, University of Melbourne.

Printed Primary Sources

Argus.

Commonwealth of Australia, *Parliamentary Papers*, 1904, Volume 2, Part 1.

Speculum: A Journal of the Melbourne Medical Students.

The Thirty-Seventh Annual report of the Committee of Management of the Melbourne Benevolent Asylum and list of subscriptions and donations for the year 1886 (Melbourne: Sands and McDougall, 1887).

Victorian Parliamentary Debates, Legislative Council, 1862, Volume 8.

Victorian Parliamentary Debates, Legislative Assembly, 1910, Volume 124.

Secondary Sources

Allen, H.B., *University of Melbourne, Medical School Jubilee 1914* (Carlton: Ford 1914).

Anderson, Warwick, *The Cultivation of Whiteness: Science, Health and Racial Destiny in Australia* (Melbourne: Melbourne University Press, Carlton South, 2002).

Berry, R.J.A. and Robertson, A.W.D., *Dioptrographic Tracings in Four Normae of Fifty-two Tasmanian Crania* (Melbourne: J. Kemp, Govt. Printer, 1909).

Brown-May, Andrew, *Melbourne Street Life: The Itinerary of Our Days* (Melbourne: Australian Scholarly/Arcadia and Museum Victoria, 1998).

Buklijas, Tatjana, 'Cultures of Death and Politics of Corpse Supply: Anatomy in Vienna, 1848–1914', *Bulletin of the History of Medicine*, 82/3 (2008): pp. 570–607.

Cage, R.A., *Poverty Abounding, Charity Aplenty: The Charity Network in Colonial Victoria* (Sydney: Hale & Iremonger, 1992).

Clarke, Adele E., Shim, Janet K., Mamo, Laura, Fosket, Jennifer, Ruth and Fishman, Jennifer R., 'Biomedicalization: Technoscientific Transformations of Health, Illness, and U.S. Biomedicine', *American Sociology Review*, 68/2 (April 2003): pp. 161–94.

Conrad, Peter, *The Medicalization of Society: On the Transformation of Human Conditions and Treatable Disorders* (Baltimore: Johns Hopkins University Press, 2007).

Crombie, Isobel, *Body Culture: Max Dupain, Photography and Australian Culture, 1919–1939* (Melbourne: Images Publishing Group, 2004).

Crowther, W.E.L.H., '"1803–1876. The Passing of the Tasmanian Race", The Halford Oration', *Medical Journal of Australia* (3 February 1934): p. 148.

Davison, Graeme, 'The City-bred Child and Urban Reform in Melbourne 1900–1914', in Peter Williams (ed.), *Social Process and the City – Urban Studies Yearbook 1* (Sydney: Allen & Unwin, 1983), pp. 143–74.

Desmond, Adrian, *The Politics of Evolution: Morphology, Medicine, and Reform in Radical London* (Chicago: University of Chicago Press, 1989).

Hafferty, F.W., *Into the Valley: Death and the Socialization of Medical Students* (New Haven: Yale University Press, 1991)

Hurren, Elizabeth T., 'A Pauper Dead-House: The Expansion of the Cambridge Anatomical Teaching School under the Late-Victorian Poor Law, 1870–1914', *Medical History*, 48/1 (2004): pp. 69–94.

Hurren, Elizabeth T., 'Whose Body is it Anyway? Trading the Dead Poor, Coroner's Disputes, and the Business of Anatomy at Oxford University, 1885–1929', *Bulletin of the History of Medicine*, 82/4 (Winter 2008): pp. 775–818.

Jones, D. Gareth, 'Bequests, Cadavers and Dissections: Sketches from New Zealand History', *New Zealand Medical Journal*, 104 (1991): pp. 210–12.

Jones, F. Wood, 'The Legalization of the Study of Human Anatomy', in J.V. Barry and A.E. Coates (eds), *The Proceedings of the Medico-Legal Society of Victoria During the Years 1933–1934 and 1935–1936*, vol. ii (Melbourne: Brown Prior Anderson Pty. Ltd, 1937).

Jones, Ross L., 'The Rogers-Templeton and Pearson Royal Commissions: Contemporary Views of the 1872 Education Act', *History of Education Review*, 27/2 (1998): pp. 50–66.

Jones, Ross L., 'The Master Potter and the Rejected Pots: Eugenic Legislation in Victoria 1918–1939', *Australian Historical Studies*, 30/113 (October 1999): pp. 319–42.

Jones, Ross L., *Humanity's Mirror: 150 Years of Anatomy in Melbourne* (Melbourne: Haddington Press, 2007).

Kehoe, Mary, *The Melbourne Benevolent Asylum: Hotham's Premier Building. The Annals of Hotham*, vol. 1 (North Melbourne: Hotham History Project, 1998).

Kennedy, R., 'Poor Relief in Melbourne: the Benevolent Society's Contribution', *Journal of the Royal Australian Historical Society*, 60 (1974): pp. 256–66.

Kerr, Barbara, *The State Franchise in Victoria, 1842–2005*, Professional Intern Report, Professional Internship Program PSI3000 (Monash University and the State Parliament of Victoria, 2005).

Kevles, Daniel, *In the Name of Eugenics* (Cambridge, MA: Harvard University Press, 2001 [1985]).

MacDonald, Helen, *Human Remains: Dissection and its Histories* (New Haven: Yale University Press, 2006).

MacDonald, Helen, '"Humanity's Discards": The New South Wales Anatomy Act 1881' *Mortality*, 12/4 (2007): pp. 365–82.

MacDonald, Helen, 'A Scandalous Act: Regulating Anatomy in a British Settler Colony', *Social History of Medicine*, 20/1 (2007): pp. 39–56.

MacDonald, Helen, 'The Anatomy Inspector and the Government Corpse', *History Australia*, 6/2 (2009): 40.1–40.17.

MacDonald, Helen, 'Procuring Corpses: England's Anatomy Inspectorate, 1842 to 1858', *Medical History*, 53/3 (2009): pp. 379–96.

Mayhew, Henry, *London Labour and the London Poor: A Cyclopaedia of the Conditions and Earnings of Those that Will Work and those that Cannot Work, and Those that Will Not Work* (London: Woodfall, 1851).

McRae, Chris R., 'Reports of the Psychological Laboratory, Teacher's College. No. V. The Relation between Intelligence and Social Status', *Education Gazette and Teacher's Aid*, (20 July 1926): p. 242.

Mulvaney, D.J., 'Reflections on the Murray Black Collection', *Australian Natural History*, 23/1 (1989): pp. 66–73.

Pensabane, T.S., *The Rise of the Medical Practitioner in Victoria* (Health Research Project, Research Monograph 2, Canberra, Australian National University, 1980).

Pick, Daniel, *Faces of Degeneration: A European Disorder, c.1848–1914* (Cambridge: Cambridge University Press, 1989).

Richardson, Ruth, *Death, Dissection and the Destitute* (Harmondsworth: Penguin, 1988).

Roe, J., 'Challenge and Response: Religious Life in Melbourne, 1876–86', *Journal of Religious History*, 5/2 (December 1968): pp. 149–66.

Sappol, Michael, *A Traffic of Dead Bodies: Anatomy and Embodied Social Identity in Nineteenth-Century America* (Princeton: Princeton University Press, 2002).

Serle, Geoffrey, *From Deserts the Prophets Come – The Creative Spirit in Australia 1788–1972* (Melbourne: Heinemann, 1973).

Serville, Paul de, *Pounds and Pedigrees: The Upper Class in Victoria 1850–80* (Melbourne: Oxford University Press, 1991).

Sherington, Geoffrey, '"A Better Class of Boy" The Big Brother Movement, Youth Migration and Citizenship of Empire', *Australian Historical Studies*, 33/120 (October 2002): pp. 267–85.

Souter, Gavin, *Acts of Parliament: A Narrative History of the Senate and House of Representatives Commonwealth of Australia* (Melbourne: Melbourne University Press, 1988).

Springthorpe, J.W., *Therapeutics, Dietetics and Hygiene: An Australian Textbook* (Melbourne: James Little, 1914).

Taylor, Greg, *The Constitution of Victoria* (Melbourne: The Federation Press, 2006).

Tibbits, George, 'Slums and Public Housing in Southern Fitzroy', in Cutten History Committee of the Fitzroy History Society (eds), *Fitzroy: Melbourne's First Suburb* (Melbourne: Melbourne University Press, 1991), pp. 118–25.

Turnbull, Paul, 'Rare Work for the Professors: The Entanglement of Aboriginal Remains in Phrenological Knowledge in Early Colonial Australia', in Jeanette Hoorn and Barbara Creed (eds), *Body Trade: Cannibalism, Captivity and Colonialism in the Pacific* (Melbourne: Pluto Press, 2001), pp. 3–23.

Uhl, Jean, *Mount Royal Hospital: A Social History* (Parkville: Mount Royal Hospital, 1981).

Warner, John Harley and Edmonson, James, *Dissection: Photographs of a Rite of Passage in American Medicine, 1880–1930*, (New York: Blast Books, 2009).

Warner, John Harley and Rizzolo, Lawrence J., 'Anatomical Instruction and Training for Professionalism from the 19th to the 20th Centuries', *Clinical Anatomy*, 19 (2006): pp. 403–14.

Willingham, Allan, 'The Rise and Fall of a Fitzroy Villa', in Cutten History Committee of the Fitzroy History Society (eds) *Fitzroy: Melbourne's First Suburb* (Melbourne: Melbourne University Press, 1991), pp. 118–25.

Chapter 3

Dissection, Anatomy Acts and the Appropriation of Bodies in Nineteenth-Century Australia: 'The Government's Brains' and the Benevolent Asylum

Susan K. Martin

In July 1864 the brains of the executed murderer Christopher Harrison were the subject of a dispute between the government sheriff and Professor of Anatomy, George Halford, at the new Melbourne University School of Medicine. Halford claimed the brains were his to dissect, but the sheriff maintained they were the 'Government's brains'. The embarrassing struggle over these brains was widely reported in the Melbourne newspapers and beyond.

While this chapter concentrates on the Harrison case and the Victorian Anatomy Act, I will argue that the theft, dissections and dismemberments of bodies in the 1860s exemplify the treatment and understanding of particular sorts of bodies in Australia across the nineteenth century. Harrison was a white, middle-class executed murderer. Other bodies subject to appropriation in this period include the bodies of the indigent and unclaimed who died in the Melbourne Hospital and much later the Benevolent Asylum, and the bodies of Aboriginal people.[1] Such incidents are connected by the way in which the subordinate bodies of the people involved were understood to be available and useful to the government and its sometime extensions; in this case the uses of institutionalized science and medicine. Of course the interests of science and the state do not always coincide.

---

[1] On Aboriginal bodies see Lyndall Ryan, *The Aboriginal Tasmanians*, 2nd edn (St Leonard, NSW, 1996), pp. 214–17; Helen MacDonald, *Human Remains: Episodes in Human Dissection* (Carlton, 2005), pp. 144–9; Stefan Petrow, 'The Last Man: The Mutilation of William Lanne in 1869 and its Aftermath', *Australian Cultural History*, 16 (1997): pp. 18–44; Paul Turnbull, '"To What Strange Uses": The Procurement and Use of Aboriginal Peoples' Bodies in Early Colonial Australia', *Voices* 4/3 (1994): pp. 5–20. See also Thomas F. Tierney, 'Anatomy and Governmentality: A Foucauldian Perspective on Death and Medicine in Modernity', *Theory & Event* 2/1 (1998). Available at: http://muse.jhu.edu/login?uri=/journals/theory_and_event/v002/2.1tierney.html (accessed 3 August 2009).

Indeed the Melbourne University case pivots on a disagreement between state and medical science. Underlying the argument, however, is a shared understanding of the body as owned not by the subject, but by one or other official body.

Looking at the dissection and collection of the body parts of people who were poor, Aboriginal, criminal or insane reveals the way that fundamental cultural constructs produce not just the subjectivity of the living but that of the dead, and produce sameness (everybody is a potential body) as well as difference (of race, class, gender, etc.).[2]

Across the period covering white settlement of Australia in the late eighteenth and nineteenth centuries the dead body, in Britain and its colonies, became a new kind of object and subject, one which was intensively classed, raced and gendered, but also invested with emotional and commercial value.[3] Ruth Richardson argues, in her study of death and dissection in Britain, that the passing of the 1832 Anatomy Act was a turning point in the meaning of the body in Britain.[4] During the time of the professionalization of medicine, the rise of medical schools and the development of anatomy as a science, fresh dead bodies were in increasing demand for demonstration and experimentation. The bodies of executed murderers were available for this purpose, but execution rates were declining, and these bodies were not equally available to all. V.A.C. Gatrell points out that although execution rates were high from the second half of the eighteenth century only 20 per cent of these were for murder, and therefore subject to dissection.[5]

In Australia the first Anatomy Act was passed in Victoria in 1862, 30 years after the British Act. Before 1832 in Britain, as supply did not meet demand, a market for bodies arose which was met by the rise of an illegal trade in stolen bodies snatched from graves. In popular imagination the 'resurrection' business which existed in Britain prior to the 1832 Act was a democratic trade; that is, all bodies, of rich and poor alike, were seen as potentially vulnerable to theft. In reality this was not quite the case. The democratization lay more in the fact that

---

[2] See Helen MacDonald, 'Human Remains: Episodes in Nineteenth Century Colonial Human Dissection', PhD, Department of History, University of Melbourne (2002); MacDonald, *Human Remains*.

[3] See for example V.A.C. Gatrell, *The Hanging Tree: Execution and the English People, 1770–1868* (Oxford, 1994), pp. 225–41; Thomas Laqueur 'Cemeteries, Religion and the Culture of Capitalism', in Jane Garnett and Colin Matthew (eds), *Revival and Religion since 1700* (London, 1993), pp. 183–200; Fernando Vidal, 'Brains, Bodies, Selves, and Science: Anthropologies of Identity and the Resurrection of the Body', *Critical Inquiry*, 28 (2002): pp. 930–74; Gwenda Morgan and Peter Rushton, 'Visible Bodies: Power Subordination and Identity in the Eighteenth-century Atlantic World', *Journal of Social History*, 39/1 (2005): pp. 39–64.

[4] Ruth Richardson, *Death, Dissection and the Destitute* (London, 1987), p. 4, p. 52.

[5] Richardson, *Death, Dissection and the Destitute*, pp. 100–106; Gatrell, *The Hanging Tree*, pp. 7–9, Appendix 2. See also Michael Sappol, *A Traffic of Dead Bodies: Anatomy and Embodied Social Identity in Nineteenth-Century America* (Princeton, 2002) for the American context.

any body in good condition was worth a good price. Class and social status, age and youth, good looks and bad – the social hierarchies – were erased, except that in some instances those things which kept the individual in reduced circumstances when alive – deformity, disease, an othered racial identity, criminality, femaleness – gave them a higher value in the, or as, flesh.

The value of the body had increased in other ways by the nineteenth century. With fundamental shifts in the understanding of subjectivity in Europe, the bodies of the dead were no longer seen as empty receptacles left by the departed soul, as almost meaningless objects. At least this was the popular and official rhetoric, for example on gravestones.[6] They became subjects, still connected to the personality and meaning of the loved one lost. This feeling has been associated with the rising middle classes, and it can be read in the rise of rituals of bereavement increasingly centred around the body of the individualized loved one.[7]

In his study of changing views on the Christian doctrine of resurrection and its understanding of bodily resurrection and subjectivity, Fernando Vidal argues that the period from the end of the eighteenth century marks a shift in the understanding of the connection between the 'self' and the body, or rather it initiates a period when it is possible to think about 'having' a body. He argues, '[w]e "have" bodies only in the perspective of the post-Lockean possessive individualism that makes us their owners; objectified and distanced from our "selves", our bodies are for us things we own, not entities we are'.[8] Elizabeth Grosz identifies this as a gendered view, as well as an historical one.[9]

If we accept Vidal's arguments, then the period from the eighteenth century onwards marks a shift to the possibility of seeing the body not as self but as possession or property which would enable some of the ways of thinking, and activities involved, in the full commercialization of the supply of bodies for dissection. However Vidal also argues that this post-Lockean, Cartesian understanding is entirely contrary to the Christian view that 'rejects the possibility of a person existing otherwise than as a composite of body and soul'.[10] The period from the late eighteenth to early nineteenth century might then be seen as a cusp, with the coexistence in Western thought of at least two major, contradictory ways of understanding the body and its relation to the person. Scientific

---

6 Sarah Tarlow, *Bereavement and Commemoration: An Archaeology of Mortality* (Oxford and Malden, 1999), pp. 76–107.

7 Patricia Jalland, *Death in the Victorian Family* (Oxford, 1996); Patricia Jalland, *Australian Ways of Death: A Social and Cultural History 1840–1918* (South Melbourne, 2002); Ralph Houlbrooke (ed.), *Death, Ritual, and Bereavement* (London, 1989); Chris Brooks et al., *Mortal Remains: The History and Present State of the Victorian and Edwardian Cemetery* (Exeter, 1989), pp. 4–6; Thomas Laqueur, 'Cemeteries'.

8 Vidal, 'Brains, Bodies, Selves, and Science', pp. 935–6.

9 Elizabeth Grosz, *Volatile Bodies: Toward a Corporeal Feminism* (Bloomington, 1994), pp. 3–24.

10 Vidal, 'Brains, Bodies, Selves, and Science', p. 936.

'progress', understanding the body as a separate entity, could make use of bodies as 'disembodied' – objects detached from subjects, even though some of their searches were exactly for the physical site of a self. But at the same time, older understandings of self, including Christian understandings, contained no concept of the 'disembody' – of a person or self not composed of soul-with-body. The Christian doctrine of the resurrection was partly responsible for anxiety about mutilation of the dead body. As Vidal shows, much energy was spent contemplating the extent, if any, to which the corpse must be preserved to ensure resurrection of the body.[11]

The British 1832 Anatomy Act put an end to the lucrative business of grave robbing per se because it ostensibly removed the shortage of bodies that had given such commodity value to those of the stolen dead. It did this by providing a source of corpses, the bodies of the 'unclaimed poor', although recent research suggests the supply was not so immediate or uncomplicated as supposed.[12] As Richardson demonstrates, the problem with this apparently ideal solution to the unsavoury traffic in the dead (and the resulting nasty taint on the increasingly professional, middle-class doctor) lay in two main areas. Firstly the definition of 'unclaimed' and secondly the underlying assumptions about the values of others: the emotional and sentimental value attached by friends and relations to the bodies of the poor. The British Act did not define 'unclaimed' and this was easily interpreted as an 'economic' category. That is, if no relative emerged with money for the funeral within a stated time, the body could be classed as unclaimed, although there were very likely grieving relatives who would attend a parish funeral but be unable to pay for one, or relatives who were unaware of the death until too late. Friends who might raise the money for burial could be denied the body because of narrow, middle-class definitions of 'relations' which excluded the kinds of connections and loyalties common to the poor, but not necessarily recognized by the better-off.[13] Across this period 'middle-class values', if that is really what they can be called, spread across society, as François Barret-Ducrocq argues in relation to Victorian

[11] Vidal, 'Brains, Bodies, Selves, and Science', pp. 940ff.; Brooks et al., *Mortal Remains*; Laqueur, 'Cemeteries'; Jalland, *Death in the Victorian Family*; John C. Loudon, *On the Laying Out, Planting and Managing of Cemeteries and on the Improvement of Churchyards* (London, 1843); Tarlow, *Bereavement*, pp. 108–46; James Curl, *A Celebration of Death: An Introduction to Some of the Buildings, Monuments, and Settings of Funerary Architecture in the Western European Tradition* (London, 1993); Susan K. Martin, 'Monuments in the Garden: The Garden Cemetery in Australia', *Postcolonial Studies* 7/3 (2004): pp. 333–52, p. 336; Celestina Sagazio 'Introduction' in Celestina Sagazio (ed.), *Cemeteries: Our Heritage* (Melbourne, 1992), p. 13.

[12] Fiona Hutton, 'The Working of the 1832 Anatomy Act in Oxford and Manchester', *Family and Community History* 9/2 (2006): pp. 125–39, pp. 125–6; Helen MacDonald, 'Procuring Corpses: England's Anatomy Inspectorate, 1842 to 1858', *Medical History*, 53/3 (2009): pp. 379–96.

[13] Richardson, *Death, Dissection*, pp. 121–9, 234–5; Gatrell, *The Hanging Tree*, p. 76, p. 79; Jalland, *Australian Ways of Death*; Jalland, *Death in the Victorian Family*.

working-class sexual mores.[14] Although Thomas Laqueur sees a rise in this period of the 'humanitarian narrative' which enables the (educated) reader to empathize with the suffering body, I see as more forceful the arguments of Richardson and Gatrell which demonstrate the ability of these classes to dissociate themselves from such suffering. The wording of the Anatomy Acts (in its particular use of words like 'persons' and 'unclaimed' discussed below) is evidence of this.

The practice of 'anatomizing' hanged murderers ceased in Britain in 1832,[15] when the Anatomy Act provided its alternative source of available commodity. Richardson suggests that dissection thus became, and was viewed as, a punishment for being poor.[16] In Australia, however, murderers were not uniformly excluded from dissection after that date.

V.A.C. Gatrell, discussing middle-class attitudes to hanging, argues that towards the nineteenth century it

> seems ... to have become more necessary to insist on the 'otherness' of the hanged man or woman ... the condemned were to be defined with increasing explicitness as social others (poor people and thieves) or political others (subversives or traitors) or psychological others (monsters, murderers); and you learnt not to look at such men without shuddering. To see them as human was becoming helpfully difficult.[17]

In Australia, commodified bodies (live and dead) included Indigenous people, the bodies of criminals, and other individuals subject to the English state. A continuation and refinement of this 'othering' could be seen in relation to the understanding of the body to be anatomized, hanged or not. As we know, class categories are not produced or defined or negotiated in isolation from other social categories.[18] Thus the understanding of the poor body as a usable commodity available to the state had ramifications for, and was produced in conjunction with, the understanding of other bodies.[19] In each case, whatever was performed on the bodies of these subject individuals was frequently justified in the name of scientific advancement. In Australia as in Britain, the practice of dissection was represented as a teaching tool, and as an aspect of medical anatomical research that would advance the cause of science, and lead to breakthroughs which would benefit the poor as well as those wealthy enough to avoid dissection.[20] Likewise, the practice of treating

---

14 Françoise Barret-Ducrocq, *Love in the Time of Victoria: Sexuality, Class, and Gender in Nineteenth-Century London*, trans. John Howe (London, 1991).

15 Gatrell, *The Hanging Tree*, p. 84.

16 Richardson, *Death, Dissection*, p. 178.

17 Gatrell, *The Hanging Tree*, p. 263.

18 Anne McClintock, *Imperial Leather: Race, Gender, and Sexuality in the Colonial Contest* (New York, 1995).

19 MacDonald, *Human Remains*, pp. 9–10; Joy Damousi, *Depraved and Disorderly: Female Convicts, Sexuality and Gender in Colonial Australia* (Cambridge, 1997).

20 Richardson, *Death, Dissection*, pp. 210–15.

Aboriginal people as specimens was often not seen as requiring justification to the subjects, but was represented as advancing the cause of science.[21]

For Aboriginal people most intensely, but also for the British and Australian poor and criminal classes, the theft and appropriation of the body was a denial of property rights by a society founded on belief in capital and private property. In this it echoed the doctrine of *terra nullius*. In the same way that Indigenous colonized people were not seen to be effectively 'using' their land, and their cultural, emotional, physical attachment to it was rendered invisible or negligible, they were not seen to be fully occupying their own bodies which could then be regarded as having a use-value for the colonizing peoples. In addition this appropriation was a denial of emotional rights or investments in bodies, one's own and those of one's friends or relatives or connections; one's 'people'. Although non-Aboriginal people whose loved ones were appropriated on these terms were undoubtedly distressed, the application of this practice against Aboriginal people has had even more profound effects, as Paul Turnbull points out: 'grave robbing and body snatching's severance of the continuum of ancestral past, life in the land, death and return to the realm of dreaming has been spoken of as indistinguishable from taking the country itself'.[22]

The availability of bodies – those sorts of bodies which were understood as more valuable to science than to themselves – was a central concern in the setting up of Australia's first medical school, the Melbourne Medical School established at Melbourne University in 1862. In the first proposal drafted and submitted to University Council in 1857, Anthony Collings Brownless put at the top of his list a professor whose teaching areas included anatomy, and whose responsibilities would include being 'Conservator of the Anatomical and Pathological Museum'.[23] Item 4 called for legislative change of a very particular kind:

> That it will be necessary to obtain the sanction of the Legislature to an Anatomy Act, providing for the supply of bodies for dissection; to build an Anatomical Theatre and Dissecting Room, in the grounds of the University, and to take immediate steps for the formation of a Museum of Anatomy, and Pathology, and another of Materia Medica and Botany.[24]

In fact, the Medical School was delayed by the lack of government funding, despite appeals including Council's thrifty assertion that:

---

21 MacDonald, *Human Remains*, pp. 94–5; Turnbull, 'To What Strange Uses'; Paul Turnbull, 'Ancestors, Not Specimens: Reflections on the Controversy over the Remains of Aboriginal People in European Scientific Collections', *Electronic Journal of Australian and New Zealand History* (1995/1996): pp. 6–7; Stephen Jay Gould, *The Mismeasure of Man*, rev. edn (New York, 1981), pp. 86–7.

22 Turnbull, 'Ancestors, Not Specimens', p. 4 citing Michael Mansell.

23 K.F. Russell, *The Melbourne Medical School 1862–1962* (Carlton, 1977), p. 12.

24 Quoted in Russell, *The Melbourne Medical School*, p. 13.

> every facility for Clinical Teaching and Pathological Demonstrations is already provided by the large number of cases constantly under treatment in the Melbourne Hospital, and the number of unclaimed bodies interred at the public expense would afford greater opportunities of dissection than could be obtained at any School of Medicine in Europe.[25]

In other words the bodies of the 'unclaimed' poor were regarded as a rich unexploited resource in Melbourne, waiting to be used. In the absence of a Medical School, Brownless and the Council established the Medical Museum, gaining the hearty cooperation of the Melbourne Hospital and – at that stage – the Benevolent Asylum.[26]

By 1859 there was a resident curator for the Museum, Thomas Shearman Ralph, collecting specimens, 'anatomical and botanical, as well as pathological', with a concentration on the latter.[27] In this the university was narrowly and perhaps uncomfortably in advance of the introduction to Melbourne of such quasi-medical salacious entertainments as Kreitmayer and Wiseheart's Grand Anatomical Museum, which opened in 1861, or Jordan and Beck's Anthropological Museum, which, like the 'legitimate' university museum displayed female anatomy, but not to females.[28]

Ralph reported objections to his 'post-mortem examinations'.[29] Although Kenneth Russell's 1977 history of the Medical School is coy about what 'willingness to give every assistance in their power'[30] might mean, coming from the Melbourne Hospital, and what the Benevolent Asylum might have to do with it, it is presumably the case that the 'assistance' referred to consisted of providing bodies, body parts, and samples. In Australia, benevolent asylums were run by benevolent societies, private charitable organizations, usually managed by committees of prominent citizens, and funded primarily by donations and subscriptions from the general public. They were aimed at relieving the sick and elderly poor, often with an emphasis on the deserving poor. Although they sometimes received government financial assistance (Victorian Hansard Sessions, 5 June 1862 record a proposal to fund various Melbourne institutions, including £6,000 for the Melbourne Benevolent Asylum),[31] they were organizations

---

25 Quoted in Russell, *The Melbourne Medical School*, p. 17.

26 Ibid., p. 18.

27 Ibid.

28 Ross L. Jones, *Humanity's Mirror: 150 Years of Anatomy in Melbourne* (South Yarra, 2007), pp. 6–7, p. 26; Andrew McCann, 'Colonial Gothic: Morbid Anatomy, Commodification and Critique in Marcus Clarke's the Mystery of Major Molineux', *Australian Literary Studies*, 19/4 (2000): pp. 399–412; Mimi Colligan, 'Anatomical Museums in Melbourne 1861–1887', *Australian Cultural History*, 13 (1994): pp. 52–64.

29 Russell, *The Melbourne Medical School*, p. 19.

30 Ibid., p. 18.

31 *The Victorian Hansard containing the debates and proceedings of the Legislative Council & Assembly of the Colony of Victoria* (Melbourne, 1858–1865) 5 June 1862 vol. 1861–1862, p. 1277.

independent of government, unlike British workhouses, although many were conducted along lines similar to workhouses.[32] The Melbourne Hospital, like most early Australian hospitals, was initially set up along similar lines to English voluntary hospitals but, Ken Inglis claims, only because the government would not take responsibility for it.[33] Its mix of public and private funding made its status rather problematic for some time.[34]

The Act passed by the Victorian Parliament in Melbourne, Australia, in 1862, 'An Act for Regulating Schools of Anatomy',[35] is based on the British Act for Regulating Schools of Anatomy, 1832. In the Victorian Act, Clause V reproduces almost exactly the relevant sections of the British Act, presumably because the latter had proved itself such a brilliant form of obfuscation, and hence opened up a potentially rich source of bodies for British medical schools. As Richardson points out, this clause in the 1832 British Act removed any mention of dissection and also, by its wording, 'the clause … did not specify the social origin of its victims, except by inference'.[36]

Both Acts use the term 'Anatomical Examination', although the Victorian Act dispenses with the capitalization, thus enabling some useful confusion with post-mortem examination of a less invasive kind. The British Act states: 'That it shall be lawful for any Executor or other Party having lawful Possession of the Body of any deceased Person … to permit the Body of such deceased Person to undergo Anatomical Examination'. The Victorian Act is identical in wording except that it replaces the term 'Party' with 'person'. One might see this distinction as a further obfuscation on the part of the colonials, with their 30 years' hindsight. 'Party' carries the 'inference' of an official body, such as the workhouse. '[P]erson' seems much less official. But the Victorian Act adds a clause much later in the document (Clause XVI) which clarifies the meaning of person, 'That in order to remove doubts as to the meaning of certain words in the Act the word "person" shall

---

32 Ron Rathbone, *A Very Present Help: Caring for Australians Since 1813: The History of the Benevolent Society of New South Wales* (Sydney, 1994), pp. 13–25; David Evans, 'The Plight of the Poor in the Working-Man's Paradise', in John Pearn and Catherine O'Carrigan (eds), *Australia's Quest for Colonial Health: Some Influences on Early Health and Medicine in Australia* (Brisbane, 1983), pp. 203–12.

33 Ken Inglis, *Hospital and Community: A History of the Royal Melbourne Hospital* (Carlton, 1958), pp. 1–17.

34 Alan Gregory, *The Ever Open Door: A History of the Royal Melbourne Hospital 1848–1998* (South Melbourne, 1998), pp. 12–13.

35 'An Act for Regulating Schools of Anatomy', published as a supplement to the Victorian Government Gazette 24 June 1862 *Acts of the Victorian Parliament* CLVI [156] (Melbourne, 1862), pp. 271–4.

36 Richardson, *Death, Dissection*, p. 205. See Lord Shaftesbury's amendments replacing 'dissected' with 'anatomical examination', *House of Lords Journal* 64 10 July 1832, p. 368. History of Parliament Trust, Journal of the House of Lords. Available at: www.british-history.ac.uk/source.aspx?pubid=45.

be deemed to include any number of persons or any society whether by charter or otherwise'.[37] Hence it might be argued that the Victorian Act makes it even less evident than does the British that what was being legislated and legitimated was the provision of bodies for dissection by government and private hospitals and benevolent asylums and other institutions. The Tasmanian Anatomy Act of 1869 reverted to the use of 'party'.[38] The later South Australian Anatomy Act of 1884 makes this implication explicit in an additional clause and definition: 'The Chief Secretary may … authorise the medical officer of any public institution, supported wholly or in part by funds from the general revenue, to permit the body of any person who may die in such public institution, unless such institution shall be a public hospital, to undergo anatomical examination'.[39] 'Public Institution' is defined by an addition to clause 2 as including 'any prison, gaol, lunatic, destitute, or other asylum or hospital'.[40] In Britain at the same period, according to Fiona Hutton, such openness was inadvisable if the supply of bodies was to be kept up.[41] However, Ross L. Jones argues that the Melbourne Medical School suffered from a lack of detail in the Victorian Act, and Helen MacDonald argues that this was addressed in the New South Wales Act of 1881.[42] An *Argus* editorial from 1869 comments:

> we may remark incidentally that it is a deficiency in the Victorian Anatomy Act that it does not specify from what sources bodies are to be obtained. It is not too much to say that if bodies cannot be procured from our public institutions, the practice of 'body-snatching' will be revived.[43]

In fact the Victorian Act was merely repeating the British Act in this deliberate vagueness about the actual source of cadavers. From what evidence there is, the

---

[37] 'An Act for Regulating Schools of Anatomy', 1862 clause XVI, p. 274. The 1865 Medical Practitioners Act Part IV Schools of Anatomy, moved this clause to the first item '20. The word "person" wherever the same occurs in this Part of this Act shall be deemed to include any society whether established by charter or otherwise', *Acts of the Victorian Parliament* (Melbourne, 1857–1901), p. 308.

[38] 'Anatomy Act 1869', *The Acts of the Parliament of Tasmania* (Hobart, Tasmania 1857–1981), vol. 1, pp. 124–8; See also Helen MacDonald, 'A Scandalous Act: Regulating Anatomy in a British Settler Colony, Tasmania 1869', *Social History of Medicine*, 20/1 (2007): pp. 39–56, p. 45.

[39] 'Anatomy Act 1884', *Acts of Parliament of South Australia* (Adelaide 1858–), vol. 1, pp. 236–41, p. 238.

[40] 'Anatomy Act 1884', *Acts of Parliament of South Australia*, p. 236.

[41] Hutton, 'The Working of the 1832 Anatomy Act in Oxford and Manchester', p. 127.

[42] Helen MacDonald, '"Humanity's Discards": The New South Wales Anatomy Act 1881', *Mortality* 12/4 (2007): pp. 365–82, pp. 371–2.

[43] *Argus*, 7 August 1869, p. 4.

Melbourne Hospital, as Ross L. Jones argues in this book, provided a steady, if not adequate, supply of 'unclaimed corpses' to the Medical School.[44] In a letter to the Melbourne Benevolent Asylum from 1879, George Halford outlined his 'arrangement' with the hospital:

> The arrangement I make with the Committee of the Melbourne Hospital is that I give £ 2.0.0 for each subject. This money covers the expense of removing the body to us & subsequent burial & Clergyman's fee. I also give a similar fee to the Hall Porter who knowing who [has] & who has not friends; is the chief agent of our getting supplied; and I should be glad to give the same to any one in your institution who would take on himself the trouble of forwarding the subjects.[45]

This letter, half demand and half coaxing, was intended to encourage the Benevolent Asylum to hand over 'bodies of unclaimed persons'. As with earlier letters it does not appear to have had the desired effect.

Like the British Anatomy Act, the Victorian Act and subsequent Australian Acts exclude 'friends' or other categories from protesting or preventing 'anatomical examination'. Only the deceased person's 'surviving husband or wife or … known relative' can 'require the body to be interred without such examination'. The Victorian Act takes this further, specifying not just a known relative but 'a nearest known relative or any one or more of such person's nearest known relative being of kin in the same degree'. The meaning of this seems particularly unclear, and I have been unable to trace any legal interpretation of it. The exclusion of 'friends' had profound implications even in Britain. In Australia, in a dislocated settler-community where close living relatives may have been thousands of miles away, the exclusion of other groups from interest or rights in the body of a loved one would have been even more substantial. The Melbourne *Argus* record of the Benevolent Society Meeting of 29 July 1869, for instance, lists the deaths of six inmates whose origins are given as 'Chatham, England … Hampshire England … Cavan, Ireland … Antrim, Ireland … Ayrshire, Scotland … Gloucestershire'. This does not mean the deceased did not have local relatives, but it is suggestive of the diasporic nature of the population.[46] For Indigenous people, who could not have been more local, scattered relatives and unrecognized connections were also a problem. Richard Broome notes that by the middle of the nineteenth century Victorian Aboriginal groups, depleted in numbers by disease and dispossession, were forming new clan alliances and partnerships,[47] but even where acknowledged

---

44 Jones, *Humanity's Mirror*, pp. 82–3.

45 Letter from George Halford to J. Harcourt, Chairman of Committee, Benevolent Asylum, 21 May 1879. Melbourne University Archives. Dissections: Bodies For UM 447UL 124/18 Box 3 office # 461.

46 *Argus*, 30 July 1869, p. 5.

47 Richard Broome, *Aboriginal Victorians: A History Since 1800* (Crows Nest, 2005), pp. 91–3, p. 119.

Aboriginal kinship bonds had been formed these would often not have been recognized as Christian marriages or 'real' family ties by the dominant society. Aboriginal people who died in the Melbourne Hospital, according to one inquiry, were buried by the hospital 'in the "same way as other people who have no friends"'.[48]

As in the British Act, the Victorian Act has no stated provision for notifying the relatives of a death. This understanding of who has rights in the bodies of subordinated people seems particularly enduring. In Paul Turnbull's discussion of the 1984 Australian Archaeological Association's correspondence with the Victorian Minister for Planning and the Environment, he describes the Association as only supporting the 'disposal of remains when it could be shown that the person in question was known, and had expressed a desire not to be used for scientific purposes, or when it was the wishes of an appropriate community that remains be buried'.[49] The 'escape clause' offered to the 'unclaimed' in the British and Victorian Anatomy Acts of the nineteenth century was that the body of the deceased can be used for 'anatomical examination':

> unless to the knowledge of [the] executor such person shall have expressed his desire either in writing at any time during his life or verbally in the presence of two or more witnesses during the illness whereof he died that his body after death might not undergo such examination.[50]

The same limited set of relatives (deemed perhaps the 'appropriate community') could also prevent the practice. As Richardson points out in relation to the 1832 British Act, such provisions look good, but the likelihood of the subject's being aware of this clause and able to fulfill its requirements was low.[51] The British Act allows only 48 hours before removal of the body, but the Victorian Act specifies 12 hours, which leaves very little time to notify relatives. The later Victorian *Medical Practitioners Statute 1865*, continues to specify 12 hours.[52]

Appropriations of bodies took different forms. It may have been concern over the 1862 Victorian Anatomy Act and its use at the University of Melbourne School of Anatomy, which spurred some of the interest and controversy around the 1864 Harrison case noted above, even though the acquisition of Harrison's brains was not directly connected to the Anatomy Act at all. There was a public and embarrassing fight at the University of Melbourne about the possession of body parts, when the Professor of Anatomy, George Britton Halford, attempted to retain the brain of the executed murderer, Christopher Harrison which had been delivered to the Medical

---

48 Broome, *Aboriginal Victorians*, p. 145 citing Coranderrk Inquiry Report 1881–2.

49 Turnbull, 'Ancestors, Not Specimens', p. 2.

50 'An Act for Regulating Schools of Anatomy', 1862, V, p. 272.

51 Richardson, *Death, Dissection*, pp. 206–7.

52 *The Medical Practitioners Statute 1865*, item 27, p. 309.

School. The admonitory letter from Redmond Barry, Chancellor of the University, does not clarify who owned the body, but it is perfectly clear about who did *not*:

> It has been stated to me that instead of yielding obedience to the direction of the Law officers of the Crown you insisted on retaining the brain – asserting that Harrison had bequeathed his body to you. To me it is incomprehensible that you could have supposed it was in the power of a felon so to do.[53]

The 'felon', Harrison, had no rights according to the law as voiced by Justice Barry, not only to his living body, but to any say as to its disposition after death, though the Melbourne *Age* records Harrison as saying that 'as I should like to make a present of my body to Professor Halford, it may be given up to him'.[54] The *Argus* also states that Harrison 'wished that his body should be given to Professor Halford'.[55] One of the two men hanged with Harrison, William Carver, 'had, before his trial, objected to casts of his head, or pictures of him in the newspapers, but now he hoped it would be done, that he might serve as an example'. The *Age* claimed that such a cast was for the Waxworks, rather than the more edifying display kept by the Melbourne Gaol. There is no record of Carver offering his body parts to Halford.[56]

Christopher Harrison had been charged with the murder of his business partner after an argument on a Melbourne street in 1862. Because of his erratic behaviour and attempted suicide at the time of the murder, and his behaviour after the murder, questions were raised about his sanity. Halford wanted Harrison's brain because he believed that the man should have been spared hanging by reason of insanity. Having failed to prevent the execution he wished to prove his point by dissecting Harrison's brain afterwards.[57] The Melbourne *Age* of 5 August 1864 states that the brains and stomachs of the three executed men were delivered for examination the morning after the execution.[58] Another member of the university's staff, John Macadam, was supposed to receive and examine the brain of Harrison, but Halford obtained it and would not release it. Post-mortems had first been performed at the gaol.[59] According to Russell, a letter in *The Lancet* at the time says the brains had been delivered so that their 'cubic capacity' might be calculated.[60]

---

53 Quoted in Russell, *The Melbourne Medical School*, p. 37.

54 'Execution of Harrison', *Age*, 4 August 1864, pp. 5–6.

55 'Execution in Melbourne Gaol', *Argus*, 4 August 1864, p. 5.

56 'Execution of Harrison', pp. 5–6.

57 Ernest Scott, *A History of the University of Melbourne* (Melbourne, 1936), p. 116; George B. Halford, 'Letter to the Editor', *Argus*, 19 July 1864, p. 7; George B. Halford, 'Letter to the Editor', *Argus*, 30 July 1864, p. 7.

58 'The *Post Mortem* Examination on the Bodies of Harrison, Woods and Carver', *Age*, 5 August 1864, p. 5.

59 R.J.W. Selleck, *The Shop: The University of Melbourne, 1850–1939* (Carlton, 2003), p. 109.

60 Russell, *The Melbourne Medical School*, p. 37, no date cited.

Certainly the body of the murderer, like the bodies of the unclaimed poor and those of many Aboriginal people, was regarded not as the 'property' of the individual, or of his friends or relatives, or 'of the earth'[61] but as the usable property of the state. The skirmish in the dissecting room is arguably between 'state apparatuses'.[62] Halford had built up a collection of Aboriginal skulls at around the same time,[63] presumably also to prove his own theories, though as an anti-Darwinist he was clearly not using them to demonstrate evolution, as some were.[64] Melbourne University's anatomy department, like those of other older Australian universities, has a long history of Aboriginal body-snatching. Turnbull cites a discussion of the 1907 Melbourne Professor of Anatomy, Richard Berry having 'exhumed' the 'skulls of several Tasmanians' in his endeavour to prove Darwinism.[65]

The account from the London *Times* treats the sequence of events around Halford's acquisition of Harrison's head as an amusing Antipodean farce:

> The gaol surgeons were in consternation, and appealed to the Sheriff. The Sheriff appealed to the Attorney-General and the Minister of Justice. Law and justice were for a moment at fault, for larceny, or trover, or detinue for brains (so perishable an article) was rather a ridiculous and embarrassing subject for a Government prosecution. At length it was determined that the Sheriff, accompanied by a justice of peace and by a policeman, should proceed forthwith to the University and demand the brains. On arrival of the formidable Sheriff, 6 ft. 4 in. in height, at Professor Halford's rooms, the Professor was found surrounded by medical men and with the brain before him, the dissection then proceeding. The Sheriff, backed by the justice of the peace, the policeman, and the gaol surgeons, demanded the public property. Professor Halford asserted that the brains were his by bequest of their former owner. The Sheriff contended, with much force, that the brains were 'the Government's brains,' and that a convict on the scaffold had no property even in his own brains, to bequeath to any one. The Sheriff's law seemed to stagger the Professor, who began to treat. Finally the gaol surgeons being present, it was arranged that the dissection should proceed, and at the end the brain was pronounced perfectly healthy.[66]

---

61 Jane Wildgoose, 'Who Really Owns Our Bodies?', *Guardian*, 30 January 2001. Available at: http://society.guardian.co.uk/alderhey/comment/0,8006,431006,00.html (accessed 22 April 2004).

62 Louis Althusser, 'Ideology and Ideological State Apparatuses', trans. Ben Brewster, *Louis Althusser 1970 'Lenin and Philosophy' and Other Essays*. Available at: www.marxists.org/reference/archive/althusser/1970/ideology.htm (accessed 26 September 2011).

63 Russell, *The Melbourne Medical School*, p. 105.

64 W.A. Osborne, 'George Britton Halford: His Life and Work', *The Medical Journal of Australia*, 1/3 (1929): pp. 64–71; Turnbull, 'Ancestors, Not Specimens', p. 6.

65 Ibid., pp. 12–13.

66 'Australia: (From Our Own Correspondent) Melbourne AUG 26', *Times*, 18 October 1864, p. 9.

The Melbourne *Age* also produced a comic set piece out of the encounter, in which Halford cries, 'The Brains are mine, Sir' while the Sheriff insists they are the 'Government's brains'.[67] The Melbourne *Argus* headed one article 'The Battle of the Brains' and commented 'Time was when, if a man was hanged, he was at rest; but for this unfortunate wretch Harrison, there has been provided by the assiduous care of his friends, a punishment ten times more cruel than was ever perhaps inflicted on any murderer'.[68] This article resonates oddly with the Anatomy Act and its predecessors, as friends were excluded from the category of those who could stop dissections, and in times past *exactly* this fate would have awaited the murderer. Redmond Barry, Chancellor of the University, outraged at Halford's notion that a condemned man might retain any rights in his own body and its disposition, is perhaps most famous for presiding at the trial of heroized outlaw Ned Kelly, who received some of the same scientific data-gathering inflicted on those in this category. Death masks made of murderers including Kelly were used for phrenological examinations. Kelly's skull was certainly examined by doctors, and apparently disappeared, though it possibly spent some years as a trophy on a police desk.[69]

Such discourses are never entirely monolithic. There are always contradictions and fissures. One of these may perhaps be found in the earlier career of Redmond Barry, who was the Standing Counsel for the Aborigines through the 1840s and therefore defence counsel in the trial for murder of a group of Van Diemen's Land (Tasmanian) Aborigines, including Truganini, in 1841.[70] At the time Barry objected to 'the want of natives on the jury' and successfully saved the lives of the women by arguing, dubiously, that they were in 'slavish subjection to the men'. The men were sentenced to hang, despite some opposition.[71] Their bodies were regarded as entirely at the disposal of the authorities, but not necessarily, at this point, by Barry. One of the men, Tunnerminnerwait, was reported in the *Port Phillip Herald* at the time of their public execution as saying that '"he had three heads, one for the scaffold, one for the grave, and one for V.D. Land"'. Though ultimately impenetrable, this statement suggests a potential awareness of the commercial value placed, literally, on his head, and also a resistance to a regime which understood bodies as property, and used the bodies of those most subject to the regime in manners entirely contrary to their will and wishes.[72] Ann Galbally cites another instance where Barry apparently attempted to insert acknowledgement of Aboriginal culture and bodies before the public, at the 1866

67 'The *Post Mortem* Examination on the Bodies of Harrison, Woods and Carver'.

68 H.E.W. 'The Battle of the Brains', *Argus*, 6 August 1864, p. 5.

69 Damien Carrick and Jan Wositsky, 'Law Report: Ned Kelly's Skull', 21 May 2002. Australia: ABC Radio National.

70 Ann Galbally, *Redmond Barry: An Anglo-Irish Australian* (Carlton, 1995), pp. 55–7.

71 *Port Phillip Gazette*, 22 December 1841, p. 3.

72 *Port Phillip Herald*, 21 January 1842.

Intercolonial Exhibition. Across the same period Barry worked hard to prevent the access of women (in effect middle-class white women) to the university and the study of medicine – in part because he viewed them more as body than mind, objects rather than subjects. Galbally jokingly suggests he saw women as 'not just another species but another genus to be treated with a different set of rules and standards', as 'others' in V.A.C. Gatrell's terms, therefore.[73] Of course, although separated out and objectified in similar ways, women of a race and class able to contemplate attendance at the university were extremely unlikely to be found on the dissecting table or in a collection of bones. Eventually they would be amongst those doing the dissecting.

Redmond Barry's relationship to the available bodies of the subjugated continued to be a vexed and ambivalent one, suggestive, if not representative of dominant middle-class white understandings. He presided over the university, including its dissecting activities, and his congruent assertion of the government ownership of the dead bodies of criminals. His commissioning of portraits and casts of the heads of Aboriginal people of Victoria is more ambiguous. On the one hand, clearly, it is another way of appropriating the bodies of subject people and submitting them to the scientific gaze and use. The portraits, as Ann Galbally points out, were consistent with and potentially available for phrenological studies and theories of racial hierarchy.[74] However, according to Galbally, Barry may have resigned from his Presidency of Commissioners for the 1866 Intercolonial Exhibition because of the Commissioners' refusal to display the photographs, busts, a collection of Aboriginal materials and a study of Aboriginal languages. She suggests that the portraits were too sympathetic and therefore the other commissioners feared them 'capable of stirring up issues about the Aborigine's place in society', whereas Barry thought them an important contribution.[75]

The early resistance of the Melbourne Benevolent Asylum to providing bodies to the Medical School in the 1860s and 1870s may stand as another credible example of resistance to the objectification of 'othered' bodies. The Asylum consistently resisted or stymied requests and demands for bodies from George Halford and the University Medical School over these decades. This may in part have been caused by Halford's approach, which showed little sense of the cadavers as former people. His 1879 letter to the Benevolent Asylum opens:

> Sir,
> May I apply to you for the bodies of unclaimed persons who die in your institution. The Medical Practitioner's Act 1st June 1865 give[s] such bodies to me as a licenced teacher of Anatomy.[76]

---

[73] Galbally, *Redmond Barry*, p. 165.

[74] Galbally, *Redmond Barry*, pp. 154–6.

[75] Galbally, *Redmond Barry*, p. 151.

[76] George Halford to J. Harcourt, Chairman of Committee, Benevolent Asylum, 21 May 1879.

He also refers the Superintendent to the 1862 Anatomy Act. *Argus* accounts of 1869 Benevolent Asylum committee meetings record the committee at first acceding to a similar letter on behalf of Halford that had arrived from Dr M'Crae, Inspector of Anatomy, 'so far as the same can be done without wounding the feelings of any person living'.[77] A subsequent report of the meeting of 12 August 1869, records a petition from 402 of the inmates against this resolution. Committee member Mr Wild supported rescinding the motion and said 'he considered the committee would not be properly managing a charitable institution if they disregarded the feelings of the inmates in such a matter'. Wild proposed to move a motion that,

> in conformity with the … Medical Practitioners' Statute of 1865, a duly authenticated record of those inmates at present in the asylum who may express a desire that their bodies after death may not undergo anatomical examination be made forthwith by the visiting committee, and that in future each inmate on admission be requested to record, if they wish to do so[,] their desire that their bodies after death may not undergo such examination.[78]

The *Australian Medical Journal* records another letter from Halford to the Asylum in 1873, and describes the response with outrage. Having first declined, the Benevolent Society Committee later (and again) resolved 'That a record be kept of the names of all persons who, in the presence of the visiting Committee, or a magistrate, to be duly certified by him or them, have expressed their willingness to have their bodies transferred after death to the medical school, and that such wish be respected'.[79] It seems that the Committee of the Benevolent Society consulted the Statute as Halford had recommended, but used it to facilitate that portion of the Act which allowed a person to express 'his desire either in writing at any time during his life or verbally in the presence of two or more witnesses during the illness whereof he died that his body after death might not undergo such examination'.[80] As an article in the medical student journal *Speculum* acknowledges, 'I suppose the answer is invariably – No! as we never see any of their bodies in the dissecting room'.[81] The *Australian Medical Journal* attributes the petition produced by the Benevolent Asylum inmates to foolish sentimentalism, and the impetus of the members of the committee inciting the inmates, and of the press representing dissection 'as a kind of butchery and anatomists as brutal and unfeeling'.[82] It may have been that the Committee's middle-class sensibilities were offended by the notion of dissection, or the brusqueness of Halford's approach. However it may also have been that from more intimate weekly contact with the Asylum inmates

77 *Argus*, 30 July 1869, p. 5.

78 *Argus*, 13 August 1869, p. 5.

79 *Australian Medical Journal*, June 1873, pp. 169–71, p. 170.

80 'An Act for Regulating Schools of Anatomy', 1862, Clause V, p. 272.

81 *Speculum*, 11 (October 1887): p. 47.

82 *Australian Medical Journal*, June 1873, pp. 169–71, p. 171.

and their concerns, they formed cross-class bonds; they identified *with* them as living humans, rather than identifying them *as* potential cadavers. The brutal and unfeeling side of anatomists is perhaps evident in the continuation of the article in *Speculum*, which comments on the inmates' refusal:

> This seems a very curious proceeding. I should rather think that people who live on the bounty of the Government ought to be pleased at being able to make some return to the public who have kept them for so long.[83]

As Ross L. Jones points out, and as noted above, the Benevolent Asylum was in fact not entirely funded by the 'public purse', but independently run.[84] He notes committee member Thomas Dickson's protest against the *Argus*'s representation of the Committee. Dickson wrote in a letter to the editor,

> surely on a death-bed it would not do to ruffle the departing spirit by asking at such a crisis whether or not there was any objection to the body being 'utilised' for the living or not. I do not admit that the inmates of the Benevolent Asylum, living or dead, are the property of either the Government or the committee of management. The institution is not the same in constitution as an English poorhouse.[85]

Nevertheless the students, at least those vocal in the student journal, appear to have regarded the hospitals, the Benevolent Asylum and lunatic asylums as rightful sources of available bodies, rather than refuges for unfortunate people.[86] The fears of the Benevolent Asylum inmates were not entirely unfounded. Despite assurances from Halford that 'All is done quietly & decently',[87] Jones notes occurrences of 'meat fights' and the stealing of bones.[88] The assurance that 'the bodies of prisoners were [not] removed to the School of Anatomy' also rings a little untrue only five years after the Harrison scandal.[89]

As I have been suggesting, across the period which saw the passing of the 1832 Anatomy Act and the Australian versions of it starting with the 1862 Victorian Act, there arose and was sustained a particular understanding of non-white and non-middle-class bodies. Some version of this might be seen in an 1878 photograph of medical students at Melbourne University (see Figure 3.1).

Historian Kenneth Russell draws attention to the fact that the courtyard has a wooden floor, but not to the fact that the students are posing with two skeletons

---

83 *Speculum*, 11 (October 1887): p. 47.

84 Jones, *Humanity's Mirror*, p. 89.

85 *Argus* supplement, 10 August 1869, p. 1.

86 See also 'The Dissecting Room', *Speculum*, 11 (October 1887): pp. 12–13.

87 George Halford, Letter, 21st May 1879, Melbourne University Archives. Dissections: Bodies For UM 447UL 124/18 Box 3 office # 461.

88 Jones, *Humanity's Mirror*, pp. 84, 93–5.

89 *Argus*, 30 July 1869, p. 5.

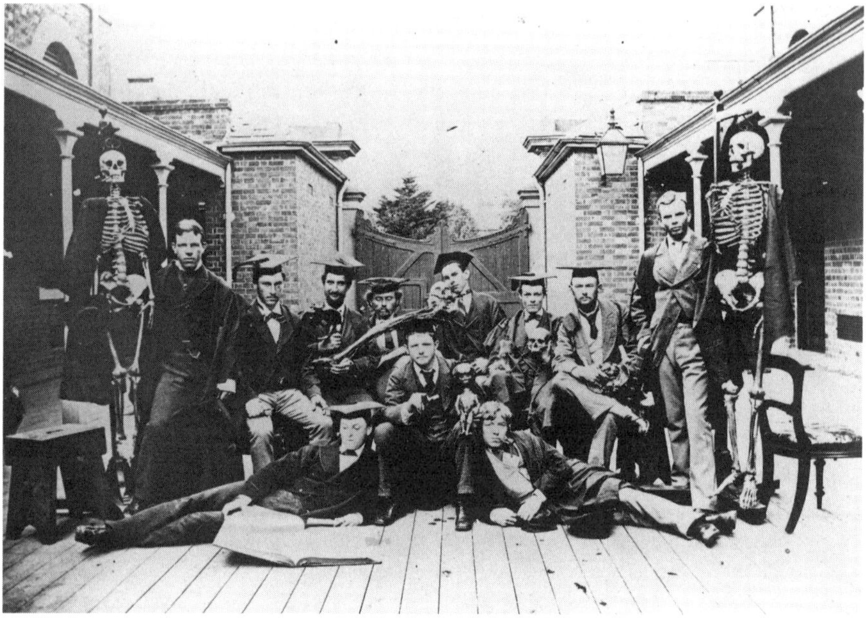

Figure 3.1 Portrait of Medical Students 1876 to 1880
Source: University of Melbourne Medical History Museum MHM00460 Series 31. 'A group of students in the courtyard of the old building in 1878'. Creator not known. Used by permission.

in gowns, and that most of the students are holding biological specimens; skulls, bones, and what appears to be a pelvis.[90] Such combinations were relatively common in Medical School photographs.[91] What is distinctive about this one is that, as the crowning feature, the central figure, identified as H. Lyons, has a mummified baby or foetus sitting on his left knee.[92] John Harley Warner and Lawrence J. Rizzolo argue that such images were 'a display of collective identity and a vehicle for emotional release enacted as a group'.[93] It is a commonplace that medical students have to become inured to death and distanced from it, in order to undertake their work. This image demonstrates this, perhaps to the extreme (although, as Warner and Rizzolo point out, such photographs may also be taken as acknowledgements of the affective dimension of dissection).

90 Russell, *The Melbourne Medical School*, p. 102.

91 John Harley Warner and Lawrence J. Rizzolo, 'Anatomical Instruction and Training for Professionalism from the Nineteenth to the Twenty-first Centuries', *Clinical Anatomy*, 19 (2006): pp. 403–14.

92 See also Adelaide University medical students (male and female) *c.*1910, reproduced in *Lumen* (Winter 2005): p. 6.

93 Warner and Rizzolo, 'Anatomical Instruction', p. 407.

In his discussion of the responses of contemporary medical students to the dissection of their subjects, Gareth Jones points out that students have more difficulty with some parts of the body than with others, and that these degrees of difficulty can be mapped according to their relation to a 'human referent', for instance, the head and face which most identify the body as an individual person.[94] I would speculate that for the 1878 students one of the things which separates the body parts from their 'human referent' is their otherness from the students. Melbourne University imported skeletons from Europe, though it appears to have acquired some locally also.[95] In both cases these skeletons would almost certainly have the same origin as the subjects of dissection – the 'unclaimed' poor who had died in 'asylums' or equivalent, and/or the racially other. The baby figure – mummy or doll, is black in the photograph, whether by original skin colour or preservation technique.

This image, taken almost 50 years after the 1832 Anatomy Act, and 16 years after the Victorian Act, demonstrates some of the separations symptomatic of, and enabled by, those Acts. In the hands of white middle-class males, the bodies of the poor and anonymous and racially other are objects, not subjects. They are equally useful to define the status and meaning of the men who hold them, and hold them away from themselves. The image's very frivolity and insouciance demonstrates the naturalization of the manner in which the practice of anatomy forged a new way of separating out middle-class white masculinity from a set of others whose primary definition was their exclusion from this category. Those who cut and collected, after 1832, were virtually never those who *were* cut and collected.

Bibliography

Printed Primary Sources

Age.
Argus.
Australian Medical Journal.
Port Phillip Gazette.
The Medical Practitioners Statute 1865 (Victoria), see: http://www.austlii.edu.au/au/legis/vic/hist_act/mps1865293/.
Speculum.
The Times.
'An Act for Regulating Schools of Anatomy'. 18 June 1862 [Repealed by Act No. 262]. *Acts of Parliament of Victoria. Title Acts of Parliament of Victoria*, 1862. Vol. CLVI [156], pp. 271–4.

94 Gareth Jones, *Speaking for the Dead: Cadavers in Biology and Medicine* (Aldershot, 2000) pp. 55ff., p. 66.

95 Russell, *The Melbourne Medical School*, p. 6; Jones, *Humanity's Mirror*, p. 72, p. 248.

Secondary Sources

Althusser, Louis, 'Ideology and Ideological State Apparatuses', trans. Ben Brewster, *Louis Althusser 1970 'Lenin and Philosophy' and Other Essays*. Available at: www.marxists.org/reference/archive/althusser/1970/ideology.htm (accessed 26 September 2011).

Barret-Ducrocq, Françoise, *Love in the Time of Victoria: Sexuality, Class, and Gender in Nineteenth-Century London*, trans. John Howe (London and New York: Verso, 1991).

Brooks, Chris, with Julian Litten, Brent Elliott, Eric Robinson, Richard Robinson and Philip Temple, *Mortal Remains: The History and Present State of the Victorian and Edwardian Cemetery* (Exeter: Wheaton in association with The Victorian Society, 1989).

Broome, Richard, *Aboriginal Victorians: A History since 1800* (Crows Nest: Allen & Unwin, 2005).

Carrick, Damien and Wositsky, Jan, 'Law Report: Ned Kelly's Skull', 21 May 2002. Australia: ABC Radio National.

Colligan, Mimi, 'Anatomical Museums in Melbourne 1861–1887', *Australian Cultural History*, 13 (1994): pp. 52–64.

Curl, James, *A Celebration of Death: An Introduction to Some of the Buildings, Monuments, and Settings of Funerary Architecture in the Western European Tradition* (London: Batsford, 1993).

Damousi, Joy, *Depraved and Disorderly: Female Convicts, Sexuality and Gender in Colonial Australia* (Cambridge: Cambridge University Press, 1997).

Evans, David, 'The Plight of the Poor in the Working-Man's Paradise', in John Pearn and Catherine O'Carrigan (eds), *Australia's Quest for Colonial Health: Some Influences on Early Health and Medicine in Australia* (Brisbane: Department of Child Health, Royal Children's Hospital, 1983), pp. 203–12.

Galbally, Ann, *Redmond Barry: An Anglo-Irish Australian* (Carlton, Victoria: Melbourne University Press, 1995).

Gatrell, V.A.C., *The Hanging Tree: Execution and the English People, 1770–1868* (Oxford and New York: Oxford University Press, 1994).

Gould, Stephen Jay, *The Mismeasure of Man*, rev. and expanded edition (New York and London: Norton, 1981).

Gregory, Alan, *The Ever Open Door: A History of the Royal Melbourne Hospital 1848–1998* (South Melbourne: Hyland, 1998).

Grosz, Elizabeth A., *Volatile Bodies: Toward a Corporeal Feminism* (Bloomington: Indiana University Press, 1994).

Houlbrooke, Ralph (ed.), *Death, Ritual, and Bereavement* (London and New York: Routledge in association with the Social History Society of the United Kingdom, 1989).

Hurren, Elizabeth T., 'Whose Body Is It Anyway? Trading the Dead Poor, Coroner's Disputes, and the Business of Anatomy at Oxford University, 1885–1929', *Bulletin of the History of Medicine*, 82/4 (2008): pp. 775–818.

Hutton, Fiona, 'The Working of the 1832 Anatomy Act in Oxford and Manchester', *Family and Community History*, 9/2 (2006): pp. 125–39.
Inglis, Ken, *Hospital and Community: A History of the Royal Melbourne Hospital* (Carlton: Melbourne University Press, 1958).
Jalland, Patricia, *Death in the Victorian Family* (Oxford: Oxford University Press, 1996).
Jalland, Patricia, *Australian Ways of Death: A Social and Cultural History 1840–1918* (South Melbourne: Oxford University Press, 2002).
Jones, Gareth, *Speaking for the Dead: Cadavers in Biology and Medicine* (Aldershot: Dartmouth, 2000).
Jones, Ross L., *Humanity's Mirror: 150 Years of Anatomy in Melbourne* (South Yarra: Haddington Press, 2007).
Laqueur, Thomas, 'Cemeteries, Religion and the Culture of Capitalism', in Jane Garnett and Colin Matthew (eds), *Revival and Religion since 1700* (London: The Hambledon Press, 1993), pp. 183–200.
Loudon, John C., *On the Laying Out, Planting and Managing of Cemeteries and on the Improvement of Churchyards* (London: Longman, Brown, Green and Longmans, 1843).
Adelaide University medical students (male and female) *c.*1910, reproduced in *Lumen* (Winter 2005): p. 6.
Martin, Susan K., 'Monuments in the Garden: The Garden Cemetery in Australia', *Postcolonial Studies*, 7/3 (2004): pp. 333–52.
McCann, Andrew. 'Colonial Gothic: Morbid Anatomy, Commodification and Critique in Marcus Clarke's "The Mystery of Major Molineux"', *Australian Literary Studies*, 19/4 (2000): pp. 399–412.
McClintock, Anne, *Imperial Leather: Race, Gender, and Sexuality in the Colonial Contest* (New York: Routledge, 1995).
MacDonald, Helen, 'Human Remains: Episodes in Nineteenth Century Colonial Human Dissection', PhD, Department of History, University of Melbourne, 2002.
MacDonald, Helen, *Human Remains: Episodes in Human Dissection* (Carlton: Melbourne University Press, 2005).
MacDonald, Helen, '"Humanity's Discards": The New South Wales Anatomy Act 1881', *Mortality*, 12/4 (2007): pp. 365–82.
MacDonald, Helen, 'A Scandalous Act: Regulating Anatomy in a British Settler Colony, Tasmania 1869', *Social History of Medicine*, 20/1 (2007): pp. 39–56.
MacDonald, Helen, 'Procuring Corpses: England's Anatomy Inspectorate, 1842 to 1858', *Medical History*, 53/3 (2009): pp. 379–96.
Morgan, Gwenda and Rushton, Peter, 'Visible Bodies: Power Subordination and Identity in the Eighteenth-century Atlantic World', *Journal of Social History*, 39/1 (2005): pp. 39–64.
Osborne, W.A., 'George Britton Halford: His Life and Work', *Medical Journal of Australia*, 1/3 (1929): pp. 64–71.

Petrow, Stefan, 'The Last Man: The Mutilation of William Lanne in 1869 and its Aftermath', *Australian Cultural History*, 16 (1997): pp. 18–44.

Rathbone, Ron, *A Very Present Help: Caring for Australians Since 1813: The History of the Benevolent Society of New South Wales* (Sydney: State Library of New South Wales Press, 1994).

Richardson, Ruth, *Death, Dissection and the Destitute* (London: Routledge and Kegan Paul, 1987).

Russell, K.F., *The Melbourne Medical School 1862–1962* (Carlton: Melbourne University Press, 1977).

Ryan, Lyndall, *The Aboriginal Tasmanians*, 2nd edition (St Leonards: Allen & Unwin, 1996).

Sagazio, Celestina, 'Introduction' in Celestina Sagazio (ed.), *Cemeteries: Our Heritage* (Melbourne: National Trust of Australia, 1992).

Sappol, Michael, *A Traffic of Dead Bodies: Anatomy and Embodied Social Identity in Nineteenth- Century America* (Princeton: Princeton University Press, 2002).

Scott, Ernest, *A History of the University of Melbourne* (Carlton: Melbourne University Press, 1936).

Selleck, R.J.W., *The Shop: The University of Melbourne, 1850–1939* (Carlton: University of Melbourne Press, 2003).

Tarlow, Sarah, *Bereavement and Commemoration: An Archaeology of Mortality* (Oxford and Malden, MA: Blackwell Publishers, 1999).

Tierney, Thomas F., 'Anatomy and Governmentality: A Foucauldian Perspective on Death and Medicine in Modernity', *Theory & Event*, 2/1 (1998). Available at: http://muse.jhu.edu/login?uri=/journals/theory_and_event/v002/2.1tierney.html (accessed 3 August 2009).

Turnbull, Paul, '"To What Strange Uses": The Procurement and Use of Aboriginal Peoples' Bodies in Early Colonial Australia', *Voices*, 4/3 (1994): pp. 5–20.

Turnbull, Paul, 'Ancestors, Not Specimens: Reflections on the Controversy over the Remains of Aboriginal People in European Scientific Collections', *Electronic Journal of Australian and New Zealand History* (1995/1996).

Vidal, Fernando, 'Brains, Bodies, Selves, and Science: Anthropologies of Identity and the Resurrection of the Body', *Critical Inquiry*, 28 (2002): pp. 930–74.

Warner, John Harley, and Lawrence J. Rizzolo, 'Anatomical Instruction and Training for Professionalism from the Nineteenth to the Twenty-first Centuries', *Clinical Anatomy*, 19 (2006): pp. 403–14.

Wildgoose, Jane 'Who Really Owns Our Bodies?' *Guardian*, 30 January 2001. Available at: http://society.guardian.co.uk/alderhey/comment/0,8006,431006,00.html (accessed 22 April 2003).

Chapter 4
Bodies of Evidence: Dissecting Madness in Colonial Victoria (Australia)

Dolly MacKinnon

When *The Argus* in Melbourne published the article 'An Ineffective Post Mortem The Result of Medical Interference' in 1900, something untoward was revealed in the press.[1] Laid before the readers was an account of potentially scandalous behaviour in the morgue at Kew Asylum. At the official coronial inquest into the death of Irish-born James B.F., aged 45, who was admitted to the Kew Asylum four days before his death, Dr William Beattie-Smith, Superintendent of the Asylum, was challenged by the Government Pathologist for the Colony of Victoria, Dr James Neild, and reprimanded by the coroner for Bourke, Mr Morrison, for examining the body before the official coroner's post-mortem was conducted. Neild exposed what could happen to asylum bodies in colonial Victoria with the following six words: 'the brain had already been examined' (see Figure 4.1). That this event had occurred was corroborated by the asylum's Warder Mercer and a Mr Murphy, M.B. who stated that the brain 'had been so interfered with by Mr Smith, F.R.C.S. [Edinburgh] that an examination by Dr Neild, F.R.C.S. [London] was impossible', and 'prevented' Neild 'from forming a just opinion of the condition of the brain' and determining the brain weight.[2] Dr Beattie-Smith's actions in conducting his own scientific enquiry had thwarted the Government Pathologist's use of this body as evidence to determine the cause of death under the law as governed by the *Coroners Act 1890* and *Coroners Act 1896*. More damning still was Neild's statement that 'this was not the first time such interference had taken place', and that Neild 'hoped that he would be pardoned for making some remarks about it'. Therefore the body of James B.F. was a contested object for these two medical men who both considered that they could not do their respective jobs properly without access to post-mortem evidence. The matter was further complicated by the fact that both men also lectured to medical students in anatomy at the University of Melbourne, and if James B.F.'s case were used for teaching by either man, its use also fell under the *Anatomy Act 1886*. The issues of post-mortems and dissection

[1] *Argus*, 18 December 1900, p. 7.

[2] Murphy had conducted the post-mortem in the case of the sudden death at Bendigo of Sarah Alice Turner, see *Argus*, 'Sudden Deaths at Bendigo', 26 November 1900, p. 9.

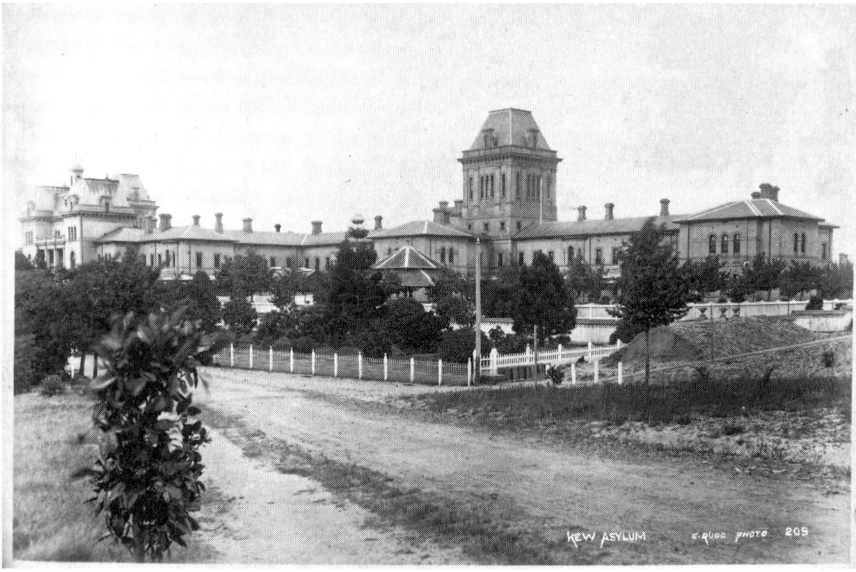

Figure 4.1 Photograph of Kew Asylum (1889–1891)
Source: By Charles Rudd, reproduced by permission from the Picture Collection, State Library of Victoria.

were contentious topics regularly discussed in the press from the 1850s to 1900. Beattie-Smith's 'medical interference' therefore highlighted the multiple uses for asylum corpses, the various statutes that governed post-mortem and anatomical examinations, and the potential conflict that could arise when a scientific quest could compete with the requirements of the law.

The legitimate quest for scientific knowledge had to be balanced with compliance with the laws of the state, and Beattie-Smith had taken advantage of his ready access to the corpse that lay in an asylum dead house. In compliance with the law, the coroner directed Neild to conduct the post-mortem on the corpse of James B.F., in the belief that the corpse would not already have been subjected to any form of internal anatomical examination. As the press reported, this was not the case. The public record remained resolutely silent, however, about what James' 'brothers' and the 'friends' who were known to have visited him during his brief days in the asylum, thought about these events.[3]

What then is the nineteenth-century pre-history of the event of Beattie-Smith and Neild in 1900? What does this history reveal about what could happen to the bodies of lunatics between 1851 and 1900 in Victoria? Which men had access to these asylum corpses, and under which law was that access determined? What

[3] *Argus*, 18 December 1900, p. 7, column 4; Public Record Office of Victoria (here after PROV) VPRS 7681/P0001/5, Discharge Register Kew Asylum (1896–1900), No. 4881, 14 December 1900; PROV VPRS24/P0000/727 Inquest James B.F., 1900.

were the links between the post-mortems conducted in the asylum dead house and dissection as part of the study of pathology and mental illness as taught at the University of Melbourne? What laws governed corpses in nineteenth-century Victoria, and to what scientific purpose and use were asylum bodies put? If an asylum body was subjected to post-mortem examination and dissection, what use – as anatomical material for teaching or as a pathology specimen for scientific research – if any, was made of the evidence to further the study of insanity within Victoria? The Beattie-Smith and Neild case of the ineffectual post-mortem highlighted the public fear of the potential scandals to be found in the asylum morgue involving scalpel-wielding doctors, and a tug of law over access to asylum corpses.

Within the history of psychiatry, patients' post-mortems are mentioned only in passing and, much like those whose bodies were dissected and their body parts harvested for science, they are missing from the existing historiography. This chapter therefore addresses these compelling absences in the history of the asylum for nineteenth-century Victoria by offering a greater understanding of the intersections between medicine, medical teaching, scientific research and the law in urban and rural asylums. The rise of nineteenth-century medical science relied upon post-mortems and dissection. This chapter charts a new direction by concentrating on what happened to asylum bodies, an issue that has not received any analytical investigation within the existing Australian literature.[4] Furthermore, while Helen MacDonald and Ross L. Jones have identified the problematic practice of access to bodies for dissection in colonial Australian public hospitals, and identified the centrality of dissection to the survival of the fledgling colonial university medical schools, it remains to examine post-mortems and dissections in the nineteenth-century asylum in Victoria.

In order to understand what happened to the bodies of lunatics in asylums we must first analyse what access medical men had to corpses within the

---

4 See Cressida Fforde, *Collecting the Dead: Archaeology and the Reburial Issue* (London, 2004), and Helen MacDonald, 'In the Interests of Science: Gathering Corpses from Lunatic Asylums', in Catharine Coleborne and Dolly MacKinnon (eds), *Exhibiting Madness in Museums: Remembering Psychiatry through Collections and Display* (New York, 2011), pp. 139–60; for general works in the Australian context see Mark Finnane, 'Asylums, Families and the State', *History Workshop*, 20/1 (1985): pp. 134–48; Stephen Garton, *Medicine and Madness: A Social History of Insanity in New South Wales, 1880–1940* (Kensington, NSW, 1988); Catharine Coleborne, 'Making "Mad" Populations in Settler Colonies: The Work of Law and Medicine in the Creation of the Colonial Asylum', in Diane Kirkby and Catharine Coleborne (eds), *Law, History, Colonialism: The Reach of Empire* (Manchester, 2001), pp. 106–22; Catharine Coleborne and Dolly MacKinnon (eds), *'Madness in Australia': Histories, Heritage and the Asylum* (St. Lucia, Qld, 2003); Catharine Coleborne, 'Families, Insanity and the Psychiatric Institution in Australia and New Zealand, 1860–1914', *Health and History*, 11/1 (2009): pp. 65–82, and Catharine Coleborne, *'Madness' in the Family: Insanity, Institutions and the Australasian Colonial World, 1860s–1914* (London and New York, 2010).

interconnected legislation that governed the legally qualified medical men who conducted post-mortems instigated by the coroner, and/or performed dissection for teaching purposes in nineteenth-century Victoria. Between 1850 and 1900 asylum post-mortems were regularly performed in Victoria under the auspices of the interconnected *Medical Witnesses*, *Medical Qualifications*, *Medical Practitioners*, and *Coroners Acts* dating from 1838 to 1896.[5] This legislation in Victoria had firmly established from 1860 onwards exactly who legally qualified medical men were, and what their coronial obligations were under the law. While Victoria enacted colonial Australia's first Anatomy Act in 1862, allowing licensed medical men in the University Medical School to hold bodies for the purposes of dissection for a period of six weeks before interment, the Act still failed to specify any public institutional sources from which corpses might be readily obtained. The *An Act for Regulating Schools of Anatomy 1862* (Victoria) did not interfere with post-mortems conducted under the coroner's jurisdiction. In 1865, the 1862 Anatomy Act was repealed in its entirety, with the whole contents being re-written instead into section 'IV Schools of Anatomy' of the *Medical Practitioners Act 1865*. The practice of anatomical examination or dissection now appeared within the *Medical Practitioners Statute 1865*, and the then highly controversial term 'Anatomy' did not reappear again as a title of a statute in Victoria until 1886. Therefore newspaper reports about parliamentary debates concerning amendments to the *Medical Practitioners Statute 1865* attracted little comment unlike the public interest that had surrounded the 1862 Anatomy Act. The removal of the contentious term 'anatomy', considered by many as synonymous with 'dissection', therefore, saw the parliamentary debates in the press pass without public comment and outrage.[6] In 1876, however, a most significant amendment was made to the *Medical Practitioners Statute 1865* Part IV that enabled all unclaimed asylum

[5] The following NSW acts governed these aspects of the Port Phillip Colony until the State of Victoria enacted its own legislation: 1 Vic. No. 3 [13 June 1838] *Medical Witnesses Act* [NSW]; 2 Vic. No. 22 [12 October 1838] *Qualifications of Medical Witnesses Act*; 8 Vic. No. 8 [23 August 1844] *An Act to amend the Medical Witnesses Act*; 9 Vic. No. 12 [27 October 1845] *An Act to amend 'Medical Witnesses Act*; 17 Vic. No. 14 [31 March 1854] *An Act relating to legally qualified Medical Practitioners* [NSW]; 24 Vic. 118 [18 September 1860] *An Act to amend an Act for legally qualified Medical Practitioners* [VICTORIA]; 25 Vic. 158 [18 June 1862] *An Act to amend the Laws relating to the Registration of Legally Qualified Medical Practitioners* [VICTORIA]; 28 Vic. 253 [9 May 1865] *An Act to Consolidate the Law relating to Coroners* [VICTORIA]; 54 Vic. 1077 [10 July 1890] *Coroners Act 1890* [VICTORIA], and 60 Vic 1455 [16 November 1896] *An Act to amend the Coroners Act 1890* [VICTORIA].

[6] As Helen MacDonald has shown for practices in Scotland, the medical lobby, with its vested interest in ensuring that the public remained entirely unaware of highly contentious amendments guaranteeing the supply of corpses to anatomy schools, encouraged parliamentarians to offer a 'silent reception' to such clauses when they were presented for debate in the parliament. As the titles of these bills did not include the term 'anatomy', there was no automatic connection with the Anatomy Act. See Helen MacDonald, 'In the Interests of Science'.

bodies, the bodies of prisoners and those who died in public institutions to be used for dissection by medical staff teaching anatomy at the University of Melbourne. In 1886, the *Medical Practitioners Statute 1865* was further amended to allow bodies for dissection to be held for a period of six months before interment, rather than just six weeks (the time period used in the English Anatomy Act of 1832), and the Act's name was changed to *The Anatomy Act 1886*. What links existed between the medical men of the asylum and the medical men teaching anatomy, studying pathology, and researching mental science that led to standoffs such as that between Neild and Beattie-Smith?[7]

Within this chapter I will be using the terms post-mortem and anatomical examination (that is dissection) in specific ways. By post-mortem I mean any internal and external anatomical and pathology examination of a patient's body after death conducted by a medical doctor as directed by the coroner or JP, under the *Coroners Acts*, as part of the official coronial inquests or inquiries. The terms anatomical examination or dissection are used throughout this chapter to describe internal surgical examinations as stipulated under the state legislation governing the practice of anatomy. The evidence discussed here serves to correct Milton Lewis's claim, in his brief discussion of the history of general paralysis of the insane in Australia, that in Victoria, asylum 'postmortems [*sic*] began to be carried out in the late 1880s'.[8] The archival evidence, the related nineteenth-century legislation in operation governing medical practitioners, the coroner's inquests and post-mortems, and anatomical examinations, as well as published medical literature for Victoria discussed in this chapter, all clearly indicate that this was not the case. Post-mortems had been conducted on lunatics in asylums and prisons in Victoria from the 1850s onwards by legally qualified medical doctors acting under the instruction of the coroner. Although the nineteenth-century pathology registers for Victoria have not survived, it is still possible to reconstruct a chronological history of asylum post-mortem and dissection practices. Nineteenth-century post-mortem notes survive in individual asylum patient casebook records, in the

---

7 For a discussion of medical education and access to corpses in England, see Elizabeth Hurren, 'A Pauper Dead-House: The Expansion of the Cambridge Anatomical Teaching School under the late-Victorian Poor Law, 1870–1914', *Medical History*, 48/1 (2004): pp. 69–94; For the regulation of anatomy in Tasmania and South Australia, see Helen MacDonald, *Human Remains: Episodes in Human Dissection* (Carlton, Victoria, 2005) and *Human Remains: Dissection and its Histories* (New Haven, 2006); Helen MacDonald, 'A Scandalous Act: Regulating Anatomy in a British Settler Colony, Tasmania 1869', *Social History of Medicine*, 20/1 (2007): pp. 39–56; For the teaching of anatomy, see Ross L. Jones, *Humanity's Mirror: 150 Years of Anatomy in Melbourne* (South Yarra, 2007); Helen MacDonald, 'The Anatomy Inspector and the Government Corpse', *History Australia*, 6/2 (2009): 40.1–40.17. For the rise of medical science in South Australia see K.N. White, 'Negotiating Science and Liberalism: Medicine in Nineteenth-Century South Australia', *Journal of Medical History*, 43/2 (1999): pp. 173–91, especially p. 174.

8 Milton Lewis, *Thorns on the Rose: The History of Sexually Transmitted Diseases in Australia in International Perspective* (Canberra, 1998), p. 71.

reports of public inquests and inquiries into asylum deaths, in legislation, as well as in the medical publications of those medical men connected with asylums in Victoria. Asylum casebook post-mortem data served simultaneous purposes within the asylum. These casebook entries were designed to record aspects of the life of the patient within the asylum under the gaze of the medical staff, and in death any physical evidence of the causes of madness in individual patients. Some post-mortems were also generated as part of coronial inquests and copied into the casebooks. Post-mortem records were 'to be available for inspection by government officials', and also used 'to act as insurance against lawsuits' as, very often, post-mortem records were used specifically to combat allegations of staff brutality and mistreatment.[9] These records were also a useful resource for the doctors as 'internal readers' within the asylum for the purposes of their own study and for the teaching of pathology.[10]

A study of the uses of asylum bodies also demonstrates how the post-mortem evidence gathered in Victoria was influenced by developments in the study of pathology and the links to medical training that warranted such scientific investigation in the first place. The descriptions of the state of brain tissue of lunatic patients who died in prisons and asylums in post-mortem evidence from coronial inquests from the 1850s in Victoria also suggests we should question assumptions that mid-nineteenth-century medical references to causes of death, that included terms such as died of a 'softening of the brain', were simply generic labels for mental illness that had no basis in post-mortem pathology. While there were cases in which the cause of death of a lunatic was attributed to a softening of the brain without any examination of the brain taking place, there were also cases where brain tissue was recorded and described in detail. Furthermore, the practice of pathology was evident in the language of asylum statistics published in the annual reports. In Victoria in 1869, for example, four years after the enactment of the *Coroners Act 1865* that made it compulsory to perform post-mortems on all asylum deaths, there were 128 deaths recorded in public asylums: of which 26 patients (17 men and nine women) had died of inflammation and other diseases of the brain, softening and tumours; and 21 patients (eight men and 13 women) had died of various thoracic diseases.[11] Asylum doctors knew their patients inside and out. What is more, annual reports travelled around the globe, and staff collected statistical and qualitative accounts gleaned from anatomical examinations as grounds for comparison regarding rates of disease. For example, copies of the annual lunacy reports for Victoria for the years 1870 and 1884, as well as the

[9] For a very brief discussion of post mortems see Jonathan Andrews, 'Case Notes, Case Histories, and the Patient's Experience of Insanity at Gartnavel Royal Asylum, Glasgow, in the Nineteenth Century', *Social History of Medicine*, 11/2 (1998): pp. 255–81, and especially p. 267.

[10] Andrews, 'Case Notes, Case Histories', p. 267.

[11] Victorian Parliamentary Papers (hereafter VPP), vol. 2 (1870), Annual Report for Asylums 1869, p. 10, Table 3.

Royal Commission into Asylums for the Insane and Inebriate (1884–1886), were sent to the Library of the Royal Edinburgh Asylum in Scotland, while copies of British asylum reports and inquiries were held in the Victorian Parliamentary Library and asylums. Therefore annual reports gathered from around the colonial world allowed asylum superintendents to place their populations, post-mortem findings, and population statistics, within a global context.

In order to trace the history of post-mortem and dissection practice in the asylums in Victoria between 1850 and 1900 it is important to understand where and in what conditions the insane were housed in public institutions during this period. The problem of adequately housing lunatics plagued the Colony of Victoria (created in 1851) in the second half of the nineteenth century, as it had done its predecessor the Port Phillip District (1838–1850), part of the Colony of New South Wales. From 1848 until 1867 lunatics were housed either in gaols, or in the single state Lunatic Asylum at Yarra Bend. The first decade of inquest post-mortem records for Victoria from 1851 is dominated by inquests into the deaths of lunatics in the prison system, with very few asylum inquests recorded. This was because while the coroner was legally required to conduct an inquest into all prison deaths, this was not mandatory for asylums under the *Coroners Act 1865* in Victoria. In 1852–1853, for example, the doctors at the Yarra Bend asylum refused to do an autopsy on a female patient named Hastings who had died after being transferred from a Melbourne gaol.[12] The inquiry revealed that had Hastings died in the prison there would automatically have been a coronial inquiry involving a post-mortem, but as she had died in the asylum the decision was made by the Colonial Surgeon not to conduct a post-mortem. If a post-mortem did occur, asylum doctors were in the habit of conducting them themselves.

As the Victorian population rapidly expanded between 1850 and 1900 through the gold rush and waves of immigration, a new public asylum system rapidly developed, to house the rising numbers of insane.[13] The government constructed eight public asylums of which four were urban and four were rural: Yarra Bend (1848–1925),[14] Collingwood Receiving House (1868–1873), Kew (1872–1988), Kew Cottages (1887–2008), Ararat (1867–1993), Beechworth (1867–c1990s),

---

12 VPP (1852/3), vol. 2, *Report from the Select Committee of the Legislative Council on the Yarra Bend Lunatic Asylum, together with Proceedings of the Committee, Minutes of Evidence and Appendix*, pp. iv–v.

13 William Henry Archer, 'The Colony of Victoria Being a Brief Statistical Sketch', in *Catalogue of the Victorian Exhibition, 1861: With Prefatory Essays, Indicating the Progress, Resources, and Physical Characteristics of the Colony, by W.H. Archer, Ferd. Mueller, E. Brough Smyth, Professor Neumayer, Fred. McCoy, A.R.C. Selwyn, and W.M. Birkmyre* (Melbourne, 1861), p. 70 and p. 90.

14 With a colonial population of just over half a million people, in 1861 Yarra Bend contained 351 male and 245 female patients, the government having spent over £104,067 on improving the buildings and grounds. Archer, 'The Colony of Victoria', p. 70 and p. 90; VPP (1870), vol. 2, p. 5, Annual Report for Asylums 1869.

Ballarat (1877–1878) and Sunbury (1879–*c*.1993). By 1904 the resident population in rural and urban asylums had reached 4,389 patients (2,276 men and 2,113 women).[15] Overcrowding was a recurring problem, resulting in lunatics still being housed at times in metropolitan and regional gaols, but there was substantial capital investment by the government in response to medical lobbying. But rising rates of lunacy were a common problem across the British Empire, and in 1870, for example, Edward Paley, Inspector of Asylums for Victoria, and a member of the Medico-Psychological Association (UK) was able to place Victoria's levels of insanity into a global context. He was optimistic about the colony's standing, for while the rates of insanity between 1859 and 1869 had increased, he argued:

> this result is inevitable in a new colony, where the large majority of the population consists of healthy adult immigrants, in whom and whose families the natural amount of insanity cannot be developed until a complete generation has elapsed from the time of their arrival and settlement.[16]

Victorian asylums still had 'reason for congratulations' for:

> in spite of the many causes which might be expected to produce a more than ordinary amount of insanity, such as the solitary life of shepherds, habits of intemperance, and sudden reverses of fortune, especially among the mining population, the ratio of lunacy still remaining lower than in Great Britain and Ireland.[17]

The relatively low number of medical staff in these overcrowded public institutions struggled to provide even the basic medical treatment required, let alone further the study of mental science. The result was three major public inquiries into Victoria's asylums in which the issues of post-mortems and anatomical investigations were also raised. These inquiries – the Yarra Bend Asylum Inquiries and libel case (1852–1853, 1858–1859 and 1862); Kew Asylum Inquiry (1876); and the Royal Commission into Asylums for the Insane and Inebriate (1884–1886) – centred on the adequacy of the administration, the treatment of patients and included discussions of the scientific merits of post-mortems and anatomical examinations. Each investigation proved a catalyst for the gradual legislative change governing access to asylum bodies, post-mortems and dissection.[18] The first *Lunacy Act* for

---

15 This does not include the 257 patients on probation, boarded out or held in a lunacy ward of a regional hospital. VPP (1905), vol. 3, Part 1, p. 603, Annual Report for Hospitals for the Insane 1904.

16 VPP (1870), vol. 2, p. 5, Annual Report for Asylums 1869.

17 VPP (1870), vol. 2, p. 5, Annual Report for Asylums 1869.

18 *A Report of the Inquiry into the Management of Yarra Bend Lunatic Asylum [1858–59], as described in the Nine Days' Trial of the Action for Libel Bowie v. Wilson. Held in the Supreme Court, Melbourne, from Wednesday, May 28, to Friday, June 6, 1862* (Melbourne,

Victoria was proclaimed in 1867, but post-mortems were covered by the *Coroners Acts*.[19] In 1876 an amendment to the *Medical Practitioners Statute 1865*, specified that all unclaimed bodies from asylums, prisons and other public institutions were then permitted to be used for the purposes of dissection in order to further medical education in the state. Prior to this there were rare instances of individuals in public institutions who actually requested their brains be dissected after death, such as the case of Christopher Harrison, a murderer executed in Melbourne gaol in 1864, that is discussed elsewhere in this volume. Furthermore, the need for lunacy reform was championed largely by the agitation of the Medical Board of Victoria that resulted in the Royal Commission into Asylums for the Insane and Inebriate (1884–1886) which included, amongst its findings, a brief discussion of the function, procedure and potential to be gained from conducting post-mortems in the asylum. These findings and debates about reform coincided with the reworking and proclamation of the *Anatomy Act 1886*. Two years later when the *Lunacy Amendment Act 1888* was proclaimed it expressly stipulated that on the death of a patient 'in addition to any notice respecting such death as required by any law now or hereafter in force relating to the registration of deaths', the superintendent of the asylum was required automatically to inform the coroner of the district, and 'send through the post office in a registered envelope a notice of such death to the relation or one of the relations named in the statement (if any) subjoined to the order for admission of such patient'.[20] If no relatives were known or recorded, then the unclaimed bodies were legally available for medical science.

Medical men conducting post-mortems and dissection on nineteenth-century asylum patients under the laws of the state increasingly attempted to claim a scientific basis for the cause of death from mental disease. But there were limited opportunities for scientific research even though the teaching of anatomy at the University of Melbourne had begun as early as 1855 – seven years before the proclamation of the Anatomy Act in 1862.[21] Technically, between 1850 and 1862, only qualified medical men acting on behalf of the coroner had access to asylum corpses. The 1862 Anatomy Act, however, also enabled any medical man conducting a post-mortem on behalf of the coroner to extend that scientific scrutiny to include dissection for the purposes of teaching medical students. Initially, the

---

1862); *Report of The Board Appointed to Inquire into Matters Relating to the Kew Lunatic Asylum, Taken Together with the Minutes of Evidence and Appendix* (Melbourne, 1876); *Royal Commission into Asylums for the Insane and Inebriate Report* (Melbourne, 1886).

[19] 31 Vic. No. 309, *An Act to Consolidate and Mend the Law Relating to Lunatics* [6 September 1867] [VICTORIA], and this act then repealed the following acts relating to the custody and care of lunatics, the majority of which were legislated by New South Wales between 1843 and 1849, and applied to the state of Victoria until 1867: 7 Vic. No. 14 [NSW, 1843], 9 Vic. No. 4 [NSW, 1845], 9 Vic. No. 34 [NSW, 1846], 13 Vic. No. 3 [NSW, 1849], and the Act passed in Victoria, 16 Vic. No. 8 [VICTORIA 1852].

[20] 52 Vic. No. 986 *Lunacy Amendment Act* (1888), section 51.

[21] Jones, *Humanity's Mirror*, p. 4.

number of medical students undertaking dissection at the University of Melbourne from 1863 was very small, totalling just four male students. Over the course of the next 20 years, however, the numbers increased dramatically. In 1872 there were 20 male students. The legislative response to medical lobbying came in 1876 in the form of an amendment to the *Medical Practitioners Act 1865* to specify a supply of unclaimed bodies for the purposes of dissection from the asylums, prisons and other public institutions. By 1879 the number of students studying dissection had reached 58, with the sharpest increase occurring in the year 1882 and 1883 when the numbers rose from 78 to over 100.[22] This placed even greater pressure on the demand for corpses.

During the Royal Commission into Asylums for the Insane and Inebriate (1884–1886), Soloman Iffla, an alienist trained at Glasgow, who was a JP and Official Visitor to Kew Asylum, was asked 'are the bodies of deceased inmates in any way utilized for scientific purposes, such as examination of their brains?' He replied that he was 'not aware what is done to their bodies'. He did, however, 'have no doubt that students may go there sometimes and perform dissections, where the bodies are not claimed'. When asked 'Is this not exceptional?', he replied 'I believe it is … students do occasionally go there, but they are not at all utilized to the extent they might be'.[23] A year after the Royal Commission findings, in 1887, this problem of a shortage of bodies was further exacerbated when the first women were admitted into the university medical school. Segregated dissecting rooms were created – one for women and one for men – doubling the pressure on the already crippling demand for corpses for dissection.[24]

Nineteenth-century medical men, however, who conducted post-mortems for any Coronial or Justice of the Peace inquests, had ready access to asylum corpses. Dr James Neild recalled in 1886 that he had conducted 900 'post mortems examinations on those dying insane' in the asylum over a 20-year period.[25] By 1898 as chief of the pathology staff at the Melbourne Morgue he had made 'upwards of 5,000 post mortems'.[26] The issue of variable access to corpses for the different but related purposes of post-mortem and scientific enquiry, and dissection for teaching, clearly created some tensions within the medical fraternity.

For the District of Port Phillip and Colony (from 1901, State) of Victoria between 1848 and 1904 a total of 9,708 asylum patients died (6,422 men and 3,286 women) offering plenty of potential for further medical research into the

22 *Victorian Parliamentary Debates* (hereafter *VPD*), Legislative Council, 29 June 1886, p. 464.

23 *Royal Commission into Asylums* (1886), pp. 396–7.

24 Jones, *Humanity's Mirror*, p. 91, p. 92 and p. 94.

25 *Royal Commission into Asylums* (1886), p. 459.

26 *The West Australian*, 15 December 1898, p. 7, 'A Post-Mortem Surprise: Discovery at the Kew Asylum a Nail in a Woman's Head'.

pathology of madness.[27] During the Royal Commission into Asylums for the Insane and Inebriate (1884–1886), there were calls to expand the coronial post-mortem to include much greater use of microscopic investigation. The Royal Commission also 'recommended … honorary medical staff … be appointed in connection with each asylum, and that each member of such staff should undertake to pay a given number of visits to the asylum every year … The outside medical practitioner would be a valuable auxiliary to the asylum Superintendent regarding general practice, and the Superintendent could give the general practitioner many valuable opportunities of studying remarkable cases of brain disease'.[28] But 15 years later, as the Report into Lunacy Reform in Victoria in 1901 articulated, precious little was being made of the post-mortem data collected, and only a select number of asylum medical men appeared to have access to this data. This report recommended 'higher rates of pay' and the opening up of 'some positions … to women practitioners'.[29] Yet the nineteenth-century asylum was entirely the preserve of medical men who were either resident asylum medical officers, such as Beattie-Smith, or medical men called in to conduct post-mortems under the *Coroners Act*, such as Neild.

Furthering the study of the nineteenth-century pathology of madness was clearly of interest to some colonial medical men who worked in or were connected with asylums on behalf of the coroner. A growing body of international medical literature discussing the brain and body as an essential focus of scientific inquiry was based on the findings of pathology over the course of the second half of the nineteenth century. As Andrew Scull suggests, performing post-mortems offered another way 'to minimize the amount of time' medical men 'were forced to spend in the unpleasant and disturbing company of (live) patients'.[30] Doctors in Victoria like Beattie-Smith and Neild, who were themselves published authors, were well aware of the influential medical works including John G. Fleming's *Remarks on the Pathology and Treatment of Ramollissement of the Brain: A Probationary Essay Submitted to the Faculty of Physicians & Surgeons of Glasgow* (Glasgow, 1833), Adam Addison's 'On the Pathological Anatomy of the Brain in Insanity' published in the *Journal of Mental Science* (1862), and Thomas Clouston's article calling for better individual patient histories with the aim of improving treatment regimes published as 'The Medical Treatment of Insanity' in the *Journal of Mental Science* (1870).[31]

---

27 VPP (1905), vol. 3, Part 1, p. 603, Report for the Hospitals for the Insane 1904, Table VI.

28 *Royal Commission into Asylums* (1886), p. 29.

29 VPP (1901), Lunacy System in Victoria: Reports of the Master-in-Lunacy and the Inspector of Lunatic Asylums on the defects of the lunacy system in Victoria, p. 14.

30 Andrew Scull, *The Most Solitary of Afflictions: Madness and Society in Britain 1700–1900* (New Haven and London, 1993), p. 263.

31 Thomas Clouston, 'The Medical Treatment of Insanity', *Journal of Mental Science*, 16 (1870): pp. 24–30.

Evidence of the familiarity colonial doctors had with influential medical literature exists in the terminology medical men in Australia used and the references they cited in their own inquest notes and publications. One of the earliest public inquest records in Victoria is for a lunatic prisoner, James S. from Barwon Gaol, Geelong, who according to William Cook's post-mortem, died in 1856 of 'brain disease'.[32] James S.'s remains were then buried in an unknown grave at the Geelong Eastern Cemetery.[33] One of the earliest asylum post-mortem cases is that of Joseph L., aged 40, who died at Yarra Bend Asylum from a 'softening of the Brain' in 1857.[34] The terminology of John G. Fleming's work is reflected in the post-mortem examination of a 'remanded lunatic', Thomas D., aged 50, who died in the Melbourne Eastern Gaol in 1857, with the cause of death ascribed to 'Ramollissement du cerveau'.[35] Medical literature had a practical application. Post-mortems also formed a major component of medical teaching in Britain, and colonial medical schools, and influential teaching studies included John Haslam's, *Observations on Madness and Melancholy* (1798), A.L.J. Bayle's, *Nouvelle Doctrine des Maladies* (Paris, 1825), Rudolph Virchow's and Benno Reinhard's new journal *Archiv für pathologische Anatomie und Physiologie und für klinische Medizin* (*c.*1849), and Virchow's own *Post-Mortem Examinations with Especial Reference to Medico-Legal Practice*, translated by T.P. Smith (1896).[36] By 1893, George H. Savage's fourth edition of his clinical manual on insanity, candidly observed that 'among several thousand patients in Bethlem [Hospital, London], I have only met, *post mortem*' one who displayed a particular form of brain disease.[37] Savage's well-illustrated study was exposing the major reliance on examining and dissecting the dead, as well as the frustration medical men encountered because of the limitations such examinations presented in generating tangible evidence of the causes of insanity.

The frontiers of mental science stretched across the globe. For Victoria, the earliest publication of asylum post-mortem findings was the 'Report of Post-mortem

---

[32] PROV VPRS 24/P0000/33 Inquest James S., 1856.

[33] Geelong Cemeteries Trust, Register 115159, 18 June 1856, Geelong Eastern Cemetery, UNK*XX**X (see: www.gct.net.au).

[34] PROV VPRS 24/P0000/45 Inquest Joseph L. 1857.

[35] PROV VPRS 24/P0001/43 Inquest Thomas D., 1857.

[36] John Haslam's *Observations on Madness and Melancholy* (London, 1798); A.L.J. Bayle's, 'Recherches sur les Maladies Mentales' presented to the Faculty of Medicine in Paris on 21 November 1822 and *Nouvelle Doctrine des Maladies* (Paris, 1825) regarding theories of insanity and the creation of the categorization of moral and physical forms of insanity; and Rudolph Virchow's journal *Archiv für pathologische Anatomie und Physiologie und für klinische Medizin* published in Berlin from the mid-nineteenth century onwards, and his *Post-Mortem Examinations with Especial Reference to Medico-Legal Practice*, trans. T.P. Smith (Philadelphia, 1896).

[37] George H. Savage, *Insanity and Allied Neuroses: Practical and Clinical*, 4th edn (London, 1893), p. 389.

Examinations at the Yarra Bend Asylum, 1861–62' by James T. Rudall, FRCS. that appeared in the *Australian Medical Journal* (1862).[38] Rudall (*c.*1828–1907), FRCS. [London], was a medical doctor in general practice, who conducted post-mortems for the coroner from *c.*1859 onwards, and between 1866 and 1901 he was also an examiner in Pathology and Physiology at the University of Melbourne.[39] Rudall used notes from the Yarra Bend asylum post-mortem registers – which are no longer extant – for the 21 post-mortems he had conducted on behalf of the coroner – 16 men and five women – over a 12-month period between August 1861 and August 1862.[40] Rudall was 'impressed … with the value of *facts* in morbid anatomy, as helping to the construction of a rational pathology', but he conceded that 'the circumstances under which these examinations have been made, were often by no means favourable for minute pathological investigation'.[41] He was not the only colonial doctor to hold such views. Repeated calls for the improvement of pathology facilities are a feature of nineteenth-century asylum reform in Victoria, first with Rudall in 1862, in the Royal Commission (1884–1886), and again in 1895 in the *Australian Medical Journal*.[42]

In February 1864, two years after Rudall's article, Thomas Allan, LFPSG, the Resident Surgeon at the Yarra Bend Lunatic Asylum, read his paper to the Medical Society of Victoria. His study 'On the General Paralysis of the Insane' was based on the case histories and post-mortem findings of 52 patients who died in Yarra Bend in 1863, which he then published in the *Australian Medical Journal* in March 1864.[43] The paper cited the works of John Haslam (1764–1844) the apothecary of Bethlam Hospital in London, as well as Louis-Florentin Calmeil (1798–1895), on the history of insanity. Allan provided an account of the development and variety in symptoms as he saw it based on the male patient case histories at Yarra Bend including post-mortem findings that '[furnished] no clue to the peculiar symptoms during life'.[44] He also stated that there were no

[38] James T. Rudall, 'Report of Post-mortem Examinations at the Yarra Bend Asylum, 1861–62', *Australian Medical Journal*, 7, (October 1862): pp. 252–8; I am grateful for Dr Lee-Ann Monk's research assistance regarding the *Australian Medical Journal* material used in this article.

[39] 'Rudall, James Thomas (*c.*1828–1907)', *Australian Dictionary of National Biography*, 6 (1976): pp. 70–71.

[40] My research into publications relating to post mortems discussed here, and that I have located in the *Australian Medial Journal* for the nineteenth and twentieth centuries forms the basis of a separate research project currently investigating the scientific literature relating to madness in Australia.

[41] Rudall, 'Report of Post-mortem Examinations', pp. 252–7, p. 252.

[42] See 'Conference of Medical Staffs of the Hospitals for Insane', *Australian Medical Journal*, 20 October (1895): pp. 470–72.

[43] Thomas Allan, 'On the General Paralysis of the Insane', *Australian Medical Journal*, 9 January (1864): pp. 67–78.

[44] Allan, 'On the General Paralysis', p. 77.

cases of general paralysis in women in Victoria. Rudall's and Allan's papers were just two of over 40 publications my research project has found by medical men (asylum doctors and coroners) in Victoria published in *The Australian Medical Journal* relating to the study and treatment of cases of insanity and intellectual disability between 1857 and 1900. In addition, in 1869 James T. Rudall published his English translation of Jacobus Loderwijk Conradus Schroeder van Kolk's (1797–1862) *The Pathology and Therapeutics of Mental Diseases* (Melbourne: Samuel Mullen, 1869).

Some of the colonial doctors connected with asylums in Victoria also belonged to prestigious global organizations such as the 'Medico-Psychological Association' that included members such as Daniel Hack Tuke – formerly of the Retreat at York, Henry Maudsley, a former president of the association, Professor of Medical Jurisprudence, University College, and former Medical Superintendent of the Royal Lunatic Hospital – and Dr T.S. Clouston, the editor of the *Journal of Mental Science*, and influential Physician Superintendent of the Royal Asylum, Morningside, in Edinburgh, and the first lecturer in Mental Science at the University of Edinburgh. Members of the Association from outside the United Kingdom and Ireland included medical superintendents from Jamaica, Assam in the East Indies, the Cape of Good Hope, Bombay, North America, Nova Scotia, and Australian colonies. The Australian representatives included Frederick Norton Manning, Inspector of Asylums for New South Wales, and Medical Superintendent of Gladesville, near Sydney, and Edward Paley, the Medical Superintendent of Yarra Bend Asylum in Victoria. Connections were also forged through international medical education as many Victorian asylum doctors were trained in overseas medical schools in England and Scotland, whilst some were also trained locally in Melbourne.

For example, Beattie-Smith, who was born in England, was a graduate of the University of Edinburgh, and was taught by the internationally renowned Dr Thomas Clouston. Beattie-Smith came to Victoria in 1881, worked in the Victorian asylum system at Ararat and Kew Asylums, and taught at the University of Melbourne from 1899 until 1907. In January 1888, in his capacity as the Secretary of the Psychological Medicine session at the Inter-Colonial Medical Congress of Australasia, he offered a paper on the Scottish boarding out system for asylum patients, which was adopted in the *Lunacy Amendment Act 1888* in Victoria.[45] These proceedings were discussed in D. Hack Tuke's 'Colonial Retrospect' published in the *Journal of Mental Science* in 1889, and also reported

---

[45] 'Special Correspondence, Australia', *British Medical Journal*, 1/1477 (20 April 1889): p. 912; 'Intercolonial Medical Congress, Melbourne, 1889', *British Medical Journal*, 2/1477 (22 September 1888): p. 679. See also W. Beattie Smith, 'Removal of Horny Growth From Wrist', *British Medical Journal*, 1/1015 (12 June 1880): p. 886; Bryan Gandevia, 'Neild, James Edward (1824–1906)', *Australian Dictionary of National Biography*, 5 (1974), pp. 327–39.

in the *British Medical Journal*.[46] Beattie-Smith resigned from the public asylum system and worked in private practice from 1902 until his death in 1921, and he left a substantial bequest of £1,000 to fund the annual Beattie-Smith Memorial Lecture in Mental Sciences.[47] James Neild on the other hand was born in England, but was a University of Melbourne medical graduate (1864), as well as a Fellow of the Royal College of Surgeons [London]. He conducted post-mortems for the coroner, worked as a coroner, and also lectured in Forensic Medicine at the University of Melbourne between 1865 and 1904.[48] Neild was the editor of the *Australian Medical Journal* between 1862 and 1879, and in 1888 published an article 'On the Immunity of the Insane from Physical Pain in Organic Diseases, and in Injuries which, in the Sane, are accompanied by Much Bodily Suffering'.[49] As part of one of his presentations to the Medical Society of Victoria meeting he exhibited the foreign objects, including a fork, which he had collected during post-mortem examinations of patients at Kew Asylum. As he stated 'the case is only one of some hundreds which I have made … where there was evidence of disease or injury, which in the sane would have occasioned much suffering, but, which had caused neither pain nor inconvenience' in the insane.[50] Neild's post-mortems were also widely reported in the press. An article about his 'grim trophy' – a nail in a woman's head – taken from the skull of Elizabeth Hamilton, a deceased inmate from Kew Asylum, reflected the fascination the public and medical fraternity had with tales of medical curiosity, and was reported in the Melbourne *Age* and also the Western Australian press in 1898.[51] In 1891 the *British Medical Journal* informed its readers that Neild had also been instrumental with Dr McCreery, the Medical Superintendent of Kew Asylum, in taking 'the first steps towards the formation of a Neurological Society' in Victoria, and 'McCreery informed the meeting that all the medical officers of the asylums in Victoria had notified their intention of joining'.[52] Asylum corpses were central features of scientific enquiry in both the medical literature and popular press of nineteenth-century Victoria. Yet asylum bodies could still fall into a liminal space in practice somewhere between the legislation governing the coroners, medical practitioners and anatomy, and lunacy.

46 D. Hack Tuke, 'Colonial Retrospect', *Journal of Mental Science* 35 (1889): pp. 124–9; 'Special Correspondence, Australia', *British Medical Journal*; 'Intercolonial Medical Congress, Melbourne, 1889'.

47 E. Cunningham Dax, 'Smith, William Beattie (sic) (1854–1921)', *Australian Dictionary of National Biography*, 11 (1988): pp. 664–5.

48 Gandevia, 'Neild'.

49 James Edward Neild, 'On the Immunity of the Insane from Physical Pain in Organic Diseases, and in Injuries which, in the Sane, are accompanied by Much Bodily Suffering', *Australian Medical Journal* 15 February (1888): pp. 54–8.

50 Neild, 'On the Immunity of the Insane', pp. 54–8.

51 *West Australian*, 15 December (1898): p. 7, 'A Post-Mortem Surprise'.

52 'Proposed formation of a neurological society', *British Medical Journal*, 1/1586 23 May (1891): p. 1148.

Colonial doctors kept specimens harvested from the post-mortem examinations they conducted, as these specimens provided the only comparable evidence before the development of large collections of medical slides in the late nineteenth century. This was in keeping with the British, North American and European practices. For example, Rudolph Virchow, who revolutionized post-mortem practice during the nineteenth century in Europe, had a personal museum collection of over 23,000 specimens, while the University of Melbourne Anatomy Museum in 1898 had some 5,000 specimens, of which a significant proportion had come from Professor George Britton Halford's own collection shipped with him from England.[53] The potential for the harvest of body parts through post-mortems and dissection was possible because body parts were not covered in any of Victoria's legislation. Recent work by Cressida Fforde and Helen MacDonald's work for the Parkside Asylum in South Australia and for other colonies demonstrates that some Chinese and Aboriginal asylum patients' bodies were specifically harvested for private and public museum collection both within Australasia and overseas.[54] Twenty years earlier and pre-dating the proclamation of the 1862 Anatomy Act, inquiries into Yarra Bend Asylum revealed disturbing allegations of the multiple uses made of asylum bodies between 1852 and 1860.

The public read startling accounts of what could happen to the living and dead in a lengthy series of inquiries that by 1862 culminated in a libel case before the courts, that included allegations by a Dr Carr regarding his treatment as a patient. Allegations of endemic malpractice emerged that included dubious post-mortems conducted by asylum doctors with the assistance of juries made up of asylum attendants that exonerated the asylum from any wrongdoing regarding a patient's death. Unsettling allegations emerged about what could happen to dead bodies and body parts once any post-mortem had been conducted. Samuel Wainwright, an asylum attendant, said when he went 'into the keeper's room … in the pannikin there was a man's brains, brought from the dead-house and left there'.[55] Wainwright added, 'I was looking for a pannikin to drink with, and reaching this down, smelt what it contained. [Attendant] Goode said – "It's old So-and-so's brains" (I forget whose). Dr [Robert] Bowie [the doctor in charge of the asylum] told me to bring them'.[56]

---

53 Jones, *Humanity's Mirror*, p. 73, pp. 247–8.

54 Fforde, *Collecting the Dead;* MacDonald, 'In the Interests of Science'. See also Catharine Coleborne, 'Exhibiting Madness: Material Culture and the Asylum', *Health and History*, 3/2 (2001): pp. 104–17.

55 *Votes and Proceedings of the Legislative Assembly, Session 1860–1861*, vol. 2., Appendix C. Evidence taken before the Select Committees of The Lunatic Asylum During Sessions 1858–9 and 1859–60, p. 48.

56 *Report of the Inquiry into the Management of the Yarra Bend Lunatic Asylum* (1862), p. 18; I am grateful to both Dr Lee-Ann Monk (for alerting me to this reference about the brain in the dish), and Professor Elizabeth Malcolm (for our discussion about 'the body tree').

A former patient, Mr Robert Coates, claimed that there were 'portions of bodies hanging on the trees until the stench was so sickening and offensive that we could scarcely bear the place ... There were skulls and portions of skulls lying about the garden. They were afterwards taken, and put into the dead-house, and that box was subsequently taken away'.[57] Dr Bowie countered Wainwright's account by clarifying that: 'There never was a skull lying about the grounds. There were two or three which I had collected in the deadhouse, intending to present them to the Museum; but as they found they had no room, I buried them.'[58] Collecting and exhibiting potentially significant and curious asylum items was clearly of interest to Dr Bowie as he had entered 'a mosaic table, made of colonial woods' and 'photographic views of [the] Asylum and Patients' as exhibits from Yarra Bend Asylum in the Victorian Exhibition in 1861.[59] As for the 'bodies hanging on the tree' Bowie's response to Coates' claim is more enigmatic: 'There never were any anatomical preparations of my own on the boughs of trees'.[60] We are left wondering if we should read this statement as that there were no specimens on the tree at all or rather that those specimens that were there did not belong to Dr Bowie. Collecting was a medical man's prerogative, and, some 20 years later, James Neild was to display to the Medical Society of Victoria 'the German silver dinner fork, seven and a half inches long and weighing one ounce and three quarters' that he had 'found' in 'the body of Julian Smith, aged 36' during 'a *post mortem* examination on September 23rd, 1887' at the Kew Asylum.[61] The Yarra Bend Inquiries' evidence does not offer any answer to this specific conundrum about whose medical specimens were allegedly hanging on the Yarra Bend body tree, but it did offer some insight into who else had access to asylum bodies.

More shocking than the allegations surrounding Dr Bowie and his collection of skulls, was the startling revelation that asylum attendants were 'operating' on dead bodies. Mr Robert Coates, a patient resident in Yarra Bend Asylum between 1856 and 1858 was asked 'have you ever seen *post-mortem* examinations conducted there?'[62] He replied 'I don't know what you call them, but I have seen the mangling of bodies carried on there'. Coates, recounting what attendants had told him, stated:

---

57 *Report of the Inquiry into the Management of the Yarra Bend Lunatic Asylum* (1862), p. 16; *Votes and Proceedings of the Legislative Assembly, Session 1860–1861*, vol. 2., Appendix C. Evidence taken before the Select Committees of The Lunatic Asylum During Sessions 1858–9 and 1859–60.

58 *Report of the Inquiry into the Management of the Yarra Bend Lunatic Asylum* (1862), p. 81.

59 *Catalogue of the Victorian Exhibition, 1861*, p. 264, Item 406.

60 *Report of the Inquiry into the Management of the Yarra Bend Lunatic Asylum* (1862), p. 81.

61 Neild, 'On the Immunity of the Insane', pp. 54–8.

62 *Report of the Inquiry into the Management of the Yarra Bend Lunatic Asylum* (1862), p. 16.

> Goode and Johnson were the principal persons engaged in dissecting bodies. On one occasion Goode told me that in consequence of O'Donoghue [an attendant and former patient] being drunk and mangling bodies, he should have to complain of him. On that occasion [Goode said] I locked up O'Donoghue, but he got out of the window of his room, went down to the dead-house, and commenced operating himself.[63]

Such activities predated the 1862 Anatomy Act, and attendants were not legally permitted to conduct post-mortems under either the coronial legislation or the related medical practitioners laws. Their actions were also clearly seen to flout public decency regarding appropriate ways of dealing with the dead. The Yarra Bend evidence therefore offers an insight into who may also have been preparing asylum bodies, as well as conducting these internal surgical examinations and the dismembering of asylum bodies – the asylum doctor, and some of the asylum attendants – within the asylum dead house. Nothing more was said about the matter in 1862. There was an increasing role for attendants in post-mortems though, for in 1910 strict asylum regulations were drawn up to set out the specific duties of morgue attendants that included the cutting of the scalp and sawing of the skull in preparation for the doctors to remove the brain for examination. The legislation governing anatomy, coroners and medical practitioners enacted between 1862 and 1865, however, made plain that in the eyes of the law dead bodies should only be in the hands of medically qualified men for the coronial post-mortems or for teaching anatomy at the University of Melbourne.

The public rightly feared the risk of medical malpractice, as there were well-publicized cases of colonial medical men found in possession of asylum corpses that had been subjected to dissection or, as the public understood it, butchery. This fear was further fuelled by infamous early nineteenth-century international cases such as that of Burke and Hare in Edinburgh, that linked the study of medicine with the dubious practices of obtaining bodies. The actions of medical men had to be closely scrutinized. The *Coroners Act 1865* and *Coroners Amendment Act 1869* made it the duty of the asylum in law to conduct a coronial inquest into any patient 'who dies suddenly or in prison or while detained in any lunatic asylum', but in 1870 an *Argus* editorial warned of the need for inquests into every death within the asylum, calling on readers to 'remember how well established were the reasons for inducing legislation to determine that in future an inquest should always be held upon the bodies of deceased lunatics'.[64] While the British and Australian legislation, as Helen MacDonald has shown elsewhere, was intended to safeguard a corpse from

63 Ibid., p. 16.

64 28 Vic. No. 253, Coroners Act (1865), pp. 179–80; *Argus*, 28 December 1870, p. 4 f, Editorial.

illegal dissection, medical men could navigate a course for obtaining bodies and body parts for dissection.[65]

Many members of the medical fraternity saw unclaimed bodies in publicly funded institutions as an untapped scientific or teaching resource. It is clear that medical men believed that paupers who were unable to pay for their upkeep in public institutions should, by the subjection of their bodies to dissection, give back, in kind, to science through the potential discoveries uncovered through dissection. The Medical School at the University of Melbourne had attempted in 1870, and again in 1873, without any success, to establish such a relationship with the Melbourne Benevolent Asylum, whereby unclaimed corpses could be sent to the university for the purposes of dissection under the *Medical Practitioners Act 1865*, Section IV, School of Anatomy. But on each occasion the Benevolent Asylum inmates objected and members of the Benevolent Asylum committee prevented this from happening.[66] As the English born Ephraim L. Zox, a prominent member of the Jewish community, successful businessman, and a conservative MP for East Melbourne 'observed 97 and half per cent of the inmates had, according to the return of the committee, objected to their bodies being given up for anatomical purposes' in 1870. Zox then 'suggested that the bodies of criminals who died in goals and suicides should be absolutely devoted by law to those purposes'.[67] In 1873, English-born George B. Halford, who had studied medicine in England and Scotland, and was Professor of Anatomy at the University of Melbourne, bitterly responded to Zox's suggestion that he should access bodies from asylums and prisons for teaching dissection, declaring that 'In prisons and lunatic asylums *post mortem* examinations are made, which render the bodies almost useless to us'.[68] Halford was well versed in the mortuary practices of asylums having worked at Liverpool Asylum before migrating to Australia.[69] The University of Melbourne Medical School, faced with increasing numbers of students attending dissection classes, needed to secure a supply of corpses.

This lack of specified sources of corpses in law changed in July 1875 when the Irish-born, Anglican, MP for East Bourke Boroughs, Mr George Higinbotham, introduced a Bill into the Victorian Parliament to amend the *Medical Practitioners Act 1865* so that the bodies of those who 'died in a public institution, supported wholly or in part by the State' were 'to undergo anatomical examination, unless such person had, before death, expressed a wish to the contrary, or one of his surviving relatives required the body to be interred without such examination'.[70]

---

65 Helen MacDonald, 'Procuring Corpses: The English Anatomy Inspectorate, 1842 to 1858', *Medical History*, 53/3 (2009): pp. 379–93, especially p. 380 and pp. 388–9.

66 *Argus*, 2 July 1873, p. 7b [Letter].

67 *Argus*, 27 May 1870, p. 7, 'Benevolent Asylum'.

68 *Australian Medical Journal*, June (1873): p. 170, cited in Jones, *Humanity's Mirror*, p. 82.

69 I am grateful to Ross L. Jones for this information.

70 *VPD*, Legislative Assembly, 15 July 1875, p. 715.

Mr R.H. Lock, the Member of the Legislative Assembly (MLA) for Grenville, stated the Bill 'was framed solely in the interests of medical science, and he did not see that there could be any objection to it'. Furthermore, 'the existing law provided only two means whereby bodies could be obtained for *post mortem* [that is dissection or anatomical] examinations. One was by the sanction of relatives; the other was by the express request of a person made during the illness of which he might afterwards die'.[71] Either way the clear intent was to provide the shortest possible time – 12 hours – in which families could attempt to prevent the state-sanctioned use of asylum bodies. Lock added that 'the object of the Bill was to allow the bodies of those who died while in legal custody to become subjects for *post mortem* [meaning dissection] examinations where no objection had been given'.[72]

The ensuing debate surrounded the key issues of informing the family and friends of a patient's death and ensuring that bodies were properly buried. Mr Thomas Cope (the MLA. for Normanby who was born in England and educated by a Protestant non-conformist uncle) objected because it seemed to him that bodies 'might be handed over for anatomical examination without the friends or relatives of the deceased knowing anything about the matter'. Furthermore, 'the object of the measure seemed to be merely to enable medical gentlemen to practice upon the bodies of deceased persons for their own improvement or instruction'.[73] Sir Henry John Wrixon (the Irish born M.L.A for Belfast, Victoria), disagreed and 'considered the measure most useful, inasmuch as it would enable medical men to perfect themselves in their particular study'. He entirely supported the clause enabling 'a person or their family to object to this process' and felt that 'that feeling was respected in the clause'. But Mr William Witt (M.L.A. for the Murray District) considered 'there were many individuals in public institutions who strongly objected to be subjects for *post mortem* examinations' and indicated he felt post-mortems and dissection were necessary only 'in cases where person died of obscure diseases'. He concluded that 'patients would be reluctant to enter hospitals' if their wishes were not complied with.[74]

As to the disposal of bodies after dissection, Mr R. De Bruce Johnstone (M.L.A. for Geelong West) 'had been given to understand … it was not an unusual practice to bury two bodies in the one coffin', and 'was it fair or proper that persons, when following the remains or a relative to the grave, should be called upon also to follow the remains of someone else?'[75] Assurances were sought and given about what actually became of the body after dissection, and that bodies were 'decently

71 *VPD*, Legislative Assembly, 15 March 1876, pp. 2495–6.

72 *VPD*, Legislative Assembly, 15 March 1876, p. 2496.

73 *VPD*, Legislative Assembly, 15 March 1876, p. 2496.

74 *VPD*, Legislative Assembly, 15 March 1876, p. 2496.

75 *VPD*, Legislative Assembly, 15 March 1876, pp. 2495–6.

interred in consecrated ground, or in some public burial ground in use for persons of that religious persuasion'.[76]

One issue of great concern raised by Mr Wrixon was 'that it might not be generally known such a law was in existence' and he proposed 'a copy of the Bill being hung up in every institution to which the measure applied'.[77] The members of the Legislative Assembly were in agreement with Mr John Alexander Macpherson (M.L.A. for Dundas) that publicly displaying the Act in Lunatic Asylums 'would have an injurious effect upon the patients in those establishments' and 'might produce an excitement that would be most undesirable'.[78] In a vote of 28 'Ayes' defeating '20 Noes' asylums were exempt from having to display the Act.

Therefore in April 1876, the law governing the supply of bodies to the University of Melbourne for the purposes of dissection was finally prescribed, and the *Medical Practitioners Statute 1865* was amended to authorize:

> the Chief Medical Officer the Inspector-General of Penal Establishments the Inspector of Lunatic Asylums or any resident or honorary medical officer connected with any public institution supported wholly or in part by funds from the general revenue to permit the body of any person who may die in such public institution to undergo anatomical examination, in some recognized school of medicine or public institution ... a printed copy of this Act shall be posted in the entrance hall or other conspicuous place of every such penal establishment or public institution except lunatic asylums.[79]

If the family of an asylum patient could not be contacted within 12 hours of the death, then that asylum body could legally be subjected to an 'anatomical examination'. There was the potential for delay with asylum authorities having to inform inmates' families. While this was potentially easier for those families that lived within the locale of asylums, the state's 12-hour time limit offered little comfort to those families who lived considerable distances away. Some families were aware of what might happen should a family member die, even though the Act was not publicly displayed anywhere in the asylum hall, while others would have been entirely unaware.

From the perspective of asylum practices regarding a family's refusal or consent to a post-mortem, the inquiry into the death of Philip Benison as part of the Inquiry into Kew Asylum (1876), and the discussion between asylum attendant Morrison and Benison's brother and sister-in-law in the Kew Asylum

---

76 *VPD*, Legislative Assembly, 15 March 1876, p. 2495.

77 Ibid., p. 2496.

78 Ibid., p. 2497.

79 39 Vic. 527 [7 April 1876] An Act to amend the 'Medical Practitioners Statute 1865'.

morgue is most revealing.[80] The asylum casebook recorded Benison as a single man, suffering from mania, who had lost touch with his family and friends.[81] But this was not true. Benison did have family living close by the Kew Asylum. They had seen him only days before his sudden death, and during the official inquiry in March 1876 into his death, they gave eloquent testimony about their reasons for not wanting a post-mortem to be conducted in the first instance. At the time of Benison's death, no coronial inquest or post-mortem was conducted, even though it was required under the *Coroners Act 1865* and *Coroners Amendment Act 1869*.

In the Kew Asylum, morgue attendant Morrison, who had been on good terms with the patient, asked Rebecca Benison if she was 'perfectly satisfied that he had been kindly treated?' She agreed he had. Morrison then 'said as good as that there was no necessity for a *post mortem*; why would we have him cut and butchered'.[82] Dr W.L. Watkins, the asylum medical man who had pronounced Benison dead thought Morrison did not 'have any right to say anything about it'.[83] Yet attendants regularly prepared these bodies for the medical men who conducted the post-mortems. Was Morrison simply attempting to cover the tracks of his fellow attendants – Trinnear and King – and their alleged rough treatment of the patient that emerged in newspaper reports in the weeks after Benison's death? Might the science of a post-mortem reveal foul play? Or was Morrison, who was on good terms with Benison, simply trying to avoid what he knew was the fate of other patients in the asylum morgue? Was Dr Watkins simply defending the right of medical men to conduct post-mortems and anatomical examinations under the state laws?

What emerged was that Benison's relatives had not taken the appropriate steps to prevent a post-mortem under the *Coroners Act*, which would have required them to contact the coroner Mr Candler directly.[84] Even if this request to the coroner by the family had been made, the coroner could still require a post-mortem, overriding the family's wishes, in the case of a suspicious death. Furthermore, the family were also entirely unaware of any allegations of brutality at the hands of the attendants until they appeared later in the press.[85] Therefore as Rebecca Benison had no suspicion of foul play at the time she viewed the body, she merely said 'No' to a post-mortem, believing Morrison's claim that the dark discoloration stretching from the face, down the neck to the chest on the visible portion of Benison's body exposed by the sheet was merely evidence

---

80 VPP, *Report from the Board Appointed to Inquire into Matters relating to the Kew Lunatic Asylum; together with the Minutes of Evidence and Appendix* (hereafter *Report into Kew Lunatic Asylum*) (1876), p. 749.

81 PROV VPRS 7395/P1, Unit 2, Kew Asylum Male Casebook, p. 146.

82 VPP, *Report into Kew Lunatic Asylum* (1876), p. 749 and p. 1087.

83 VPP, *Report into Kew Lunatic Asylum* (1876), p. 1087.

84 PROV VA 2840 Kew Asylum, VPRS 7398/P1, Unit 2, Kew Asylum Male Casebook, 146.

85 *Argus*, 31 March 1876, p. 7d.

of the corpse 'changing'.[86] When the Inquiry asked Rebecca Benison directly, 'Did you come in and request a *post mortem* not to be made?', her answer was clear and unequivocal: 'I did not, I was surprised to be asked such a question, because I never thought they would have asked me.'[87] Dr Watkins was quizzed on the procedures for preventing a post-mortem: 'Would you be surprised if the evidence was that no further statement was made by friends, except to an attendant by whom the post mortem was prevented? –I should be very much surprised'. But on hearing about the alleged rough handling the family then came to be in favour of a post-mortem.[88] What is clear is that Benison's body had not been internally examined prior to the family viewing in the morgue. At the time Benison's brother volunteered that 'He [Philip Benison] was as sweet as a roach when I saw him', and Mrs Benison when asked by Dr Watkins 'You did not smell his inside?' replied 'No'.[89] While a sheet carefully draped over a corpse may disguise evidence of internal examination from the unsuspecting eyes of grieving family members, the disclosure of olfactory evidence could inform a medically informed inquest of the potential evidence to the contrary, hence the specific questions levelled at the family.

The official medical scrutiny – in the form of an exhumation and post-mortem – afforded Benison had one resolute purpose, which was to exonerate the asylum authorities from any blame. On the morning of 30 March late in the summer of 1876 Benison's decomposing body was exhumed from the Old Melbourne Cemetery on the government's authority, some two months after his death and burial.[90] At precisely 2:30 that afternoon and 'in the presence of Mr Thomoson, F.R.C.S.', Dr Girdlestone, 'a skilled practitioner altogether unconnected with the asylum', began his post-mortem.[91] After the post-mortem Benison's body was committed once more to the grave. The smudge on the asylum's medical reputation was removed by the publication in the *Argus* of Dr Girdlestone's detailed notes. But the physical state of a rapidly decomposing body prevented the cause of death – of 'fatal syncope [that is failure of the heart's action], from disease of the heart' – originally attributed by Dr W.L. Watkins in a 'cell in the [asylum] hospital' from being questioned or confirmed.[92] No mention was made of the state of Benison's brain or any symptoms of insanity it may have revealed, but suffice to say that 'It is satisfactory to the Board [of Inquiry] to be able to state, as it must be to the public at large to know, that it has been proved beyond a doubt that Benison could

86 VPP, *Report into Kew Lunatic Asylum* (1876), pp. 1087–8.

87 VPP, *Report into Kew Lunatic Asylum* (1876), pp. 1087–8.

88 VPP, *Report into Kew Lunatic Asylum* (1876), p. 748.

89 VPP, *Report into Kew Lunatic Asylum* (1876), p. 749, p. 1087–9.

90 *Argus*, 30 March 1876, p. 5a Thursday.

91 VPP, *Report into Kew Lunatic Asylum* (1876), p. 749.

92 VPP, *Report into Kew Lunatic Asylum* (1876), pp. 749, 1088 and 1192, Appendix II Mr T.M. Girdlestone's Report 31 March 1876.

not have been subjected to the alleged ill-treatment shortly before his death'.[93] Benison's case reported in the press made public the feelings of the family, and also the purposes of post-mortems.[94]

Some families clearly feared that the body of a loved one was likely to be at risk of a post-mortem and dissection within the walls of the colony's asylums, even though asylums were required under law from 1876 to inform families of the death. For example, the family of Donald M., a 33-year-old poor labourer from West Geelong who was admitted to Kew Asylum in July 1900, went to great lengths, writing on two separate occasions, to secure the return of his body. Donald's family comprised his mother and three brothers – Dougald, John and Alexander – and his wife Flora and their three small children.[95] Based on the content of her notes, Flora feared something. In a postcard dated 2 November 1900 sent directly to the medical superintendent – Dr William Beattie-Smith – she made her family's plea: 'Please send word when Donald M. dies to John M. … Lower Hawthorn, also to the [Geelong] address on this card as I am most anxious to get the Remains'.[96] Clearly not convinced that her wishes were acknowledged, Flora wrote a second missive to 'Dr Smith' stating clearly and unequivocally that 'I wish you to wire me as soon as Donald M. dies as I will bring his body to Geelong'.[97] Donald's cousin was also confined in Kew Asylum, which may explain why the family was so insistent about this as they might have already had knowledge of what might happen to unclaimed bodies within the asylum.[98] Flora's wishes were written into Donald's casebook – a very unusual practice – next to the pro forma information regarding any family. Her address details were updated once and contained the note that she 'will bury privately'.[99] Her fears were justified, for one month later, in December 1900, the *Argus* reported the criticisms of the Government Pathologist, Dr Neild and Coroner Morrison levelled at Dr Beattie-Smith's dissection of James B.F.'s brain at the Kew Asylum. It is unclear how vigorously the asylum attempted to ensure contact with family members for living patients let alone the dead. Surviving asylum records are far from complete, making it impossible for us to reconstruct exactly what happened in every postmortem case. Furthermore there was little uniformity across the various asylums.

In 1880 Edward Paley, in his role as Inspector, for example, found a mixed bag when it came to post-mortem procedures in the three asylums under his purview.

---

93 VPP, *Report into Kew Lunatic Asylum* (1876), p. 749.

94 *Argus*, 31 March 1876, p. 7 d.

95 PROV VPRS7456/P0001/47 Admission Warrants, Male and Female, Kew Asylum, 1900.

96 PROV VPRS7456/P0001/47 Admission Warrants, Male and Female, Kew Asylum, 1900.

97 Admission Warrants, Male and Female, Kew Asylum, 1900.

98 Admission Warrants, Male and Female, Kew Asylum, 1900.

99 PROV VPRS 7398/P0001/Unit 16, vol. 3 Kew Asylum Male Casebook, 1899–, pp. 123 and 381.

At Beechworth Asylum, Paley observed that where 'the deaths have been from ordinary causes. A magisterial inquiry is held in every case but there is no coroner's inquest nor any post-mortem examination, unless the medical superintendent gives notice to the coroner that there appears to be necessity for an extended investigation'.[100] Paley added that 'The practice at other asylums in the colony is to have a *post mortem* examination on every deceased patient; and I think it highly desirable that this practice should be resumed here or altered elsewhere, so that there may be, at all events, uniformity of procedure throughout the department'.[101] For Paley, the consistency in procedure and the paperwork it generated was the primary concern, rather than whether or not this meant that a post-mortem had to be performed on every patient. For Ararat Asylum, Paley reported that 'the deaths have been from ordinary causes, and call for no special comment. The police magistrate (or in his occasional absence a justice of the peace) holds an inquiry into the cause of every death, a post-mortem examination being made by a medical man unconnected with the asylum; but the practice of summoning a jury has been discontinued in consequence, as Dr McCreery informs me, of instructions issued to the police magistrate by the Crown Law Department'.[102]

Public scrutiny was periodically focused on public institutions through various scandals and inquiries that involved post-mortems and dissection. Regardless of the volume of post mortems being conducted within the asylums in Victoria, major criticism was still levelled at the Lunacy Department as a result of the Royal Commission into Asylums for the Insane and Inebriate (1884–1886). The issue was the lack of training in mental sciences that medical students received within the university curriculum, resulting in them being ill prepared for the demanding nature of the work including post-mortems within the asylum. Furthermore, the Melbourne Coroner, Dr Richard Yould, was scathing about the lack of 'practical experience' gained by medical men in Victorian asylums.[103] Dr John William Springthorpe – a medical graduate of the University of Melbourne, and the first Australian graduate given membership of the Royal College of Physicians – who had also been a member of the Lunacy Department, considered that, 'it seems to me that practically no systematic series of scientific observations in lunatic asylums is conducted: and practically no original scientific investigations'.[104] Furthermore, while annual reports were published, Springthorpe added that 'I do not know of any original papers that have come from asylums, or any scientific discoveries or reforms such as might be, considering the facilities we have'.[105] From as early as

[100] VPP (1880–1881), vol. 4, Annual Report 1880, p. 32.

[101] VPP (1880–1881), vol. 4, Annual Report 1880, pp. 28 and 32.

[102] VPP (1880–1881), vol. 4, Annual Report 1880, p. 28.

[103] Royal Commission into Asylums (1886), p. xxxv.

[104] Royal Commission into Asylums (1886), p. xxxvi; Bryan Egan, 'Springthorpe, John William (1855–1933)', *Australian Dictionary of National Biography*, 12 (Melbourne, 1990): pp. 38–9.

[105] Royal Commission into Asylums (1886), p. xxxvi.

1862, however, papers were being published and presented, but the fundamental problem remained that there was an inability to find microscopic evidence because of the time constraints governing post-mortem examinations and a lack of suitable equipment and facilities. The evidence of post-mortem practice in Australia in the 1880s, offered at the Royal Commission into Asylums for the Insane and Inebriate (1884–1886) by Dr J.A. Beattie, who had worked in the Asylums in Victoria from 1879 to 1881, before moving to employment in the Health Department in New South Wales, however, clearly indicates that colonial medical men were well versed in what constituted 'microscopic investigation'.

> First, the head is opened for the purposes of psychological investigation. I speak now, of course, of a man dying of some disease of the heart, or any other viscus – this would be subjected to a *post mortem* examination on the ordinary lines – but, with regard to his cerebral symptoms, the gross weight of the brain and membranes, the condition of the arterial vessels, the blood supply, and also the ventricles and other portions of the brain, would be all investigated; the weight of the brain taken, the gross weight, and any gross lesion detected would be entered in a register, or in the surgeon's *post mortem* book. The microscopic investigation would follow, the brain being prepared, steeped in bi-chromate of potash or some other chemical agent, and subjected to microscopical examination.[106]

For Dr John W. Springthorpe, however, a medical man, who had only been very briefly employed in the asylums in Victoria, and interestingly not at the time he gave evidence to the Royal Commission, the Lunacy Department lacked direction through a suitably qualified medical man from 'home' [United Kingdom] to combat 'the comparative absence of scientific spirit in the colony'.[107] While medical opinion was divided, the findings of the Royal Commission into Asylums for the Insane and Inebriate (1884–1886) in Victoria concluded:

> We know of no better rule than that existing of holding *post mortem* examinations on the bodies of all patients who die in the hospitals for the insane, and would not have it disturbed in principle under any pretence whatsoever. The only change that it might be desirable to make would be to direct some arrangement to be made whereby the *post mortem* would be conducted in succession by all the medical men in each district willing to undertake the duty. We think that it ought to be made an invariable rule that the *post mortem* examination should be conducted by an outside medical man and by one of the asylum medical staff.[108]

The public and asylum interests were represented respectively. The asylum medical officer should:

---

106 Royal Commission into Asylums (1886), p. 561.

107 Royal Commission into Asylums (1886), p. xxxvi.

108 Royal Commission into Asylums (1886), p. xiv.

> make a careful examination of the brain and nervous system, and, indeed, of the whole body, for scientific purposes, entering the result of his observations in a book kept for the purpose. The extent of the microscopical examination would of course be directed by the specialist [described as an alienist from 'home'] whose engagement we suggest elsewhere.[109]

Very rarely does the view from within the colonial Victorian asylum mortuary appear in the historical record in Victoria, but in addition to Benison's case in the Kew Inquiry (1876), the state of the Ararat Morgue was commented upon by an Official Visitor to the Asylum in June 1879. Conditions were of such concern to the Justice of the Peace, J Tobin that he wrote to J Grant at the Law Office:

> I beg to bring under your notice the totally inadequate and disgraceful building used as a Morgue at this Lunatic Asylum. It is only fit for a pig stye and I am sure that if the matter is brought under your notice that you will take measure [*sic*] to have a suitable House erected for [the illegible] purpose.[110]

"What had happened to the bodies in the morgue that made Tobin decide to act? What we do know is that between January and June 1879, 18 people – two women and 16 men – had died within the asylum and their bodies were transferred to the asylum morgue and subjected to post-mortems. What actually happened to those bodies and body parts is unrecorded, but for Tobin the condition of the morgue was clearly of a disturbing nature. Neatly glancing over the issue of Tobin's concerns about the state of the morgue, Paley instead focused on Tobin's conflicts of interest. Tobin was a JP who could conduct inquests in the absence of the coroner, a contractor to the asylum, and also an Official Visitor. In order for Tobin to remain an Official Visitor, he was required to resign his contract." Nothing more was said about either the conditions in the morgue, nor who was contracted to build the new morgue.[111] Plans for a morgue had already been drawn up, but a lack of funds had prevented its construction (see Figure 4.2). Tobin's letter appears to have got momentum going regarding the construction of the new purpose-built dead house in the 1880s.[112]

---

[109] Royal Commission into Asylums (1886), p. xiv.

[110] PROV, VA 475 Chief Secretary's Department, VPRS 3991/P Inward Registered Correspondence II, Unit 1080, File 1879/Q5416, letter, J P Tobin to J M Grant, 14 June 1879. My thanks to Dr Lee-Ann Monk for her expertise with the Chief Secretary's correspondence files in locating this material.

[111] PROV, VPRS 3991/P Inward Registered Correspondence II, Unit 1080, File 1879/Q5416, letter, J P Tobin to J M Grant, 14 June 1879.

[112] Allom Lovell and Associates Pty Ltd, *Aradale Ararat Conservation Analysis Prepared for Department of Treasury and Finance Victorian Government Property Group* (Melbourne, 1996), pp. 59–60.

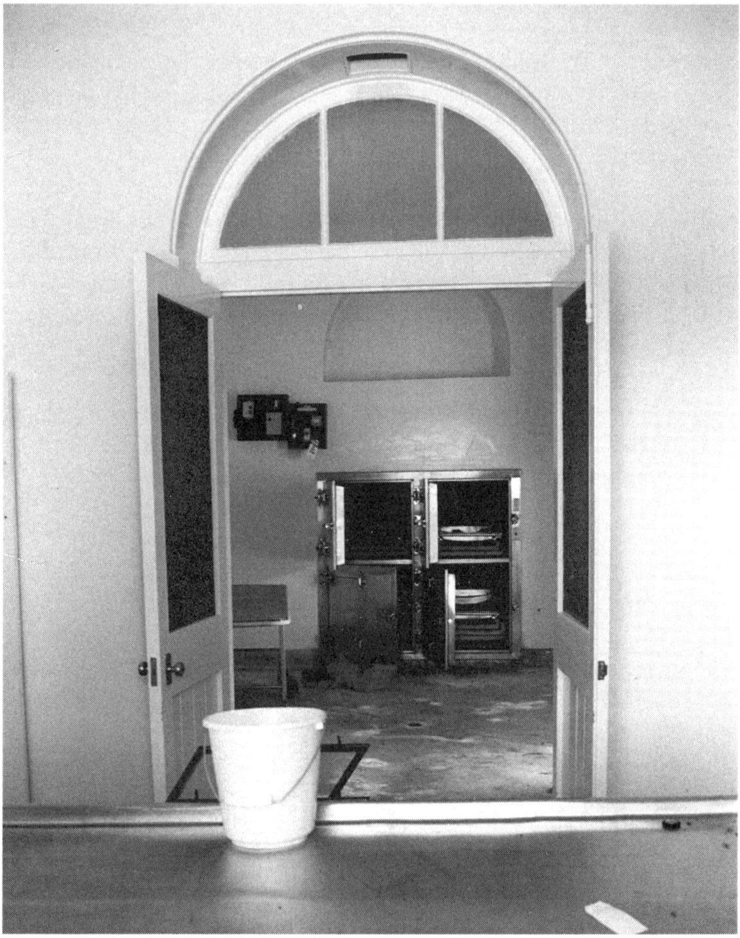

Figure 4.2 Photograph of the interior of the *c.*1881 Ararat Asylum Morgue (regional Victoria) showing the modern dissection table and refrigerated cadaver store

Source: Photograph by Peter Lovell of Lovell Chen Architects & Heritage Consultants, 1996. Used by permission.

The asylum morgue built in 1868, between the *Coroners Act 1865* and its amendment in 1869, survives at Beechworth Asylum.[113] The nineteenth-century morgue for Kew Asylum has not survived.

[113] Allom Lovell and Associates Pty Ltd, *Mayday Hills Hospital Beechworth Conservation Analysis Prepared for Victorian Government Department of Finance Assets Management* (Melbourne, 1994), pp. 92–5.

Conclusion

The *Argus* newspaper's report of the fate of James B.F.'s body and brain at the hands of Dr Beattie-Smith on the Kew Asylum mortuary table only 96 hours after his admission by family and friends in 1900, and the public criticism of Beattie-Smith's actions by Dr Neild, Government Pathologist, and Coroner Morrison, alerted the public once more to the dark spectre of the actual uses of asylum bodies. Within the medical fraternity, asylum doctors were not always held in high regard and the pursuit of scientific evidence to prove the physical manifestations of madness was one positive to be gained from what many medical men considered a fruitless appointment.[114] Nineteenth-century asylums were increasingly seen to be self-governing and self-sufficient institutions, and amongst the service buildings that included the kitchen, scullery, stores, boilers, engine houses, administration, laundry and washhouses, was the mortuary. The journey from life to death for some unclaimed asylum patients' bodies from 1876 onwards involved the body being legally removed from the ward or hospital to the morgue where it was subjected to a post-mortem and anatomical examination before being committed to a grave. The statistical evidence gathered from the post-mortem examination of brains and dissections then filled annual reports and medical publications between the 1860s and the 1890s, and, some physical evidence quite probably filled specimen jars, the display of skeletal remains, and medical slides.

For the scientific study of insanity therefore, asylum brains and bodies were considered essential elements in attempting to answer the pressing medical questions regarding the physical traces and manifestations of madness. Asylum doctors were well placed to do such research under the nineteenth-century *Coroners Acts* and the *Anatomy and Medical Practitioners Acts*. From the 1850s, colonial Victoria's medical progress was demonstrated by the changing terminology found in the State Inquest Records that used such terms as 'brain disease', 'Ramollissement du Cerveau', and 'softening of the brain' tissue as causes of death for asylum and prisoner lunatics in the state.[115] By the 1870s sub-categories under the heading 'cranial and spinal' causes of death appeared. The statistical use of the findings of pathology championed the scientific nature and potential progress of such research. In Victoria, post-mortems were a feature of the asylum casebook records, discharge registers and inquests from the 1850s onwards until the introduction of the Pathology Register system at the end of the nineteenth century.

The case study evidence discussed here brings in the roles and opinions of the family, and in one case their dealings with asylum attendants and doctors regarding their discussions, about whether or not a patient's body should be 'cut

---

114 Scull, *The Most Solitary of Affiliations*, p. 263, footnote 145.

115 PROV VPRS 24/P0000/33 Inquest James S., 1856; PROV VPRS24/P0000/43 Inquest Thomas D., 1857; PROV VPRS 24/P0000/45 Inquest Joseph L., 1857.

and butchered' in the morgue. The case of Philip Benison also demonstrates that families who did not automatically want a post-mortem conducted, might have reconsidered their decision if they had been made aware of any allegations of brutality that emerged later in the press. If they had been fully aware of the circumstances surrounding Benison's death then they indicated they would have considered making a legitimate call to the powers of science in the form of a post-mortem to determine whether the asylum had been ultimately responsible for this patient's death. Equally, public inquiries and coronial post-mortems could be used as scientific evidence to exonerate the asylum staff and administration from blame. This chapter has shown how, by analysing the evidence found in the interconnecting legislation, newspapers reports, and where possible family accounts, asylum bodies were subjected to post-mortems and anatomical examinations throughout the nineteenth century. My purpose in reconstructing this practice has been to piece together some of the missing parts that make up a history of what happened to bodies in nineteenth-century asylums in Victoria, allowing me to fill the gap in the historiography regarding a prevalent pathology practice that sought to detect in the brains and bodies of diseased patients evidence of madness within the colonial asylum.

Finally, in 1901, a year after the James B.F.'s medically interfered-with post-mortem case demonstrated the tug of laws over an asylum corpse, the report for Lunacy Reform in Victoria, lamented that 'the valuable material of the post-mortems and entries in the case books' continued to be 'wasted, and no one except the medical officer of the Asylum profits by the large and varied experiences'. The problem lay in the limitations of 'the knowledge of the general [medical] practitioner' which 'is mainly of a scholastic character, and the appointee to a medical post in the asylums comes to his work nearly always thus sparsely equipped'. What was needed were 'clinical clerks attached to each asylum selected from the University ranks, and better methods in the asylums of facilitating the practical study of mental diseases', and that 'some of the positions should be open to women'.[116] But these were the first of many calls for reform that would revolutionize pathology in mental health during the next 60 years of the twentieth century. That revolution would build on the body of nineteenth-century evidence of post-mortem and dissection. These practices were shaped by the laws of the state, and the local and international medical men who implemented them in the asylum morgues, often in their dual roles on behalf of the coroner, and as teaching staff of the University of Melbourne. Asylum bodies were valuable sources of evidence in the evolution of the study of mental science in nineteenth-century Victoria.

[116] VPP (1901), Lunacy System in Victoria, p. 14.

Bibliography

Manuscript Sources

Geelong Cemeteries Trust, Victoria Register 115159.
Victorian Public Record Office VPRS 24.
Victorian Public Record Office VPRS 2840.
Victorian Public Record Office VPRS 3991.
Victorian Public Record Office VPRS 7395.
Victorian Public Record Office VPRS 7398.
Victorian Public Record Office VPRS 7456.
Victorian Public Record Office VPRS 7681.

Printed Primary Sources

Allan, Thomas 'On the General Paralysis of the Insane', *Australian Medical Journal*, 9 January (1864): pp. 67–78.

Archiv für pathologische Anatomie und Physiologie und für klinische Medizin 1850–1900.

Australian Medical Journal 1862–1900.

Argus 1870–1900.

Bayle, A.L.J., *Nouvelle Doctrine des Maladies* (Paris, 1825).

British Medical Journal 1880–1900.

Catalogue of the Victorian Exhibition, 1861: With Prefatory Essays, Indicating the Progress, Resources, and Physical Characteristics of the Colony, by W.H. Archer, Ferd. Mueller, E. Brough Smyth, Professor Neumayer, Fred. McCoy, A.R.C. Selwyn, and W.M. Birkmyre (Melbourne, 1861).

Clouston, Thomas, 'The Medical Treatment of Insanity', *Journal of Mental Science*, 16 (1870): pp. 24–30.

'Conference of Medical Staffs of the Hospitals for Insane', *Australian Medical Journal*, 20 October (1895), pp. 470–72

Haslam, J., *Observations on Madness and Melancholy* (London, 1798).

'Intercolonial Medical Congress, Melbourne, 1889', *British Medical Journal*, 2/1477 (22 September 1888): p. 679.

Journal of Mental Science 1870–1900.

Neild, James Edward, 'On the Immunity of the Insane from Physical Pain in Organic Diseases, and in Injuries which, in the Sane, are accompanied by Much Bodily Suffering', *Australian Medical Journal* (15 February 1888): p. 54–8.

'Proposed Formation of a Neurological Society', *British Medical Journal*, 1/1586 (23 May 1891): 1148

A Report of the Inquiry into the Management of Yarra Bend Lunatic Asylum [1858–59], as described in the Nine Days' Trial of the Action for Libel Bowie v. Wilson. Held in the Supreme Court, Melbourne, from Wednesday, May 28, to Friday, June 6, 1862 (Melbourne, 1862).

Report of The Board Appointed to Inquire into Matters Relating to the Kew Lunatic Asylum, Taken Together with the Minutes of Evidence and Appendix (Melbourne, 1876).

Royal Commission into Asylums for the Insane and Inebriate Report (Melbourne, 1886).

Rudall, James T., 'Report of Post-mortem Examinations at the Yarra Bend Asylum, 1861–62', *Australian Medical Journal*, 7, (October 1862): pp. 252–8.

Savage, George H., *Insanity and Allied Neuroses: Practical and Clinical*, 4th edn (London, 1893).

Smith, William Beattie, 'Removal Of Horny Growth From Wrist', *British Medical Journal*, 1/1015 (12 June 1880): p. 886.

'Special Correspondence, Australia', *British Medical Journal*, 1/1477 (20 April 1889): p. 912.

Statutes of the State of New South Wales 1838–1845.

Statutes of the State of Victoria 1854–1900.

Tuke, D. Hack, 'Colonial Retrospect', *Journal of Mental Science* 35 (1889): pp. 124–9

The Western Australian 1898.

Victorian Parliamentary Debates 1860–1900.

Victorian Parliamentary Papers 1852–1901.

Virchow, Rudolph, *Post-Mortem Examinations with Especial Reference to MedicoLegal Practice*, trans. T.P. Smith (Philadelphia, 1896).

Votes and Proceedings of the Legislative Assembly of the Parliament of Victoria 1860–1861.

Secondary Sources

Allom Lovell and Associates Pty Ltd, *Mayday Hills Hospital Beechworth Conservation Analysis Prepared for Victorian Government Department of Finance Assets Management* (Melbourne: Allom Lovell and Associates Pty Ltd, 1994).

Allom Lovell and Associates Pty Ltd, *Aradale Ararat Conservation Analysis Prepared for Department of Treasury and Finance Victorian Government Property Group* (Melbourne: Allom Lovell and Associates Pty Ltd, 1996).

Andrews, Jonathan, 'Case Notes, Case Histories, and the Patient's Experience of Insanity at Gartnavel Royal Asylum, Glasgow, in the Nineteenth Century', *Social History of Medicine*, 11/2 (1998): pp. 255–81.

Coleborne, Catharine, 'Exhibiting Madness: Material Culture and the Asylum', *Health and History*, 3/2 (2001): pp. 104–17.

Coleborne, Catharine, 'Making "Mad" Populations in Settler Colonies: The Work of Law and Medicine in the Creation of the Colonial Asylum', in Diane Kirkby and Catharine Coleborne (eds), *Law, History, Colonialism: The Reach of Empire* (Manchester: Manchester University Press, 2001), pp. 106–22.

Coleborne, Catharine, 'Families, Insanity and the Psychiatric Institution in Australia and New Zealand, 1860–1914', *Health and History*, 11/1 (2009): pp. 65–82.

Coleborne, Catharine, *'Madness' in the Family: Insanity, Institutions and the Australasian Colonial World, 1860s–1914* (London and New York: Palgrave, 2010).

Coleborne, Catharine and MacKinnon, Dolly (eds), *'Madness in Australia': Histories, Heritage and the Asylum* (St. Lucia, Queensland: Queensland University Press, 2003).

Fforde, Cressida, *Collecting the Dead: Archaeology and the Reburial Issue* (London: Duckworth, 2004).

Finnane, Mark, 'Asylums, Families and the State', *History Workshop*, 20/1 (1985): pp. 134–48.

Garton, Stephen, *Medicine and Madness: A Social History of Insanity in New South Wales, 1880–1940* (Kensington, New South Wales: University of New South Wales Press, 1988).

Hurren, Elizabeth, 'A Pauper Dead-House: The Expansion of the Cambridge Anatomical Teaching School under the late-Victorian Poor Law, 1870–1914', *Medical History*, 48/1 (2004): pp. 69–94.

Jones, Ross L., *Humanity's Mirror: 150 Years of Anatomy in Melbourne* (South Yarra, Victoria: Haddington Press, 2007).

Lewis, Milton, *Thorns on the Rose: The History of Sexually Transmitted Diseases in Australia in International Perspective* (Canberra: Australian Government Publishing Service, 1998).

MacDonald, Helen, *Human Remains: Episodes in Human Dissection* (Carlton, Victoria: Melbourne University Press, 2005).

MacDonald, Helen, *Human Remains: Dissection and its Histories* (New Haven: Yale University Press, 2006).

MacDonald, Helen, 'A Scandalous Act: Regulating Anatomy in a British Settler Colony, Tasmania 1869', *Social History of Medicine*, 20/1 (2007): pp. 39–56.

MacDonald, Helen, 'The Anatomy Inspector and the Government Corpse', *History Australia*, 6/2 (2009): 40.1–40.17.

MacDonald, Helen, 'Procuring Corpses: The English Anatomy Inspectorate, 1842 to 1858', *Medical History*, 53/3 (2009): pp. 379–93.

MacDonald, Helen, 'In the Interests of Science: Gathering Corpses from Lunatic Asylums', in Catharine Coleborne and Dolly MacKinnon (eds), *Exhibiting Madness in Museums: Remembering Psychiatry through Collections and Display* (New York: Routledge, 2011), pp. 139–60.

Scull, Andrew, *The Most Solitary of Afflictions: Madness and Society in Britain 1700–1900* (New Haven and London: Yale University Press, 1993).

White, K.N., 'Negotiating Science and Liberalism: Medicine in Nineteenth-Century South Australia', *Journal of Medical History*, 43/2 (1999): pp. 173–91.

Chapter 5
A Judicious Collector: Edward Charles Stirling and the Procurement of Aboriginal Bodily Remains in South Australia, *c*.1880–1912

Paul Turnbull

Over the past decade, a number of historians of late nineteenth- and early twentieth-century Australia have shown that, arguably more than in comparable settler societies, material and moral progress to nationhood was envisaged as dependent on ensuring the biological integrity and potential of an evolutionarily advanced white social body.[1] They have also shown how, within Australian settler culture, the concept of race and belief in the fundamentality of safeguarding white racial purity gained much of their existential concreteness through the experiences of the continent's Indigenous inhabitants being interpreted as an object lesson on the dreadful consequences of racial decay.

What is more, Warwick Anderson has shown how scientists and doctors located in both urban and tropical Australia between 1880 and 1930 prominently intervened in contemporary debates on immigration policy, settler health in the tropics, national hygiene and child health, so infusing hopes and fears for the future of white Australia with ideas and arguments generated by scientific investigations of Aboriginal racial distinctiveness and evolutionary genealogy.[2] Anderson has

---

1 See especially Russell McGregor, *Imagined Destinies: Aboriginal Australians and the Doomed Race Theory, 1880–1939* (Melbourne, 1997); Warwick Anderson, *The Cultivation of Whiteness: Science, Health and Racial Destiny in Australia* (Melbourne, 2002); Alison Bashford, *Imperial Hygiene: A Critical History of Colonialism, Nationalism and Public Health* (London, 2004); and Marilyn Lake and Henry Reynolds, *Drawing the Global Colour Line: White Men's Countries and the Question of Racial Equality* (Melbourne, 2008).

2 Anderson, *The Cultivation of Whiteness*. To date Anderson has largely focused on the anthropological activities of scientists active in Australia during the 1920s and 1930s, highlighting in particular their construal of Aboriginal people as archaic Caucasians and the destabilizing consequences this had for notions of white racial destiny that had progressively gained credence from the mid-nineteenth century onwards. He has been less concerned to explore the activities, ideas and arguments of locally-based medico-scientific investigators of Aboriginal ancestry and racial inheritance predating 1900.

suggested these men can be fairly characterized as 'out of the way intellectuals' who rarely referred 'to allegedly "key" figures and concepts in racial thought'. As to the science they produced, Anderson suggests that it amounted to little more than 'mid-level, mundane theorizing [of a kind] that commonly occurs when one does science or practices medicine in a society a long way from Europe'.[3]

My concern in this chapter is to examine the collecting of Aboriginal bodily remains and the associated anthropological interests of one such scientist: Edward Charles Stirling (1848–1919), the Cambridge-educated professor of physiology at the University of Adelaide and director of the South Australian Museum from 1884 to 1912.

From the early 1890s, Edward Stirling extended the collecting ambitions of the South Australian Museum to acquiring Aboriginal crania and other skeletal remains. In doing so he became one of a number of Australian-based medico-scientific researchers who, by the turn of the twentieth century, had given Aboriginal skeletal remains, as Philip Jones has well described it, 'the status of circulating [intellectual] capital among museums and universities, similar to that accrued by particular natural history species and fossils during the nineteenth century'.[4]

Beneficiaries of Stirling's efforts in securing Aboriginal remains included leading metropolitan British anatomists of the turn of the twentieth century, who were interested in mapping the evolutionary genealogy of the human species. However, Stirling's principal ambition was to build the future scientific capabilities of the South Australian Museum. By the early 1920s, the legacies of his long directorship were widely seen to include the creation of one of the world's most anthropologically significant repositories of human crania, numbering around 800 specimens.[5]

In what follows, I attempt to place Stirling's collecting of Aboriginal bodily remains in the context of contemporary evolutionary science. For what appears in his writings, surviving correspondence and records of the South Australian Museum suggests that the impetus for Stirling's encouraging the collecting of Aboriginal remains by the museum was his coming to see certain morphological peculiarities in Aboriginal bones of potentially important significance in reconstructing humanity's evolutionary past.

Admittedly, what Stirling wrote about these peculiarities tends to add weight to Anderson's assessment of Australian-based medico-scientific figures active prior to the 1920s. Even so, Stirling's activities and ideas still merit closer scrutiny. For one thing, it seems clear that he was not so constrained by an intellectual tyranny of distance in conversing with metropolitan scientific peers

---

[3] Ibid., p. 3.

[4] Philip Jones, 'A Box of Things': Ethnographic Collectors and the South Australian Museum, 1830s–1930s. Unpublished PhD Thesis, University of Adelaide, 1997, p. 276.

[5] Aleš Hrdlička, 'Catalogue of Human Crania in the United States National Museum Collections', *Proceedings of the United States National Museum*, 71 (1928): pp. 4–82.

as we might imagine. But more importantly, even though Stirling can be seen to have been a largely derivative thinker, who rehearsed ideas and arguments having wide credence within contemporary metropolitan scientific circles, how he interpreted and represented these ideas and arguments provides useful insights into how racialized perceptions of Aboriginality gained cognitive strength within late nineteenth- and early twentieth-century Australian settler society through scientific collecting and interpretation of Indigenous bodily remains. Indeed, as I show in this chapter, Stirling's efforts through the 1890s, to enlist police, other government officials and pastoralists in remote regions of central and northern Australia in procuring remains, reveal that disturbingly symbiotic connections existed between the racialized construal of Aboriginality, the collecting of remains and frontier violence. Stirling's correspondence with these collectors moreover contains a wealth of observation and utterance that throw into question the adequacy of recent revisionist claims that frontier violence was never a systematic phenomenon. It attests to how profoundly race determined the social and ontological categories structuring settler reactions to Aboriginal people.[6]

Evolution in the Adelaide Museum

While Stirling began encouraging the collecting of Aboriginal bodily remains in a methodical fashion in the early 1890s, his motivation is best understood by first taking account of the growing significance of evolutionary biology in the life of the museum over the previous two decades.

From the mid-1870s, close and mutually supportive relations were forged between museum staff and leading scientific personnel of the new University of Adelaide. Ralph Tate (1840–1901) was an influential figure in aligning the museum and university's scientific aspirations. An energetic researcher in various fields of geology and zoology, Tate was appointed to the new university's foundational chair in natural science in 1875.[7] He was to champion the creation within the museum of collections specifically designed to foster research into Australia's natural history. Tate was also instrumental in the university being granted two seats on the Museum and Library Board in 1879.

Tate's vision of harmonious co-evolution of the museum and university teaching and research was shared by Edward Stirling (1848–1919). Born in Strathalbyn in South Australia, Stirling was a talented young surgeon and lecturer in physiology who began teaching at the University of Adelaide soon after settling

[6] See especially Keith Windshuttle, *The Fabrication of Aboriginal History, Volume One: Van Diemen's Land 1803–1847* (Paddington, NSW, 2002).

[7] A.R. Alderman, 'Tate, Ralph (1840–1901)', *Australian Dictionary of Biography, Volume 6* (Melbourne, 1976), pp. 243–4.

permanently in the colony in 1881.[8] By the end of that year, Stirling was one of the university's nominees to the Museum and Library Board. By 1884, he had been appointed to the directorship of the museum, which he was to hold in an honorary capacity for the first 11 years of a near 40-year tenure, during which he was greatly to shape the evolution of the museum's collecting ambitions.

One of Stirling's first actions on his appointment to the Museum and Library Board was to join with Tate in persuading fellow board members that, as the teaching of medicine as well as natural science would soon commence at the university, the museum should follow the lead of those of its British and European counterparts, similarly co-located with universities in creating series of teaching specimens, comprising 'skulls, articulated skeletons and dissections illustrating the most important classes of animals, which shall effect facilities for study of students of zoology and comparative anatomy'.

On the resignation in 1882 of Frederick Waterhouse, the museum's first and long-serving curator, Tate and Stirling proved influential voices in securing the appointment of Johann Wilhelm Haacke (1855–1912) as Waterhouse's successor. Haacke was an experienced curator abreast of the latest developments in European museology, who had begun his scientific career assisting Ernst Haeckel (1834–1919), the great German biologist and champion of Darwin.[9]

With Tate and Stirling's backing, Haacke began putting the museum's collecting on a firmer, more systematic scientific basis. He sought to implement the latest techniques for field preservation and subsequent wet and dry curation of natural history specimens. During Waterhouse's years as curator, field collectors had been contracted when funds allowed, usually on the basis of payment for the number and value of specimens they secured. The Museum and Library Board were persuaded by Haacke to employ a full-time field collector and to expand the number of staff skilled in preserving and cataloguing of specimens.

However, Haacke knew that things had not changed since the days of his predecessor in one important respect. The museum's financial health continued to depend greatly on the colony's political elite being convinced of the usefulness of its collections in fostering South Australia's economic and social development. Hence one of Haacke's first recommendations as curator to the Museum and Library Board was that the museum's 'mineralogical and geological collections be made as complete as it seems desirable before any large additions are made to the zoological and ethnological collections'. Ethnological collecting was not ignored. Rather, Haacke, much as Waterhouse had done, sought donations of artefacts, purchasing individual items when the price was modest or the item so ethnologically interesting as to justify its purchase. He also added to the museum's ethnological holdings by exchanging Indigenous

---

8 Hans Mincham, 'Stirling, Sir Edward Charles (1848–1919)', *Australian Dictionary of Biography, Volume 6* (Melbourne, 1976), pp. 200–201.

9 Report on the Progress of the Museum … May 1882, State Records of South Australia [hereafter SRSA] GRG 19/168/1881–1888.

South Australian artefacts, sent for display at international expositions, with other museums.[10]

Even so, Haacke, Tate and Stirling were conscious that ethnological collecting was becoming imbued with new intellectual significance due to the rapid and widespread assent Darwin's theory of evolution had gained in European medico-scientific circles since the early 1860s. All three were keenly aware that new connections were being drawn between bodily morphology and forms of material culture. Tate had long been interested in what bodily and artefactual traces of prehistoric life might reveal about humanity's deep past. He was a member of the London Anthropological Society, which had been co-founded in 1863 by James Hunt, an admirer of the controversial racial anatomist Robert Knox.[11] In the summer of 1865, Tate had joined Hunt in superintending the excavation of ancient grave mounds on the Shetland island of Unst.[12] The outcomes of this investigation were discussed at a meeting of the Anthropological Society later that year, prompting discussion on the resemblance between stone implements in recent finds in the Loire district of France, with Tate suggesting that further investigation of the morphology of a skull unearthed in one mound might shed light on the origins of these ancient inhabitants of the Shetland isles.

As Tate's involvement in the life of the South Australian Museum grew, he sought the help of a growing circle of friends and scientific colleagues in enriching the museum's ethnological collections, readily acting as a go-between for those he persuaded to sell 'articles of native industry' at mutually agreeable prices.[13] Quite likely, Tate saw the value of these artefacts to be at least in part what they might contribute to knowledge of human prehistory, in view of archeological discoveries in central and western Europe since the late 1850s of morphologically variant human skeletal remains amidst distinctive forms of material culture. Certainly, he was aware of the interest that Aboriginal skulls and skeletal material were generating in metropolitan European medico-scientific communities. For by the early 1880s, the museum was receiving requests from leading European museums

---

10 In February 1882, for example, Haacke reported that artefacts exhibited in Melbourne had been exchanged for a range of Melanesian and Maori objects with Sydney's Australian Museum (SRSA GRG 19/168/1881–1888).

11 On Hunt and key members of the London Anthropological Society's racial thought and involvement in the procurement and investigation of Indigenous Australian remains, see Paul Turnbull, 'British Anthropological Thought in Colonial Practice: the Appropriation of Indigenous Australian Bodies, 1860–1880', in Bronwen Douglas and Chris Ballard (eds), *Foreign Bodies: Oceania and the Science of Race 1750–1940* (Canberra, 2008), pp. 205–28.

12 James Hunt and Ralph Tate, 'On the Archaic Anthropological of the Zetland Isles …', *Journal of the Anthropological Society of London*, 4 (1866): pp. xv–xviii.

13 SRSA GRG 19/424/1882.

and other scientific institutions for help in procuring 'skulls of natives in exchange for other objects'.[14]

Haacke was likewise greatly interested in the implications of evolutionary theory for reconstructing the course of human natural history. Despite recommending to the museum's governing board that priority be given to ensuring the comprehensiveness of its geological and mineral collections, he began purchasing anthropoid ape specimens soon after being confirmed in his position as curator. Moreover, within his 'geological' purchases of comparative fossil specimens were casts of ancient human remains, such as the Neanderthal skull and the 'Guadeloupe skeleton' – mineralized post-cranial remains acquired by the British Museum that were found encased in what was thought to be extremely ancient limestone strata.[15] By late 1882, Haacke had begun inquiring of settlers and government officials interacting with Aboriginal peoples in remoter parts of the colony and the Northern Territory as to the possibilities of securing not only Aboriginal artefacts, but skulls and skeletons.

After Haacke's resignation in 1884, Stirling assumed the directorship of the museum. He and Tate similarly found themselves needing to be strategic in their ethnological purchasing. Various items that would have enhanced the capacity of the museum to educate the university's students and the colonial public as to advances in knowledge of human evolutionary history could not be purchased. In February 1885, for example, they declined the offer of Robert von Schlagintweit, Professor of Geography at the University of Giessen, to sell the museum copies of 50 life-size gypsum facial castes of 'characteristic types of races' that von Schlagintweit and two of his brothers had obtained when travelling in Asia and undertaking geological surveys for the British East India Company in the mid-1850s.[16] In April the following year, August Saupe, a local sculptor whom Haacke had previously commissioned to produce hand-coloured casts of fish specimens, approached the Museum offering the originals of 'two life size figures of aboriginal natives belonging to the Macleay Tribe … executed … in plaster of Paris and painted in their natural colour' that he had created for the South Australian exhibit at the 1886 London Colonial Exhibition.[17] But the asking price of 55 guineas was beyond the museum's means. In November that same year, Stirling and Tate were forced to turn down the offer of James White (1861–1918), a young English sculptor newly

[14] One of the earliest of such requests was from Ferdinand von Hochsteller (1829–1884), director of Vienna's Imperial Natural History Museum (Hochsteller to Waterhouse, 24 February 1880, SRSA GRG 19/168/1881–1888).

[15] Report of the Progress of the Museum, July 1881, SRSA GRG 19/168/1881–1888.

[16] SRSA GRG 19/424/1885.

[17] SRSA GRG 19/424/1886. As yet there is no comprehensive study of the creation of plaster facial casts and wax models derived from casts of Aboriginal people's remains for colonial museums and exhibitions; but see Jane Lydon's discussion of Charles Summers's life-cast busts of Coranderrk Aborigines, created for the Intercolonial Exhibition of 1866, in *Eye Contact: Photographing Indigenous Australians* (Durham, NC, 2005).

arrived in Sydney, to sell them a group of wax models derived from 'plaster casts of living Aborigines … finished, with the skin marking carefully preserved, & in various attitudes, illustrating the habits of the natives'.[18] White claimed to have secured orders from other museums, but needed more to enable him to create and sell the figures at a mutually attractive price. Funds could not be spared, though on Tate's suggestion, White was informed the museum would 'bear his offer in mind should they be able to avail themselves of it in future'.[19] Similarly, offers of prehistoric European artifacts were refused as being 'somewhat outside the present scope of the Museum'.[20]

Stirling and Tate were nonetheless successful in securing other items that would prove valuable in illustrating advances in evolutionary science. They acquired higher primate skeletons through Edward Gerrard (1810–1910), then one of London's leading taxidermists and dealers in natural history specimens, who specialized in the sale of comparative osteological specimens to museums in Europe, North American and British settler colonies.[21] Gerrard, from whom the anti-Darwinian director of the Melbourne Museum, Frederick McCoy (1821–1899), had purchased three gorilla skins and skeletons in 1865,[22] was aware he was dealing in specimens much sought after by colonial museums, regardless of what weight they gave Darwin's ideas. Accordingly, the prices Gerrard charged were high. Moreover, inflating the prices he could ask for chimpanzee and gorilla specimens by the later 1880s was the growing use of firearms by peoples living in the vicinity of their habitats to shoot them for food. Still, Stirling was able to take receipt of both chimpanzee and gorilla skeletons and skins due to Gerrard being willing to accept Australian fauna as part payment, though not without complaining of the difficulty of finding buyers for them.[23] Stirling also had luck in obtaining by 1886 specimens of proboscis monkey and three orang-utan skeletons through the British government resident of Sarawak.[24]

By the late 1880s Stirling and Tate were in a stronger position to convince the Museum and Library Board to support their engaging in more extensive and systematic ethnological collecting. In late 1888, Stirling had sent Amandus Zietz (1840–1921), the Museum's chief preparator, to Sydney and Melbourne's museums, ostensibly to arrange for more regular exchanges of specimens. Yet Zietz was clearly tasked with also assessing the strengths and weaknesses of their

---

18 SRSA GRG19/424/1886.

19 Ibid.

20 Ibid.

21 SRSA GRG 19/424/1882; also GRG19/424/1886. On Gerard's career, see P.A. Morris, *Edward Gerrard & Sons: A Taxidermy Memoir* (Ascot, 2004).

22 See Barry Butcher, 'Gorilla Warfare in Melbourne: Halford, Huxley and Man's Place in Nature', in R.W. Home (ed.), *Australian Science in the Making* (Cambridge, 1988), pp. 153–69.

23 SRSA GRG19/424/1886.

24 Ibid.

collections, and was to report that in both institutions holdings of both Australian fauna and ethnology were far weaker than expected. The ethnological collection of Sydney's Australian Museum he found 'very poor'.[25] Despite the efforts of its curator, Edward Pierson Ramsay, it had proved impossible to replace the many Australian artefacts among the more than 3,000 items displayed within the museum's Garden Palace that had been destroyed by fire in September 1882.[26]

In Melbourne, Zietz judged what he saw of its museum's ethnological collection as at best 'fair' and neither properly arranged nor labelled. It seemed unlikely it would be able to obtain further Aboriginal Victorian ethnological specimens.[27] Zietz also learnt (probably from Ramsay) that the Queensland Museum was actively collecting Aboriginal material in the northern and western regions of the colony.

It seemed that despite the obstacles the South Australian Museum had encountered since its earliest years, its ethnological holdings could justly 'be considered as one of the most valuable in Australia'. Moreover, the development of pastoralism and mining in the Northern Territory under South Australia's administration presented opportunities for the museum to enlist the help of police, other frontier officials and cattle station managers so as to enable it to become the premier institution for the study of southern and central Australian ethnology.

Over the next eight years, the museum was able, despite financial constraints, to collect ethnological material on a more systematic and ambitious scale. By 1896 Stirling could delight in having supervised the creation of a 'fine ... collection from Central Australia'.[28] By this time Stirling had for several years also been actively encouraging the collecting of Aboriginal skulls and skeletal material.

Stirling and Aboriginal Morphology

What roused Stirling's interest in procuring remains as well as ethnological artefacts was his coming to think that cranial and other morphological traits within the Aboriginal population of southern and central Australia had an intriguing evolutionary significance. Two things appear to have crystallized his thinking in this regard. The first was his being struck sometime in 1888–1889 by what appeared to be a 'marked resemblance' between a South Australian cranium recently donated to the museum and the cast of the Neanderthal skull that Haacke had purchased in 1881.[29] When Stirling visited England in 1891–1892 he took with him casts of this

[25] Zietz to Stirling, 12 November 1888, SRSA GRG19/424/1888.

[26] On the fire see Ronald Strahan, *Rare and Curious Specimens: An Illustrated History of the Australian Museum, 1827–1979* (Sydney, 1979), p. 39.

[27] Zietz to Stirling, 12 November 1888, SRSA GRG19/424/1888.

[28] Edward Charles Stirling, *Report on the Work of the Horn Scientific Expedition to Central Australia, Part IV. Anthropology* (Melbourne, 1896), p. 4.

[29] Anon., 'Obituary of Sir Edward Charles Stirling', *Transactions of the Royal Society of South Australia*, 43 (1916): p. 1.

Aboriginal cranium, one of which he gave to Alexander Macalister (1844–1919), then professor of anatomy at the University of Cambridge. Macalister, an admirer of Darwin interested in the evolutionary significance of rudimentary organs in human and primates,[30] judged it 'the most Neanderthaloid skull that he had seen'.[31]

The second thing was Stirling's coming to believe there was a further 'curious point of resemblance between palæolithic man and the modern Australian aboriginal'. This was 'the shape of the tibia or shin-bone' which in each race appeared 'markedly flattened'.[32]

Stirling and his colleague Archibald Watson (1849–1940), then professor of anatomy at the University of Adelaide, had at first thought this flattening of the tibia (platycnemia) was a pathological condition commonly afflicting Aboriginal people of southern and central Australia. Yet in England Stirling had learnt that what seemed identically platycnemic tibia had been found not only in other human populations generally thought to be 'lower races' in the continuum of human evolution, but also 'with varying frequency in different localities, in those of ancient man'.[33] Indeed, all the tibia of the so-called Cro-Magnon skeletons – discovered in 1868 in limestone cliffs of the Vézère river valley in the Dordogne region of France, and estimated as having occupied the region during the Upper Pleistocene – appeared to be platycnemic.[34]

On his return to Adelaide in mid-1892, Stirling set about carefully examining what Aboriginal tibia his museum and the university medical school held, finding 'nearly all of them [to be] more or less platycnemic'.[35] By early the following year, he had sought through the colony's newspapers to enlist the help of settlers in outlying parts of the colony and the Northern Territory in locating burial places. A number were happy to oblige, one suggesting that stockmen on several Barkley Tableland stations knew of 'many … disturbed examples such as would rejoice the heart of Mr Stirling'.[36]

Ancient Europeans, Aborigines and the Significance of Race

In September 1893, Stirling gave a public lecture in conjunction with the meetings in Adelaide of the Australasian Association for the Advancement of Science. The lecture offered a lively account of Europe's earliest human inhabitants. Moreover,

30 A. Macalister, 'Review of Works on Life and Organisation', *Dublin Quarterly Journal of Medical Science*, 50 (1870): pp. 112–23.

31 E.C. Stirling, *Prehistoric Man* (Adelaide, 1893), p. 12.

32 Ibid., p. 12.

33 Ibid., p. 12.

34 Stirling, *Horn Scientific Expedition*, p. 19.

35 Ibid., p. 20.

36 C. Hemphill to Stirling, 5 January 1893, South Australian Museum Archives, Stirling Papers, AA. 309, Box 5, Item 263.

Stirling could not resist the opportunity of sharing with his audience his discovery of the presence of Neanderthaloid cranial characteristics and platycnemic tibia in the modern Aboriginal population, and his belief that it proved 'we have about us in the Aboriginal races an almost exact counterpart of the most ancient men [in Europe] whose remains have come to light during recent years'.[37]

Stirling further spoke of these morphological affinities as raising an interesting question: how had Europe's most ancient human inhabitants eventually become 'a race which can claim a Shakespeare or a Newton', while in Australia their 'almost exact counterpart' had not only 'remained practically unchanged through long ages', but also seemed 'doomed to speedy extinction'. Yet he pleaded being unable to explore this question and still adequately achieve the stated aim of his lecture, which was to summarize what the earliest 'indubitable evidence' suggested Europe's paleolithic inhabitants had been like.[38]

Even so, Stirling's account of paleolithic life in Europe went some way towards answering why that continent should have witnessed the gradual emergence of advanced civilization while Australia's autochthonous people had seemingly experienced evolutionary stasis. For he was to draw extensively upon the work of the idiosyncratic Darwinian paleontologist William Boyd Dawkins (1837–1929) and follow him in representing human prehistory as essentially a story of racial struggle and supersession.

A protege of Thomas Henry Huxley (1825–1895), Dawkins had secured the professorship of geology at Manchester's Owen College for two decades in 1874 on the strength of his research into Pleistocene mammals.[39] However, by the time of Stirling's lecture, Dawkins's reputation in scientific circles now owed much to two books and numerous articles published over the previous two decades in which he sought to reconstruct the course of European prehistory from the increasing flow of discoveries concerning early human occupation made in ancient river terraces and cave deposits.[40]

Dawkins believed that prehistoric Europe had seen the successive displacement and likely extermination of racially distinct peoples by physically and intellectually superior types. The earliest of these races, whose arrival in the Middle Pleistocene Dawkins believed was marked by the presence of distinctively worked stone tools in river gravels, had been displaced in the Upper Pleistocene by at least two different races of cave-dwelling people, the latter possessing superior stone and bone tools suggesting they lived much like modern Inuit hunter-gathering bands.

---

37 Stirling, *Prehistoric Man*, p. 2.

38 Ibid., p. 2.

39 Geoffrey Tweedale, 'Dawkins, Sir William Boyd (1837–1929)', in H.C.G. Matthew and Brian Harrison (eds), *Oxford Dictionary of National Biography* (Oxford, 2004). Available at: www.oxforddnb.com/view/article/32750 (accessed 29 April 2009).

40 William Boyd Dawkins, *Cave Hunting: Researches on the Evidence of Caves Respecting the Early Inhabitants of Europe* (London, 1874); *Early Man and His Place in the Tertiary Period* (London, 1880).

Excavation of these peoples' dwelling places further seemed to indicate that by the end of the Paleolithic era they had been forced into the northern regions of the continent by new waves of migrants, the last being 'Aryan' peoples who through the Neolithic era had arrived from the east to establish themselves as the ancestors of modern Europeans.

Stirling was drawn to Dawkins's depiction of ancient Europe as the scene of ancient racial struggles that probably entailed not just the displacement, but the extermination of peoples less fitted for survival: so much so that he could declare himself convinced there was no doubt that these Inuit-like peoples of the late European paleolithic era were 'overwhelmed and annihilated by … advancing hordes of neolithic invaders'. Indeed, Stirling spoke of this ancient racial antipathy having a modern analogue in 'the same feelings as have always existed between the Eskimos and Red Indians, terror and defenceless hatred being met by ruthless extermination'.[41]

Stirling's attraction to this agonistic racialist vision of humanity's deep past may have also reflected his sharing Dawkins's scepticism about one key aspect of Darwinian theory: the idea that nature was a self-regulating arena of competition, in which individuals within a species exhibiting variations favoring their survival and reproduction were 'naturally selected' by prevailing environmental conditions. For Dawkins was one of numerous scientific contemporaries of Darwin who could accept his theory of evolution in its positing new species with greater fitness for survival arose through speciation, but believed that especially in man favourable variants of physical form and intellectual capability had not arisen through natural selection, but were the result of a creative, divinely originating force at work in the bodily economy purposely guiding the course of evolution.[42]

Stirling might have been inclined to think likewise, perhaps agreeing with his senior Cambridge colleague, Alexander Macalister, that there were two fundamental parts to the human mind:

> one the seat of the passions, desires, and appetites … identical with that of the lower animals … the other … which has no correlate in the lower animals, the seat of the moral sense, and the religious feelings … which no evolution can account for.[43]

If so, this may explain why in his lecture Stirling was to distance himself from Dawkins's suggesting the origins of modern European civilization lay in the

---

41 'Dr Stirling on Prehistoric Man', *Adelaide Advertiser*, 23 September 1893.

42 Adrian Desmond, *Archetypes and Ancestors: Palaeontology in Victorian London, 1850–1875* (London, 1982), pp. 181–2.

43 A. Macalister, 'Review of the *The Descent of Man*', *Dublin Quarterly Review of Medical Science*, 52 (1871): 150, cited David N. Livingstone, 'Science, Site and Speech: Scientific Knowledge and the Spaces of Rhetoric', *History of the Human Sciences*, 20/2 (2007): pp. 71–98, p. 78.

easterly migration and spread of Neolithic 'Aryan' peoples. Possibly Stirling thought the morphology of ancient European skulls was indicative of a higher power having produced the modern peoples of Europe from more locally originating racial types.

In 1894 Stirling participated in the Horn Expedition to the McDonnell Ranges of the Northern Territory. Named after its sponsor, William Austin Horn (1841–1922), a wealthy South Australian mining magnate and pastoralist, the expedition comprised scientists with a range of expertise from the universities of Adelaide, Melbourne and Sydney. The goal of the expedition was to undertake a comprehensive survey of the geology, biology and Indigenous peoples of the region. Stirling was charged with directing the expedition's anthropological work.

Among other members of the expedition was the Oxford trained evolutionary biologist, Baldwin Spencer (1860–1929). Born in Manchester, Spencer had left Oxford in 1887 to take up the foundation chair of biology at the University of Melbourne, becoming internationally regarded by the turn of the twentieth century as the foremost authority on the anthropology of Aboriginal Australia.[44] Historians have tended to focus on how the Horn Expedition provided Spencer with an 'anthropological apprenticeship', while endorsing the view of Spencer and other members of the expedition that Stirling's fieldwork proved disappointing.[45] John Mulvaney, for example, has observed that Stirling's 'observations on Aboriginal subjects were few and scrappy'.[46] Much has also been made of the fact that Stirling's report on the expedition's anthropological work required Spencer's editorial intervention and was published only after the addition of observations by Frank Gillen (1855–1912), the outback postmaster whom Spencer had first met on the expedition and who was destined to become his invaluable fieldwork partner over the next two decades.

Even so, one section of the Horn Expedition's anthropological report stands out in terms of focus and attention to detail. This is Stirling's documenting the prevalence of platycnemic tibia amongst Aboriginal people of the McDonnell Ranges. He was to write that when the expedition

> came into more frequent contact with the blacks, I was surprised to find that the tibiæ of a considerable number of them, both males and females, adults

---

[44] On Spencer's life and remarkable achievements, see D.J. Mulvaney and J.H. Calaby, *'So Much That Is New'. Baldwin Spencer 1860–1929: A Biography* (Melbourne, 1985).

[45] See D.J. Mulvaney, '"A Splendid lot of Fellows": Achievements and Consequences of the Horn Expedition', in S.R. Morton and D.J. Mulvaney (eds), *Exploring Central Australia: Society, the Environment and the Horn Expedition* (Chipping Norton, NSW, 1996), p. 8; also Howard Morphy, 'More than Mere Facts: Repositioning Spencer and Gillen in the History of Anthropology', in ibid., pp. 135–48.

[46] D.J. Mulvaney, '"A Splendid lot of Fellows"', p. 6.

> and young, presented the same peculiar bent conformation, the associated platycnemia being apparently also well marked.[47]

If Stirling needed further proof that the typical form of platycnemic anterior curvature he had found in Aboriginal tibia was an 'evolutionary modification of form' he had it. The lack of resemblance of this curvature to those in tibia known to have been caused by tuberculosis or similar diseases strongly suggested to him that it could have only one origin. It had arisen from 'the Australian native … [being] perpetually on the tramp, either in the pursuit of game or in the course of his wandering life'.[48]

Building a Collection

Stirling seems not to have continued investigating tibial or other Aboriginal morphological peculiarities on returning from the Horn Expedition. Possibly believing that further research on Indigenous evolutionary genealogy required larger numbers of morphological representative specimens, he now focused on encouraging the donation of crania and other skeletal remains by fellow medical practitioners, police and other frontier officials in remote regions of South Australia and the Northern Territory.[49] By 1895 he had several times accompanied museum employees on short 'body snatching' trips to burial places.[50]

Stirling may well have had his shortcomings as an anthropological observer of Aboriginal life-ways and culture, but he was well aware of the distress desecration of ancestral burial places caused. During his 1891–1892 visit to England, he had enlisted the help of his elder brother, John Lancelot Stirling (1849–1932) in instructing museum employees to procure and send him several complete skeletons for British scientific institutions. They were to obtain these skeletons in secrecy from a burial place with numerous graves that appears to have been on a pastoral station leased by the Stirling family on the Mundi Mundi Plains of central western New South Wales. The nature of Stirling's request and the fact that the two brothers evaded seeking the Museum and Library Board's approval of the venture caused alarm. Robert Kay, the board's long-time secretary, advised that approving the exhumations would have to await Stirling's return from England. The board, he informed the Stirlings, believed the matter 'too delicate' and thought the museum staff tasked with procuring the remains not to 'have judgment enough', in Kay's words, 'to be trusted in a rather delicate matter as any row or squabble might

47 Stirling, *Horn Expedition*, p. 19.

48 Ibid., p. 20.

49 Various items of correspondence relating to the acquisition of Aboriginal remains are to be found in SRSA GRG 19/424/1892–1895.

50 See Stirling to Baldwin Spencer, 9 January 1895, Walter Baldwin Spencer Papers, 1880–1929, Museum Victoria, MS 29/10.

I suppose have grave consequences'.[51] John Stirling responded that his brother would regret being unable to present skeletons to his metropolitan colleagues, assuring Kay that the museum's men would not be putting themselves at any risk. Even so, he conceded that he did not want any of his employees to assist them, lest Aboriginal workers on the holding learn of the desecration. As he explained to Kay:

> The reason for our Station people not desiring to appear in the matter is merely from the fact of our employing a good many natives and our men doing anything in the matter would probably make them shy of remaining where their last resting place may be disturbed.[52]

What weight doubts as to the morality of exhuming these skeletons had in the board's refusing Stirling's request is unclear. As surviving museum correspondence shows, there were officials and settlers in outlying regions of the colony and the Northern Territory willing to aid the museum who saw nothing immoral in sending the museum skeletal remains that had been exposed by erosion or found in the wake of land clearing. But as Stirling knew from other letters he received, there were also those collectors who could not engage in or condone 'rifling any known graves'.[53]

Even so, Stirling was able to enlist the help of a number of frontier police, other government officials and pastoral settlers in securing Aboriginal skulls and skeletons through exhuming graves. William George Stretton, for example, served in the Territory as mounted policeman from the late 1860s until joining the Customs Department in 1887. In August 1894, he wrote to Stirling from Borroloola of having secured 'the bones of the huge native I mentioned some time ago', adding that although he had been unable to obtain all the smaller bones of the skeleton, he would be able to get the museum a second 'perfect specimen later on'.[54]

The most active of Stirling's skeletal collectors during the 1890s was Paul Foelsche (1831–1914), sub-inspector in charge of the Northern Territory's mounted police. A keen amateur naturalist and skilled photographer, Foelsche had regularly sent the museum specimens of local flora and fauna since taking up his posting to Port Darwin in 1870. Over the years he had also become fascinated by the life-ways and culture of the Larrakia and other peoples whose land he policed. Foelsche had periodically sent the museum Aboriginal skulls he had come across on his patrols since the early 1880s; but with Stirling's encouragement his contributions during the 1890s became more regular and extensive. In 1894, for example, Stirling was delighted to receive the skulls of six Malay fishermen

51 SRSA GRG 19/14/16.

52 SRSA GRG 19/424/1892.

53 Thomas McCallum to Stirling, 4 June 1899, SRSA GRG 19/4/1899.

54 W.G. Stretton to Stirling, 6 August 1894, SRSA GRG 19/424/1894.

allegedly killed by Aborigines together with four Aboriginal skulls.[55] Foelsche also proved willing to assist other Territory police in sending the museum remains they acquired by steamer out of Port Darwin.[56]

Yet Stirling was wary of incurring moral censure should the extent to which police had participated in the collecting of remains become more widely known. In 1898, he thought it wise to inquire of South Australia's Commissioner of Police, whether he had any objection to naming Paul Foelsche 'as a donor in many cases of native skulls'. 'Personally I do not', Stirling declared, though admitting that he was concerned that 'there might be those who, on sentimental or other grounds, would say that members of the Force should not thus occupy themselves'.[57] For his part, the Commissioner was agreeable so long as it was made clear that Foelsche had done so as a civilian.[58]

As John Mulvaney has observed of Stirling's involvement in the Horn Expedition, his sympathies were overwhelmingly with the pastoralists of the McDonnell region whose cattle were frequently being speared. He was to downplay the brutality with which station employees and mounted police punished cattle killing in his contribution to the expedition's anthropological report, declaring himself 'glad to bear witness to the humanity and even the kindliness with which the natives are now treated by the present settlers'. Hence one can understand Stirling's reticence about drawing attention to police complicity in procuring remains, especially when he knew himself to be the indirect beneficiary of frontier violence. In November 1896, for example, Stirling wrote to the South Australian police commissioner asking whether any of his officers could identify the place where an Aboriginal man known as 'Pompey' had been killed. His skull had come to the museum with no information beyond his allegedly having been 'shot by the Police some years ago'. The commissioner made inquiries, with the result that Stirling was forwarded a report from William Henry Willshire (1852–1925),[59] a mounted constable who had gained widespread notoriety for his indiscriminate violence while serving in various parts of central Australia between 1884 and 1895. Willshire advised that there had in fact been three men named 'Pompey who came to their death in my time in the far north'. One, Willshire recalled, had been a 'big strapping young nigger man' who in 1884 was tracked by his patrol after killing cattle in the vicinity of Mount Stuart north of Alice Springs and shot dead resisting arrest. A second 'Pompey' had been shot the same year by his patrol on Undoolya Station to the east of Alice Springs after allegedly killing 'a little civilized black boy' kept by the station manager. The third bearing the name had been employed on the Victoria River Downs station, from which he had run

55 SRSA GRG 19/424/1894.

56 See, for example, W.G. Stretton to Stirling, 6 August 1894, SRSA GRG 19/424/1894.

57 Stirling to Madley, Commissioner of Police, 6 August 1898, SRSA GRG/19/4/1890–1898.

58 Madley to Stirling, 10 August 1898, SRSA GRG/19/4/1890–1898.

59 Willshire to G.L. Reid, 4 December 1896, SRSA GRG5/2/1896/203.

off with a man known as 'Jimmy … with firearms and joined the wild natives'. Willshire wrote that the men had been killed by 'the wild niggers' and he had gone out and recovered the firearms, adding that:

> some few months after when the bodies of Pompey & Jimmy had sufficiently dried I went out and brought both their sculls [*sic*] in and buried them in my garden at Gordon Creek, as the Late John Watson Manager for Goldsborough, Mort & Co. stated that he wanted Pompey's scull for a spittoon.[60]

Perhaps the most disturbing instance of police involvement in the collecting of Aboriginal bodily remains in the wake of frontier violence is that recounted in a letter Stirling received in January 1899 from Ernest Charles Cowle, a mounted constable stationed at Illamurta Springs, near Tempe Downs. Earlier that month, a miner had been speared near Alice Springs. The alleged spearer had been tracked and caught, but when the constable in charge of the tracking party fastened a chain to his leg the man had struck him down with his manacled hands and run, only to be shot dead. Cowle informed Stirling that he had read 'a garbled account' of the shooting which had occurred close to where he had recently been camped, so his patrol had sought out the body. 'I thought of the penis for you', Cowle wrote, 'but it was too diseased to handle & would have been rotten before I could get to the station next day, in fact this is what has occurred on each of the late troubles'.[61]

Valuable Scientific Capital

By the turn of the twentieth century the South Australian Museum had acquired nearly 200 Aboriginal crania, around a dozen near or full skeletons and probably a hundred or so other kinds of bone. Stirling had also seen to it that the museum was equipped with cranial and anthropometric measuring instruments favoured by British and European researchers.

However, Stirling appears to have become resigned by this time to the size and likely future rate of expansion of the collection making its value primarily use by researchers pursuing large-scale comparative investigations of Aboriginal morphology across the various holdings of Australian and overseas museums and medico-scientific institutions. Possibly the anatomist and anthropologist Wilhelm Krause (1833–1910), then head of Berlin's prestigious Anatomical Institute, confirmed to Stirling that therein lay the collection's value when he visited the museum to measure its crania in 1897.[62] But regardless

60 Ibid.

61 Cowles to Stirling, 21 January 1899, SRSA GRG 19/4/1.

62 See Wilhelm Krause, 'Anthropologische Reise nach Australien', *Zeitschrift für Ethnologie*, 29 (1897): pp. 508–58. Krause's Adelaide visit was probably arranged by Archibald Watson, who had once been his pupil.

of what Krause made of the collection, Stirling seems to have been already inclined to think that as much was to be scientifically gained by his passing on remains of particular morphological interest he received to leading British anatomists engaged in investigating the evolutionary genealogy of the human species.

Stirling had occasionally given crania to British medico-scientific colleagues since as early as 1882.[63] Now he not only sent them skulls and casts of crania in the museum, but also with the aid of local medical colleagues several complete heads preserved in spirits, two of which were carefully dissected during 1896–1897 at the University of Cambridge by W.H.L. Duckworth (1870–1956), a talented young anatomist who soon afterwards became the university's first lecturer in physical anthropology.[64]

Stirling had reason to be discreet about this latter initiative as the heads were procured during post mortems on Aboriginal people dying in one of the colony's hospitals or benevolent asylums. He was not contravening the legislation then governing anatomy teaching and post-mortem dissection in South Australia, which as professor of physiology at Adelaide University he had actually co-drafted in 1884 with the colony's chief justice. In common with other medical men of his time, Stirling could lawfully remove and use scientifically interesting bodily structures discovered during post-mortem dissection as he saw fit, unless the deceased, their relatives or friends had exercised their right under the Anatomy Act to deny him consent to do so.[65] Rather, Stirling was conscious that his moral reputation in Adelaide society could easily fall victim to the fear and disgust which dissection had long generated in the popular imagination, should his post-mortem removal of whole heads become publicly known. Moreover, from the middle of 1903 onwards he had good reason to be discreet due to the public outcry caused by the post-mortem anthropological harvesting of heads and other bodily structures by his medical colleague and Adelaide's city coroner, William Ramsay Smith (1859–1987).[66] In the eight years he remained director of the museum, Stirling took care to counsel would-be collectors that Aboriginal remains should be 'judiciously collected for you would naturally not wish to create a scandal'.[67]

---

63 *Cambridge University Reporter*, 22 May 1882, p. 576.

64 *Cambridge University Reporter*, 4 June 1897, p. 1037.

65 See Edward Charles Stirling, 15 September, Evidence taken by the Board of Inquiry into Charges against Ramsay Smith, City Coroner, 1903, SRSA GRG24/67, p. A7.

66 Helen MacDonald details the scandal provoked by Ramsay Smith in analysing the aims and outcomes of the resulting South Australian government inquiry into Smith's treatment of corpses, in 'The Anatomy Inspector and the Government Corpse', *History Australia*, 6/2 (2009): 40.1–40.17.

67 Stirling to Arthur Hardy, 4 April 1910, GRG19/11/2.

Hopes Unrealized: The Swanport Discovery

By 1910, Stirling was in his early sixties, and beginning to contemplate retiring from the museum's directorship. He still looked to expand the museum's skeletal holdings; although as he lamented when seeking two skulls from his long-time medical colleague, Archibald Watson, his ambition was now no more than the hope that the museum would acquire 250 Aboriginal crania in his lifetime.

In April the following year, however, swamp reclamation work by South Australia's lands department at Swanport, on the lower Murray River, disturbed a large ancestral burial place of the Ngarrindjeri people. Stirling was quick to send museum personnel to the site only to learn that most of the skeletons exposed had either been 'promiscuously thrown into a hole' or shoveled up with soil then tipped onto the adjacent river bank. Despite retrieving as many bones as possible, 'the individual identity of the skeletons so handled was unfortunately lost'.[68] Worse, nothing like the number of skeletons broken up were subsequently uncovered.

In spite of this setback, the burial place was agreed to be a remarkable discovery that under the supervision of museum personnel quickly increased the institution's number of Aboriginal crania to more than 500.[69] Possibly, it also led Stirling to think that further reclamation work in the lower Murray region might well yield other sites with large numbers of burials, giving researchers associated with the museum the means to investigate comprehensively Ngarrindjeri morphology and evolutionary ancestry. At any rate, three months after the Swanport discovery, Stirling spoke before the Royal Society of South Australia of his hoping to investigate the remains 'from a craniological, osteological and pathological point of view'.[70]

However, Stirling did not embark on any such comprehensive study. He consulted various local and European researchers skilled in anthropometric techniques, and supervised the museum's acquisition of relevant publications it did not yet hold and the purchase of various new osteometric instruments.[71] But these intellectual resources lay unused as Stirling confined himself to investigating matters falling comfortably within his pre-existing (largely non-metrical) medico-scientific interests and areas of expertise. What work he did on the Swanport bones was to determine whether they could be taken together with historical evidence as proving that Ngarrindjeri and other Aboriginal peoples had been the victims of

---

[68] Edward Charles Stirling, 'Preliminary Report on the Discovery of Native Remains at Swanport, River Murray; with an Inquiry into the Alleged Occurrence of a Pandemic among the Australian Aboriginals', *Transactions and Proceedings and Report of the Royal Society of South Australia*, 35 (1911): 4.

[69] Jones, 'A Box of Things', p. 290.

[70] Stirling, 'Preliminary Report', p. 42.

[71] Stirling's correspondence with Australian-based and European anthropometric experts and related material is preserved in the South Australian Museum Archives, Stirling Papers, AA. 309, Box 2, Folders 2–3.

one or more smallpox epidemics in the century or so prior to European settlement in South Australia.

Stirling's surviving papers and correspondence provide no clues as to why he did not undertake or encourage other museum personnel to further investigate the Swanport remains. It could have been that what preparatory reading he did left him unwilling to immerse himself in this late stage of his career in cranial or other avenues of anthropometric investigation, which by this time had evolved into highly technical pursuits marked by disagreement and debate amongst its leading practitioners. Further, he may possibly have become aware of growing doubts within contemporary metropolitan British scientific circles as to whether the morphology of the human head and limbs could in fact be used to map human racial diversity and evolutionary genealogy. As Nancy Stepan has observed, though many British scientists continued to believe metric analysis of crania and limb bones would yield insights into racial affinities and differences until well into the late 1930s, there were various influential evolutionary biologists and anatomists who by the time of the Swanport discovery were convinced that the human head and limbs were so susceptible to variation in response to specific environmental conditions as to render them useless as markers of racial type or evolutionary ancestry.[72]

Regardless of whether Stirling's failure to investigate the Swanport remains as he initially planned stemmed from these or other more mundane reasons, he was to take no further active interest in investigating Aboriginal morphology or pathology until his death in 1919. Though it is clear enough that he saw the museum's skeletal collection as one of his principal contributions to colonial science.

Today Stirling's contribution to how race, nation and aboriginality were discursively construed in late nineteenth- and early twentieth-century Australia seems unremarkable. His inquiries into Aboriginal morphology were more informed by interaction with metropolitan scientific authorities than we might think; but what he had to say about Indigenous bones – notably when using them to draw affinities between the inhabitants of Europe's deep past and Aboriginal Australians – amounted to little more than a rehearsal of what by the 1890s had long been commonplace in metropolitan British scientific circles.

However, Stirling's use of remains arguably deserves closer consideration than it has hitherto gained. For it stands as a telling, if minor, illustration of how Aboriginal remains were used by a colonial scientist who commanded great authority by virtue of his positions within Adelaide's university and museum, to verify that the future of Australian nationhood depended on safeguarding an evolutionary inheritance that, as Stirling put it, was responsible for Britons becoming 'a race which can claim a Shakespeare or a Newton'.[73] The parallels he drew between ancient European and contemporary Aboriginal societies especially

[72] Nancy Stepan, *The Idea of Race in Science: Great Britain, 1800–1960* (London, 1982), pp. 91, 102.

[73] Stirling, *Prehistoric Man*, p. 2.

served to underscore the lesson for a young settler society progressing to nationhood that human history was in essence a drama of racial struggle and supersession. Moreover, in Stirling's correspondence with those in frontier districts who helped him procure remains, we see how this racialized vision of history further paralleled, and was easily interpreted as giving scientific substance to and morally justifying, settlers and agents of colonial governance resorting to and condoning violence as a means of ensuring peaceful coexistence with Aboriginal peoples in frontier regions. In their conversations concerning the Aboriginal dead, we find much by way of observation and utterance on the part of Stirling's collectors disclosing that they too saw themselves as engaged in an evolutionary struggle, in which Aboriginal people were construed as destined to suffer racial extinction.

Bibliography

Manuscript Sources

Museum Victoria, Walter Baldwin Spencer Papers, 1880–1929, MS 29/10.

South Australian Museum Archives, Stirling Papers, AA. 306.

SRSA: State Records of South Australia, Records of the Public Library, Museum, and Art Gallery (formerly the South Australian Institute) 1855/6–1940, GRG 19.

SRSA: State Records of South Australia, Evidence taken by the Board of Inquiry into Charges against Ramsay Smith, City Coroner, 1903, GRG24/67.

Theses

Jones, Philip, 'A Box of Things': Ethnographic Collectors and the South Australian Museum, 1830s–1930s. PhD Thesis, University of Adelaide, 1997.

Printed Primary Sources

Adelaide Advertiser.

Anon., 'Obituary of Sir Edward Charles Stirling', *Transactions of the Royal Society of South Australia*, 43 (1916): p. 1.

Cambridge University Reporter.

Dawkins, William Boyd, *Cave Hunting: Researches on the Evidence of Caves Respecting the Early Inhabitants of Europe* (London: Macmillan, 1874).

Dawkins, William Boyd, *Early Man and His Place in the Tertiary Period* (London: Macmillan, 1880).

Hrdlička, Aleš, 'Catalogue of Human Crania in the United States National Museum Collections', *Proceedings of the United States National Museum*, 71 (1928): pp. 4–82.

Hunt, James and Ralph Tate, 'On the Archaic Anthropological of the Zetland Isles …', *Journal of the Anthropological Society of London*, 4 (1866): pp. xv–xviii.
Krause, Wilhelm, 'Anthropologische Reise nach Australien', *Zeitschrift für Ethnologie*, 29 (1897): pp. 508–58.
Macalister, Alexander, 'Review of Works on Life and Organisation', *Dublin Quarterly Journal of Medical Science*, 50 (1870): pp. 112–23.
Stirling, Edward Charles, *Prehistoric Man* (Adelaide: Privately Printed, 1893).
Stirling, Edward Charles, *Report on the Work of the Horn Scientific Expedition to Central Australia, Part IV. Anthropology* (Melbourne: Melville, Mullen and Slade 1896).
Stirling, Edward Charles, 'Preliminary Report on the Discovery of Native Remains at Swanport, River Murray; with an Inquiry into the Alleged Occurrence of a Pandemic among the Australian Aboriginals', *Transactions and Proceedings and Report of the Royal Society of South Australia*, 35 (1911): pp. 4–46.

Secondary Sources

Alderman, A.R., 'Tate, Ralph (1840–1901)', *Australian Dictionary of Biography, Volume 6* (Melbourne: Melbourne University Press, 1976), pp. 243–4.
Anderson, Warwick, *The Cultivation of Whiteness: Science, Health and Racial Destiny in Australia* (Melbourne: Melbourne University Press, 2002).
Bashford, Alison, *Imperial Hygiene: A Critical History of Colonialism, Nationalism and Public Health* (London: Palgrave, 2004).
Butcher, Barry, 'Gorilla Warfare in Melbourne: Halford, Huxley and Man's Place in Nature', in R.W. Home (ed.), *Australian Science in the Making* (Cambridge: Cambridge University Press, 1988), pp. 153–69.
Desmond, Adrian *Archetypes and Ancestors: Palaeontology in Victorian London, 1850–1875* (London: Blond & Briggs, 1982).
Lake, Marilyn and Henry Reynolds, *Drawing the Global Colour Line: White Men's Countries and the Question of Racial Equality* (Melbourne: Melbourne University Press, 2008).
Livingstone, David N., 'Science, Site and Speech: Scientific Knowledge and the Spaces of Rhetoric', *History of the Human Sciences*, 20/2 (2007): pp. 71–98.
Lydon, Jane, *Eye Contact: Photographing Indigenous Australians* (Durham, NC: Duke University Press, 2005).
MacDonald, Helen, 'The Anatomy Inspector and the Government Corpse', *History Australia*, 6/2 (2009): 40.1–40.17.
McGregor, Russell, *Imagined Destinies: Aboriginal Australians and the Doomed Race Theory, 1880–1939* (Melbourne: Melbourne University Press, 1997).
Mincham, Hans, 'Stirling, Sir Edward Charles (1848–1919)', *Australian Dictionary of Biography, Volume 6* (Melbourne: Melbourne University Press, 1976), pp. 200–201.
Morris, P.A. *Edward Gerrard & Sons: A Taxidermy Memoir* (Ascot: MPM Publishing, 2004).

Morphy, H. 'More than Mere Facts: Repositioning Spencer and Gillen in the History of Anthropology', in S.R. Morton and D.J. Mulvaney (eds), *Exploring Central Australia. Society, the Environment and the Horn Expedition* (Chipping Norton, NSW, 1996), pp. 135–48.

Morton, S.R. and D.J. Mulvaney (eds), *Exploring Central Australia: Society, the Environment and the Horn Expedition* (Chipping Norton, NSW: Surrey Beatty and Sons, 1996).

Mulvaney, D.J. and J.H. Calaby, *'So Much That Is New'. Baldwin Spencer 1860–1929: A Biography* (Melbourne: Melbourne University Press, 1985).

Stepan, Nancy, *The Idea of Race in Science: Great Britain, 1800–1960* (London: Archon Books, 1982).

Strahan, Ronald, *Rare and Curious Specimens: An Illustrated History of the Australian Museum, 1827–1979* (Sydney: The Australian Museum, 1979).

Turnbull, Paul, 'British Anthropological Thought in Colonial Practice: The Appropriation of Indigenous Australian Bodies, 1860–1880', in Bronwen Douglas and Chris Ballard (eds), *Foreign Bodies: Oceania and the Science of Race 1750–1940* (Canberra: ANU E-Press, 2008), pp. 205–28.

Tweedale, Geoffrey, 'Dawkins, Sir William Boyd (1837–1929)', in H.C.G. Matthew and Brian Harrison (eds), *Oxford Dictionary of National Biography* (Oxford: Oxford University Press, 2004). Available at: www.oxforddnb.com/view/article/32750 (accessed 29 April 2009).

Windshuttle, Keith, *The Fabrication of Aboriginal History, Volume One: Van Diemen's Land 1803–1847* (Paddington, NSW: Macleay Press, 2002).

Chapter 6
The Leprosy-Affected Body as a Commodity: Autonomy and Compensation[1]

Jo Robertson

In 2005, a committee investigating the impact of segregation policies on leprosy-affected people in Japan in the period 1907 to 1996 discovered 114 foetuses from leprosy-affected women preserved in formalin and stored in leprosy sanatoria throughout the country.[2] The committee reported that these remains resulted from 'artificial abortions, natural miscarriages, and artificially-induced births'.[3] On the basis of a detailed medical examination, the committee determined that 29 of the foetuses had been more than 32 weeks of age from conception, and amongst those,

---

[1] Leprosy is still endemic in Brazil and Nepal and although the numbers of new cases are declining, approximately 250,000 new cases are detected throughout the world every year. The disease is successfully treated with multi-drug therapy and it should no longer be something to fear or to conceal. There is a long and fascinating history of stigma as well as a history of moral and also differing cultural responses to the disease. Although there is still much to be written about these aspects of leprosy, they have been touched on to some extent elsewhere and this chapter takes that field for granted. In writing about leprosy, terminology is important. I deliberately avoid using the word 'leper' unless its pejorative weight in a quotation is indispensable to the argument. The word conveys a world of meaning that has persisted in branding and ostracizing people with the disease. In an attempt to empty leprosy of this accumulated representation, in countries such as Japan and Brazil, the descriptive term 'Hansen's disease' is used as a substitute for the word leprosy, but generally 'leprosy' is used as the medical term for the disease because it is found that in telling a person they have Hansen's disease, they still have to be told that they have leprosy.

[2] Japan Law Foundation: Verification Committee Concerning Hansen's Disease Problem, 'Verification Committee Concerning Hansen's Disease Problem: Final Report' (Summary Version), p. 64. Available at: www.leprosyhistory.org/english/bulletin.htm (accessed 18 January 2010).

[3] The leprosy sanatoria in Japan are as follows: Matsuoka Hoyo-en; Tohoku Shinsei-en; Kuryu Rakusen-en; Tama Zensho-en; Suruga; Nagashima Aisei-en; Oku Komyo-en; Oshima Seisho-en; Kikuchi Keifu-en; Hoshizuka Keiai-en; Amami Wako-en; Okinawa Airaku-en; Miyaka Nansei-en. The numbers of foetuses discovered at the following sanatoria are: Oku Komyo-en, 49; Hoshizuka Keia I en, 17; Suruga, 10; Matsuoka Hoyo-en, 1; Tama Zensho-en, 35. In addition, the Research Centre for Hansen's Disease, National Infectious Disease Research Centre also held two preserved foetuses. Japan Law Foundation, 'Verification Report', pp. 65–6.

16 would have been born at 36 weeks. Therefore at least 25 per cent of the bodies could not have been the result of abortions, but must have been early induced births or natural, full-term births. Eighty per cent of the total did not bear any marks of trauma or surgical cuts so the committee concluded that some of the babies would have been born alive. Logically it seemed that those, at least, had been killed at birth. The committee speculated on what had probably happened:

> if a foetus was born alive, the question is how the life was stopped after the birth. It is extremely difficult now to speculate how it was done, but there are some cases where the only imaginable thing is, at least for some newborn babies, that workers at sanatoria were committing murders in the sense of the Penal Law. Further to this, there are several testimonies that confirm such facts.[4]

In addition to the apparent retention of bodies of neonates whose lives had been 'stopped' by medical staff, that is, almost certainly murdered at birth, there were over 2,000 pathological samples from autopsies undertaken on the bodies of those who had died in the sanatoria, with no evidence of consent having been obtained from the deceased before death, or from their relatives. Finally, in some of the sanatoria, body parts that had been obtained as a result of surgical procedures were discovered stored haphazardly in polyethylene buckets, again with no evidence that consent had been sought or obtained.[5]

The tiny bodies in formalin, which bore mute testimony to their short experience of life, represented only one aspect of the longstanding experience of leprosy-affected people in Japan that was finally brought to the attention of the Kumamoto District court in 2001 by the surviving residents of Japanese sanatoria. They demanded compensation from the government for the treatment they had experienced when segregated against their will. The judge ruled that the Leprosy Prevention Law of 1953 was unconstitutional because it had gone well beyond what was a reasonable restriction of movement for the sake of public welfare, to the extent that its unconstitutionality was already well known.[6] The government decided not to contest the case and subsequently commissioned an investigation into the segregation policy that had resulted in violations of the human rights of the people so confined. Subsequently, the especially commissioned Verification Report, which revealed the foetal remains, represented one aspect of the government's desire to redress the injustices of past policies; in addition, the sum of 1.8 billion yen (£10.4 million) was awarded to 127 former leprosy patients in compensation for their experiences.[7]

---

[4] Ibid., pp. 65–6.

[5] Ibid., p. 67.

[6] Ibid., p. 9.

[7] Tony Gould, *Don't Fence Me In: From Curse to Cure: Leprosy in Modern Times* (London, 2005), p. 374.

This chapter examines notable instances of the way in which leprosy-affected people have had to struggle for sovereignty over their own bodies, in the face of assumptions that they were research material or a resource of some kind. One of the most well-known and earliest examples occurred in Bergen, in the laboratory of Gerhard Armauer Hansen, the scientist who identified the bacillus responsible for the disease in 1873. When Hansen inoculated the leprosy-affected Kari Nielsdatter in the eye with leprous material, she attempted to defend herself physically and then legally when her grievance was brought to court. She was successful to the extent that Hansen was removed from his post at the hospital. Battles of a different sort were also fought in the Philippines for well over 50 years in the first half of the twentieth century and particularly in the 1930s over children born to leprosy-affected people at a time when these children were regarded by the League of Nations, at least, as 'particularly valuable material' for large-scale experiments.[8] The people isolated on the leprosy colony of Culion both resisted attempts to segregate men and women and so prevent them from producing children and also resisted being separated from their babies at birth; nonetheless, one child in every three was at some time or other removed from their parents. Finally the chapter will consider the case of leprosy-affected people in Japan whose calls for redress led to the exposure of the findings which raise further questions about medical and legal attitudes to leprosy well into the late twentieth century.

These examples are spread across a century and a half in different parts of the world, but it is possible to identify a persistent strand of enabling conditions which help to explain how the practices to be discussed here came to be justified. Two preconditions pertain to the specific history and aetiological status of the disease itself. Before effective medical treatment, first with sulphones in 1941, and then more conclusively with multi-drug therapy, in 1981, the disease was viewed as a disfiguring horror that did not kill its victims, but condemned them to a lifetime of isolation from society. This history of the isolation and marginalization of leprosy-affected people was determined by difficulties in understanding the disease itself, and unfortunately, compounded by early scientific discoveries about the etiology of leprosy. In 1873, Hansen identified mycobacterium *M leprae* as the bacillus consistently present in the nodes of leprosy patients, and although it was also the very first bacterium to be discovered in the human being, the bacillus still has not been multiplied *in vitro*.[9] Subsequently, much about leprosy still eludes

[8] E. Burnet, *Provisional Report Presented to the Leprosy Commission at its Meeting in Tokyo in April 1930* (CH 836/Leprosy 7), pp. 8–9; and E. Burnet, *Provisional Report Presented to the Leprosy Commission at its Meeting in Tokyo in April 1930: Consideration of Urgent Matters to which the Commission drew attention at its May Session, 1928* (CH Leprosy 7a), p. 3. League of Nations Archive, Geneva.

[9] Hansen published his findings 'Causes of Leprosy', *Norwegian Medical Society* as part of his annual report for 1873 to the Norwegian Medical Society. G.H. Armauer Hansen, 'Preliminary Contribution Respecting the Characteristics of Leprosy', *Nordiskt Medeciniskt Arkiv Band*, 1/13 (1869); 'Further Contributions towards a Knowledge of

medical investigation.[10] How it enters the body and is transmitted to others is still unknown.[11] The mysteries that surround individual susceptibility, its onset and its progress, have been instrumental in contributing to much scientific speculation. Only recently, the mapping of the genome of the mycobacterium promises to unlock some of leprosy's ancient secrets.[12] The inability of medical science to state definitively how people contracted leprosy brought public health measures against the disease to focus upon the body of the leprosy-affected person as the source of the disease. Up until the 1950s, segregation of leprosy-affected people was the most common public health measure against the disease, albeit one that occasioned vigorous debate, both medical and public.[13]

A third enabling condition, less specific to leprosy, resides in the growing status accorded to scientific medicine and the laboratory. This coincided with and was productive of a shift in the nature of the leprosy asylum from relatively neglected charitable shelters to institutions that incorporated space for medical research.[14] In

---

the Characteristic Features of Leprosy (Spedalskhed)', *Nordoskt Medicinskt Arkiv Band*, 2/16 (1870), both reprinted in Henry Vandyke Carter, *On Leprosy and Elephantiasis with plates* (London, 1874); and G.H. Armauer Hansen and C. Looft, *Leprosy: in its Clinical and Pathological Aspects*, trans. Norman Walker (Bristol, 1895).

10 Zachary Gussow, *Leprosy, Racism, and Public Health: Social Policy in Chronic Disease Control* (San Francisco and London, 1989), p. 6.

11 It is generally thought to be spread by droplet infection. J.C. Pedley and J.G. Geater, 'Does Droplet Infection Play a Role in the Transmission of Leprosy?', *Leprosy Review*, 47/2 (1976): pp. 97–102.

12 The analysis of the first complete *M. leprae* cosmid sequence was conducted in 1993. The genome sequencing project was coordinated by Stewart Cole and Bart Barrell, and supported by the Association Française Raoul Follereau, ILEP, the Heiser Program for Research in Leprosy and Tuberculosis of The New York Community Trust, the World Health Organisation, and the Institut Pasteur. See K. Eiglemeier, N. Honoré, S.A. Woods, B. Caudron and S.T. Cole, 'Use of an Ordered Cosmid Library to Deduce the Genomic Organization of *Mycobacterium leprae*', *Molecular Microbiology*, 7/2 (1993): pp. 197–206.

13 For example when the Act providing for 'the segregation and admission to public nursing homes or sanatoria of lepers' was introduced in Norway in 1885, it met with strong opposition even in medical circles and was alleged to be callous and inhumane. See Ingvald Rokstad, 'Gerhard Henrich Armauer Hansen: Address Delivered at Inauguration of the Armauer Hansen Memorial Room, February 18, 1962', *International Journal of Leprosy*, 32/1 (1964): pp. 64–70, p. 68. (The medical debates on the etiology of leprosy were subtle and complex and shifted considerably between the nineteenth century and the twentieth. See Rod Edmond, *Leprosy and Empire: A Medical and Cultural History* (Cambridge, 2006) and Michael Worboys, 'Was there a Bacteriological Revolution in Late Nineteenth-Century Medicine?', *Studies in History, Philosophy, Biology and Biomedical Science*, 38 (2007): pp. 20–42.)

14 The types of institutions in 1941 are described, in India, for example: 'There is scope for different types of institutions to meet different needs. There is the well organised sanatorium for active and infective cases of leprosy, with proper medical staff, buildings and equipment. There is the asylum for the crippled, deformed and disabled cases of leprosy,

1931, while concluding that measures for compulsory segregation were an 'odium' of the past and had been unsuccessful in dealing with the disease, the Leprosy Commission of the League of Nations distinguished between 'segregation' and 'isolation', conceding that isolation of leprosy-affected people should be carried out 'in accordance with the circumstances prevailing in the countries involved'.[15] Then marking the turn to a more scientific approach to the disease, it recommended that there should be 'at least one centre for the study of the disease, with research laboratories and special courses for the medical profession and their assistants' in every country in which leprosy existed to an important degree.[16]

Finally, there was an investment on the part of the modern state itself in addressing the problem of the disease with the full extent of its most up-to-date scientific armoury in the hope that the nation could remake itself from having a leprosy problem to being a modern research nation and a model to others.[17]

In the face of such uncertainties, just as leprosy-control measures were focused upon the leprosy-affected body, so too was the quest to unravel leprosy's mysteries intensively located in the body of the person with the disease. People were isolated and subjected to all manner of attempts, not only to cure their disease, but also to understand it. Their bodies were investigated in life and in death. Included in this overarching medical intervention, reproduction was also medicalized to the extent that rights were subordinated to medical attempts to control the disease. In Norway, for example, when ideas of the hereditary transmission of leprosy were in their ascendancy, men were separated from women and marriage was

---

in which the medical work is of less importance. There is the agricultural colony which can be established under suitable conditions and in which the patients can partly maintain themselves. All these types of institutions have a place in any comprehensive scheme of anti-leprosy work', in Government of India, Central Advisory Board of Health, *Report on Leprosy and its Control in India* (New Delhi, 1942), p. 28. My paper 'The Leprosy Asylum in India', *Journal of the History of Medicine and Allied Sciences*, 64/4 (2009): pp. 474–517 outlines the development of leprosy asylums into agricultural colonies, but the development of the asylum that also functioned as a research laboratory has yet to be written.

[15] League of Nations, Health Organisation, *The Principles of Prophylaxis: First General Report of the Leprosy Commission Geneva* (Geneva, 1931), p. 6. League of Nations Archives, Geneva.

[16] Ibid., p. 9.

[17] This was important for the international status of countries like Japan and Colombia, for example. See Susan L. Burns, 'From "Leper Villages" to Leprosaria: Public Health, Nationalism and the Culture of Exclusion in Japan', in Carolyn Strange and Alison Bashford (eds), *Isolation: Places and Practices of Exclusion* (London and New York, 2003), pp. 104–18, on pp. 105–7 and Diana Obregon, 'Building National Medicine: Leprosy and Power in Colombia, 1870–1910', *Social History of Medicine*, 15/1 (2002): 89–108. For other countries with colonial status in relation to imperial centres, such as Hawaii and the Philippines, in relationship to the United States, it was important to demonstrate that leprosy was under control for the sake of trade. See Pennie Moblo, 'Blessed Damien of Moloka'i: The Critical Analaysis of Contemporary Myth', *Ethnohistory*, 44/4 (1997): pp. 691–726.

forbidden.[18] At the same time, governments had little respect for the subtlety of the medical discussions about the contagiousness of leprosy and speculative social policies which assumed greater knowledge than existed led to more radical governmental action than the science warranted.[19] The inability of medical science to resolve questions about the value of social isolation and behavioural constraints compounded the troubled social place of the affected.[20]

Coincident with this, the overarching history of the representation of leprosy brought its full weight to bear upon the leprosy-affected person. As a modern sufferer, Stanley Stein, strikingly describes the horror of the imagination that his own diagnosis of leprosy produced:

> Leprosy! The word was not a diagnosis; it was a pronouncement of doom. My hopes and ambitions were collapsing about me. My future was in ruins. My present? A great cold emptiness …
>
> Leprosy was not just a disease – it was a stigma, a disgrace, a visitation from on high, a punishment for some dreadful sin. What had I done to bring down the wrath of God upon my head? …
>
> Despite the doctor's kindness and understanding, I left his office convinced that my life was over. I went into the street like a sleepwalker. All the myths and frightening stories I had heard about leprosy rushed through my mind, obliterating the doctor's reassuring words. I remembered old engravings of lepers carrying a bell. I recalled the scene from *Ben Hur* and the chilling cry of 'Unclean! Unclean!' as the hero's mother and sister were driven from the city.[21]

---

[18] Virchow wrote that 'one factor in the etiology of leprosy has long been established. This is hereditary transmission … It is so clear cut, and so well established as a factor, that all possible means have been employed to prevent propagation of those with leprosy. Marriage has been forbidden, and castration has been practiced among males. Such ideas prevail at the present time in Norway, where the great frequency of the inheritance factor was shown by Danielssen and Boeck, and by Conradi'. See Rudolf Virchow, 'Virchow's Leprosy from *Die Krankhaften Geschwulste*', trans. George L. Fite, *International Journal of Leprosy*, 22/1 (1954): pp. 71–9, p. 76.

[19] This ushers in a whole other dimension – the tension between public policy and medical viewpoints about the treatment of leprosy-affected people. Very often doctors argued for humane treatment of people in the face of administrative demands that leprosy-affected people be contained for the sake of the health of the general populace. These administrative and public health arguments were usually driven by public and economic pressure, even if they were couched as moral panics.

[20] Debates about classification of various forms of the disease occupied international congresses up until a classification system was devised that was based on the body's immune response to the infection. See D.S. Ridley and W.H. Jopling, 'Classification of Leprosy According to Immunity: A Five-Group System', *International Journal of Leprosy*, 34 (1966): pp. 255–73.

[21] Stanley Stein, *Alone No Longer* (Carville, 1963), pp. 23–4.

This shift in sense of self was accompanied by changes in physical appearance. The mycobacterium that causes leprosy, *M leprae*, enters and damages the peripheral nerves, but the impact of this damage can be seen upon the body, and before effective medication, hands, feet and face, parts of the body that define it and distinguish it, were irrevocably disfigured. The face, which is particularly important in establishing identity and individuality, most often revealed the damage that leprosy could do. The nose could be affected, eyes clouded over, sight was lost, eyebrows disappeared, the skin thickened with nodules, and the quality of the voice would change. Hands and feet were also progressively damaged as a result of repeated injuries to the fingers and toes arising from the loss of sensation that came about from damage to the peripheral nerves.

As leprosy, for most of its history, has been a disfiguring disease, the loss of physical identity was accompanied by a sense of loss of essential identity, of 'humanity', and consequently of legal identity. For the medieval period Carole Rawcliffe has found that, while the development and application of legislation varied, anyone 'who seemed so deformed and terrible of aspect that he or she had to be "put out of the community of mankind" … forfeited his or her rights to plead, inherit and to make contracts of any kind'.[22] So leprosy not only compromised physical identity, burdened the sufferer with a distasteful representational history, but was also accompanied by a loss of legal status.

The affected were thus victims of a poorly understood disease that nonetheless carried a heavy social stigma. A person who was diagnosed with leprosy would find a new identity awaiting them that triggered off a convergence of social, medical, scientific and legal discursive processes. Moreover, as Rawcliffe and, before her, Mary Douglas indicates, 'official attempts to separate presumed lepers [*sic*] from society tended to occur during periods of crisis, when concerns about epidemic disease, disorder and vagrancy were running high'.[23] People with leprosy have historically functioned as trigger points for social frustrations, and in the battle for autonomy over their bodies, they could usually only rely on their own efforts to obtain justice.[24] For the period in question here, the triggers included concerns as wide-ranging as scientific competition; national pride; moral policing and eugenic policy. Throughout the world, when people were diagnosed with leprosy and came to the attention of the medical and administrative authorities, they usually

---

[22] Carole Rawcliffe, *Leprosy in Medieval England* (Suffolk, UK and Rochester, NY, 2006), p. 271.

[23] Ibid., p. 253 and Mary Douglas, 'Witchcraft and Leprosy: Two Strategies of Exclusion', *Man*, New Series 26/4 (1991): pp. 723–36, p. 734. There are extensive studies of stigma, for example: Nancy Wexler, 'Learning to be a Leper: A Case Study in the Social Construction of Illness', in Elliott G. Mishler (ed.), *Social Contexts of Health, Illness, and Patient Care* (New York, 1981), pp. 169–74.

[24] Today advocacy organizations such as IDEA (International Organisation for Integration, Dignity, and Economic Advancement) promote the rights of leprosy-affected people. Available at: www.idealeprosydignity.org (accessed 2 February 2010).

came under legislation that required their removal to a place of isolation. As a result, leprosy-affected people were not only required to surrender their liberty for the greater good but, in effect, also to surrender their bodies for medical experimentation, overtly for the sake of others similarly affected, but indirectly for the benefit of the status of scientific medicine and for the good of the nation. To be afflicted with leprosy would be accompanied by a loss of other rights such as the rights over one's own body including the right to reproduce and to keep one's own children. That leprosy-affected people objected to these demands and, in a few cases, actually managed to take their protest to the law courts provides some evidence of their battle for autonomy and their refusal of attempts to objectify them as commodities fit for medical investigation.

Gerhard Henrik Armauer Hansen and Kari Nielsdatter

In 1880 court proceedings at the City of Bergen Law Courts were held against Gerhard Henrik Armauer Hansen. He was a person of standing in the Bergen and also the Norwegian community, holding the post of resident physician at Pleiestiftelsen for Spedalske Nr 1 (the Nursing Home for Leprosy, No 1) since 1868 and also the post of Medical Officer of Health for Leprosy in Norway, since 1875.[25] In 1879, Kari Nielsdatter, a woman suffering from anaesthetic leprosy, had been a resident at the leprosy hospital in Bergen for 17 years. When the medical staff were making their rounds of the hospital, she had been summoned to accompany the doctor, Gerhard Armauer Hansen, to his office because he wanted to speak to her. She must have had some idea that this was not a good situation to be in because, as she later reported it, she stood anxiously by the door in tears. There were two other doctors working there, and she was told to approach the table, where she saw that Hansen had a sharp cutting instrument in his hand which he brought up to her eye. She stated that he attempted to bring the instrument to her eye, but she covered it with one hand and pushed him back with her other hand. He stated that he made an incision in her eye with a cataract knife which he had previously used to cut a nodule from a patient with nodular leprosy. He said that he had failed at that point to inoculate material into her eye because she would not keep her eye still. One of the other doctors tried to calm her and made her sit in a chair, and it was then that leprous material was inserted under the conjunctiva of her eye. Nielsdatter pleaded with them not to inject the other eye because she was afraid that she would lose her eyesight. She also complained that the experience was extremely painful, but the other doctors, who acted as witnesses and also experts, said that an incision in an anaesthetic eye should be painless, but then admitted when questioned in the court that the only way to determine if this were indeed the case would be to check the eye in the beginning, and this had not occurred. One of the physicians was an

[25] G. Armauer Hansen, *The Memories and Reflections of Dr. G. Armauer Hansen*, trans. G.A. Hansen (Würzburg, 1976).

ophthalmologist, and he argued that the operation should not have been painful, even in a healthy eye. He believed that she reacted as she did because she was a 'nervous and hysterical subject ... due to her imagination'. She claimed that her eye had been painful for seven weeks afterwards and it had disturbed her sleep; in addition, she had not been able to read since. The doctors admitted that her eye had been inflamed afterwards, but said that she was exaggerating about the pain. One of the physicians stated that the inflammation had arisen from another eye disease, not from the inoculation.[26]

Hansen who was relatively young, at 38, but already established as a medical practitioner, admitted to the court that 'he was not justified in carrying out the operation as he had neither obtained her permission in advance, nor told her of his aim in doing it'. He stated that 'he took it for granted that the deponent would not regard the experiment from his point of view'.

Yet as far as Hansen was concerned there were important medical reasons for what he nonetheless referred to in court as the 'unjustified operation'.[27] In his search for the causative agent of leprosy, he had seen rod-shaped bodies like bacteria which would prove that the disease was transmitted by infection; whereas, the tide of medical opinion was that the disease was hereditary. In 1847, influential Norwegians, Daniel Cornelius Danielssen (who happened to be Hansen's father-in-law) and Carl Wilhelm Boeck, had published the then definitive work of the nineteenth century on leprosy on the basis that the disease was an inheritable dyscrasia of the blood. The 1867 Report of the Royal College of Physicians that surveyed the British colonies and was circulated subsequently drew on their arguments. In 1873 when Henry Vandyke Carter visited Norway from India to investigate Norwegian leprosy control methods, his *Report on Leprosy and Leprosy Asylums in Norway with References to India* was informed by this hereditarian view: 'the original investigators of the national plague in Norway came to the unanimous conclusion that the main cause of the perpetuation of leprosy is its transmission from parent to offspring',[28] but his footnotes describe his encounter with Hansen who had shown him the bacillus. The potential of Hansen's discovery was sufficient for Carter to add an expectant footnote to his report:

---

[26] Th. M. Vogelsang, 'Gerhard Henrik Armauer Hansen 1841–1912: The Discoverer of the Leprosy Bacillus: His Life and Work', *International Journal of Leprosy*, 46/3 (1978): pp. 257–332.

[27] Ibid., p. 292.

[28] Henry Vandyke Carter, *Report on Leprosy and Leprosy Asylums in Norway with References to India* (London, 1874), p. 24. Carter joined the Indian Medical Service as Assistant Surgeon in 1858 and after six months in Central India was appointed professor of Anatomy and Physiology at the Grant Medical College Bombay. He became the Principal at the Grant Medical College and also first Physician at the J J Hospital, the foremost hospital in Bombay at the time. He was also president of the Medical and Physical Society and Dean of the Medical Faculty of the University of Bombay. He retired from the Indian Medical Service in 1888.

> I take this opportunity of alluding very briefly to the latest investigations with which I have become acquainted, from their great interest and value. Dr G A Hansen of Bergen is engaged in a series of inquiries which cannot but throw much light upon the origin and nature of leprosy. These point to the parasitic origin of the disease; and by which Dr Hansen's kindness I have myself seen the minute organisms (a species of *Bacterium)* which are present in living leprous matter taken from the interior of a 'tubercle.' Should these inquiries terminate in demonstration, it would be necessary to reconsider the topics I have just mentioned … If leprosy be shown to be a specific disease … then its propagation by hereditary transmission must be very limited … as regards leprosy it is not, perhaps, impossible to understand most of the signs of supposed heredity on the ground of local infection or possible contagion. I now rejoice to hear that Dr Hansen's investigations are likely to be soon made public, because of the light they will furnish where illumination is much needed.[29]

That was in 1873 and yet six years later Hansen was still attempting to fulfil the newly influential postulates of Koch. In order to demonstrate the infectiousness of the disease, it was necessary for him 'to transfer the bacilli experimentally to animals and human beings'.[30] He had attempted unsuccessfully to transfer the disease to rabbits and, becoming convinced of the impossibility of doing this, began to try to transfer the bacilli to human subjects. This was not the first time that experimenters in Bergen had attempted to transmit the disease to themselves or others. Danielssen and several members of the hospital had previously offered themselves as subjects and, in 1857, Danielssen had even inoculated patients with syphilis and scabies.[31] Hansen was also under considerable professional pressure because there had been a public dispute about who had discovered the bacillus first. Albert Neisser had visited him in Norway and, after Hansen had shown him his discovery, had returned to Germany to publish the discovery as his own.[32] Irgens argues that Hansen was a courageous man of conviction who had to fight to demonstrate the role of the bacillus, to secure priority for his discovery, in the face of a rival claim, and to struggle to achieve practical results in order to validate his discovery.[33]

---

29 Ibid., p. 27.

30 Vogelsang, 'Gerhard Henrik Armauer Hansen', p. 292.

31 Knut Blom, 'Armauer Hansen and Human Leprosy Transmission: Medical Ethics and Legal Rights', *International Journal of Leprosy*, 41/2 (1973): pp. 199–207, p. 202 .

32 G.L. Fite and H.W. Wade, 'The Contribution of Neisser to the Establishment of the Hansen bacillus as the Etiologic Agent of Leprosy and the So-Called Hansen-Neisser Controversy', *International Journal of Leprosy,* 23/4 (1955): pp. 418–28; Th. M. Vogelsang, 'The Hansen-Neisser Controversy, 1879–1880', *International Journal of Leprosy*, 31/1 (1963): pp. 74–80.

33 Lorentz M. Irgens, 'The Discovery of *Mycobacterium leprae*: A Medical Achievement in the Light of Evolving Scientific Methods', in Lorentz M. Irgens, Yngve Nedrebo, Sigurd Sandmo and Arne Skivenes (eds), *Leprosy* (Bergen, 2006), pp. 33–9.

Thus there were larger issues at stake for Hansen which served to obscure the humanity of his subject. Nielsdatter had suffered from leprosy for many years so was not at further risk of the disease, but he admitted that in all she had been required to bear 'some pain'. He told the court that 'He was of the opinion that he was justified in this even if the subject should have some pain, because he had chosen a subject who had suffered from leprosy for many years and therefore would not be exposed to a new disease'.[34] He was confident that her concern for her vision was unfounded. He went on to explain that he was quite sure that there would not have been a loss of vision, even if a leprous nodule had developed, because he had often extirpated nodules from patients' eyes and even succeeded in saving their eyesight.

One of the larger issues at stake was that of medical science and to that was twinned the issue of national value. Hansen gestured his submission to the values of the state in its own court of law by maintaining that 'the great scientific and national importance of finding the answer to the question' had 'forced him to act as he did'.[35] The opinion of the Director General of the Norwegian Health Directorate concurred with Hansen that 'The experiment had been carried out to contribute to a question with the most important consequences for science, the nation and the patients and that it had been performed by a man who had already made considerable contributions to the question mentioned'.[36] As Zachary Gussow points out, in the nineteenth century, Norway perfected a 'rational, basic medical science approach' to leprosy.[37] This consisted of a multi-pronged approach involving national leprosy censuses, the leprosy registry, the research centre for clinical study at Lungegaard Hospital, the establishment of four asylums, the commissioning of doctors to study the disease in other European countries, and the scientific research that led to the discovery of the bacillus. Carter's report clearly indicated the standing that the Norwegian experts on leprosy were accorded by the rest of the world:

> At the present day in no other part of the world, so far as I am aware, are there equally complete, well-conducted, and successful leper-asylums as in Norway; and the physicians in charge are often eminent men, versed in modern science

[34] Vogelsang, 'Gerhard Henrik Armauer Hansen', p. 292.

[35] Ibid., p. 292.

[36] Ibid., p. 293. Leprosy control in Norway, where the disease was endemic, focused on a system of medical registration, legislation, hospitalization and research. Surveys were conducted in 1836, 1845 and 1852, and a medical superintendent for leprosy, Ove Guldberg Høegh (1814–1863), was appointed to be responsible for a national leprosy register, established in 1856. St. Jørgen's Hospital and three additional hospitals, as well as a research hospital, were dedicated to leprosy. Knowledge of the disease of leprosy entered a new era through the work of the Norwegians Daniel Cornelius Danielssen (1815–1894), Carl Wilhelm Boëck (1808–1875) and Gerhard Henrik Armauer Hansen (1841–1912).

[37] Gussow, *Leprosy, Racism, and Public Health*, p. 84.

> and of European repute. These advantageous conditions form a most striking contrast with what is known of the arrangement and direction of the lazarettos of old ... here is a decisive experiment, conducted in the eyes of watchful Europe by a nation which, though small in numbers, has yet acquired a high position in the intellectual ranks of the age.[38]

The measures adopted against leprosy in Norway occurred at a time when Norway was just starting to see itself as an emerging nation and as such had the energy to tackle social and economic problems. Gussow states that 'The history of leprosy in Norway is part of a history of Norwegian nationalism'.[39]

So in taking on Hansen, Kari Nielsdatter was taking on the emerging Norwegian nation and everything that it had staked on its international medical reputation. There is a stark and obvious contrast here between the power of Kari Nielsdatter and the medical authorities both in the court and in the hospital. Perhaps most striking is the attempt of the medical experts to use the latest psychiatric theories to discredit Nielsdatter by attributing her nervousness to hysteria and her imagination. For Kari Nielsdatter to express her sense of powerlessness, outrage and injustice, as well as to request attention to the physical damage inflicted upon her in the face of the medical authority of Hansen and his colleagues must have taken a great deal of courage.

Crucially she did find support both from her fellow sufferers as well as from the hospital pastor, Grönvold. Knut Blom, a Justice of the Supreme Court of Norway who retrospectively analysed the case, describes the process through which the complaint came to the attention of the court: 'a considerable commotion arose in the leprosy hospital after the event in question, and the pastor there reported the incident to the supervisory board. The Board interrogated the girl and also Hansen and then referred the matter to the Minister of Justice'.[40]Apparently Hansen was already unpopular with the patients mainly because of his insistence on the importance of isolation in order to prevent the spread of the disease; this incident may have provided them with a rallying point.[41] Blom even suggests that in fact the patients may have come to regard Hansen as 'the personification of the grievous fate that life and society had inflicted on them'.[42] Additionally, once Kari Nielsdatter received the support of the hospital pastor, Blom states that it would have been practically impossible for the court to dismiss the case quietly.[43] Nonetheless, in spite of this support, Kari Nielsdatter's plaintive and desperate attempts to protect herself both physically and then legally pale by comparison

[38] Carter, *Report on Leprosy*, p. 28.

[39] Gussow, *Leprosy, Racism, and Public Health*, p. 69.

[40] Blom, 'Armauer Hansen and Human Leprosy Transmission', p. 199.

[41] Ibid., p. 199.

[42] Ibid., p. 202.

[43] Ibid., p. 203.

with the power of the professional opinions that attempted to give the lie to her claims of pain and damage by expressing scepticism about her experiences.

Hansen argued that in carrying out the inoculation and in the light of earlier experiments carried out by the doctors at the hospital, he had done nothing exceptional or disturbingly novel. Blom suggests that if the previous experiments carried out by Danielssen were also carried out without consent, then there was little difference between them and those carried out by Hansen. He hypothesizes that the only reason why there had been no previous outcry against these earlier experiments may have been that no one in authority had been prepared to champion the complaints of the patients, especially as their social position would have been so weak that 'they would in fact have found it difficult to lodge a justified complaint'.[44] In his legal analysis, Blom states that while Hansen's medical colleagues 'greatly exerted themselves' to find 'extenuating circumstances for his conduct', legally there was no doubt at the time that a question of guilt was concerned: 'there is nothing in the records of the case to support the view that any of them regarded his conduct as correct'. He summarizes:

> Accordingly, I am prepared to assume that his conduct would have been acceptable in the light of the medical ethics of that period if he had first obtained the patient's consent, but that he overstepped the limit by carrying out the operation without consent, without giving the patient the necessary information, and, moreover, in spite of a certain amount of resistance on her part.[45]

The court considered the issue of consent as crucial, but the state medical authorities were prepared to split hairs on the penalty required. The opinion of the Director General of the Norwegian Health Directorate had been sought in advance of the court hearing, and he stated that the Hansen's experiment 'appeared to him to be no more radical than must be regarded as justifiable, if the patient had given him permission to carry it out, after having been told what might happen'. Given that the patient had neither advance notice nor a sense of what was involved, he was also prepared to make a very fine distinction about consent, possibly on the advice of a lawyer, stating that although the patient 'had not given her distinct permission for the operation, she had on the other hand not distinctly opposed it'. It has to be assumed, nonetheless, that this inference was derived prior to the encounter in the surgery.[46]

Happily the court heard Kari Nielsdatter's plea for justice and decided that Hansen should be deprived of his position as resident physician at the hospital and that he should pay the expenses connected with the case. We have no way of knowing how she managed the power differentials leading up to the court case.

---

44 Ibid.

45 Ibid.

46 Vogelsang, 'Gerhard Henrik Armauer Hansen', p. 292.

Neither do we know what happened to her afterwards. She seems to have received little acknowledgement of her sufferings in court and it is probably anachronistic to look for any mention of compensation for pain and damage, but to be fair, neither did she have to pay court costs. She could take satisfaction in the fact that she would no longer have Hansen around in the hospital to bother her, but we do not know how she fared with the other medical staff. The court was nonetheless mindful of what was at stake in the larger scheme of things and Hansen was permitted to continue his appointment as medical officer of health for leprosy in Norway until his death in 1912.

One of the things which Hansen undertook in this role was to attend the First International Leprosy Congress in 1897, in Berlin, where he proposed the following resolution: 'In countries in which leprosy forms foci or has great extension, isolation is the best means of preventing the spread of the disease. The system of obligatory notification and of observation and isolation, as carried out in Norway, is recommended to all nations with local self-government and a sufficient number of physicians.'[47] The congress passed the resolution on the basis of the damage that leprosy caused in a community. It was also accepted because of the perceived success of the Norwegian approach to the disease. This international attention to leprosy in Norway then connects Norwegian models of isolation with those adopted, for example, by the Americans at Molokai in Hawaii in 1866 and on Culion in the Philippines in 1906 and in Japan from 1907.

Children as Laboratory Subjects

Segregation and isolation practices varied from country to country, but from the 1890s, and following on from the first Leprosy Conference, in Berlin, in 1897, legislation was introduced in many countries to segregate leprosy sufferers.[48] The still unsolved medical problem of the mode of transmission of leprosy and the unspecified time it took to manifest itself both contributed to public health concerns and informed the diversity of responses. Institutions for segregation varied widely in character and in the degree of compulsion exerted on those who were segregated.[49] Once people with the disease were confined, the segregation of the sexes, control of sexual activity, forcible sterilization and abortion militated against the birth of children, while the question of what to do with those children who were born within the institutions was addressed with such solutions as the early removal of babies from their mothers, the establishment of orphanages,

[47] Isadore Dyer, 'The Berlin Leprosy Conference', *New Orleans Medical and Surgical Journal*, 50/6 (1897): p. 361.

[48] For legislation see the World Health Organisation, *Leprosy: A Survey of Recent Legislation* (Geneva, 1954), reprint from the *International Digest of Health Legislation*, 5 (1954): p. 6.

[49] Ibid., pp. 4–5.

organized adoptions and the training of children to work in leprosy asylums as nursing attendants and paramedical workers. As well as the practical problem of what to do with children born to the leprosy affected, there was a growing concern that leprosy might be communicated in childhood; therefore, children born to those with the disease and in primary contact with carriers of *M leprae*, were considered particularly susceptible.[50]

Culion, a remote island in the Philippines, was established in 1906, during the American occupation. It became known as the largest leprosy colony in the world and served as a prototype for mega-colonies of a similar kind elsewhere.[51] Between 1907 and 1930, 1,320 children were born there, and of these, 497 died, 688 were released to relatives and institutions, and 70 contracted leprosy before they could be released. From the mid-1920s between 70 and 80 children were born every year. From 1934 to 1938, the yearly average was 142.[52] Before the advent of the Second World War, more than 5,000 leprosy-affected people were detained there when the colony was at its height.

The policy of isolation of such large numbers of people presented the medical administrators with a logistical problem. Men and women, many of whom were young, were confined on a small island for the rest of their lives. In spite of the efforts of the authorities, the people resisted all attempts to keep them apart. The religious nursing sisters on the island kept the young women in dormitories under lock and key, and, even today, women who were taken to Culion will tell of the strict rules governing their behaviour.[53] One of the more troubling stories on Culion tells of the night in 1932 when the young men raided the women's dormitories and carried them off into the bush.[54] In another instance the women on the island were so angry at attempts to segregate them from the men, they made the Bureau of Health Director, Victor Heiser, flee in fear of his life.[55] In spite of the

50 In 1941, Robert Cochrane stated that 'leprosy is a child's disease', in R.G. Cochrane, *The Epidemiology, Pathology and Diagnosis of Child Leprosy (being the Dr Elizabeth Mathai Endowment Lectures, 1942–43, Delivered at the Medical College, University of Madras)* (Madras, 1943).

51 Cristina Verzola Rodriguez (ed.), *Culion Island: A Leper Colony's 100-Year Journey Toward Healing* (Philippines, 2003), p. 60. For critical articles on Culion see Warwick Anderson, 'Leprosy and Citizenship', *Positions: East Asia Cultures Critique*, 6 (1998): pp. 707–30, and Jo Robertson, 'Culion, the "Island of the Living Dead": Or Another Look at Leprosy and Citizenship', in Astri Andresen, Kari Tove Elvakken and Tore Gronlie (eds), *Politics of Prevention, Health Propaganda, and the Organisation of Hospitals, 1800–2000* (Bergen, 2005), pp. 8191.

52 Rodriguez, *Culion Island*, p. 81.

53 I visited Culion on several occasions notably in November 2004 and May 2006 and conducted interviews with people and nursing staff. Many of the people had been sent to the island as children, others had been born to leprosy-affected parents there.

54 Rodriguez, *Culion Island*, pp. 88–9.

55 Ibid., p. 80.

impact of leprosy on their lives, the people refused to surrender their sexual and reproductive rights.

Policies towards the newborn on the island changed over time and in response to the resources available. Before 1925, children up to six months of age were given to relatives outside the colony. The older infants and children were isolated in an institution, a children's home called Balala, just outside the colony proper, where they were looked after for five years. If, in that time, the children showed no signs of the disease, they were then adopted out. Actually, however, only about 40 children at a time were able to be accommodated in this nursery so that the great majority had to be left in the care of their parents. Generally authorities attempted to remove children at the earliest age possible. In 1925 and 1926 all non-leprous children two years of age or over were either released to relatives or transferred to the office of the Public Welfare Commissioner at Manila. In 1927, the children were removed from their parents at the age of 10 months and from 1928 all children over six months were regularly separated from their parents. Dr Casimiro B Lara, Chief Physician on Culion Island, explained to the commission that, ultimately, the plan was to remove the children at birth. This heart-rending task fell to the sisters of St Paul. Those children free of leprosy were then sent to Welfareville, in Manila, to be adopted or released to a relative.[56]

The settlement was also home to a contingent of medical people, both American and Philippine, amongst whom a growing sense of professionalization could be observed. In 1924, they organized themselves into the Culion Medical Society. The principles of its constitution reveal the aspirations of the group:

> The purposes of this society shall be to organize the physicians of the staff of the Culion Leper Colony, so that they may meet together for the purpose of free interchange of experiences and views and otherwise act together as a recognized body independent of official relationship; should there be such in this district, to bring other physicians with them for mutual benefit; and, together with the Manila Medical Society and such other local societies as may hereafter be organized in the Philippines, to form and maintain the Philippine Medical Association, thus maintaining connections with other organizations of physicians.[57]

As is evident from this statement of intent, the newly formed society saw itself connected to the Medical Society in Manila and to any other future societies within the Philippines. One of the outstanding figures to emerge at this time was an American, Dr Windsor Wade, the medical director on Culion, who became the

---

[56] Casimiro B. Lara, 'Annual Report of the Medical Section Culion Leper Colony for the Year Ending December 31, 1929', unpublished. Culion Archives, Culion Island, Palawan Group, the Philippines.

[57] From the unpublished minutes of the Culion Medical Society attached inside their record book as a Reprint from the *Journal of the Philippine Islands Medical Association* 6/10 (October 1926). Culion Archives, Culion Island, the Palawan Group, the Philippines.

editor of the new journal, the *International Journal of Leprosy*, which would serve as the main outlet for leprosy research up until 2004 and began its publishing life on Culion under the direction of Wade. Wade would be so influential that he would hold the position of President of the International Leprosy Association between the years 1946 and 1963. This core organization would make connections between medical people who were working in various parts of the world and coordinate efforts against leprosy internationally.[58] Up until the Second World War, Culion would enjoy a reputation as a premier centre for medical research into leprosy.

Early experimental work involved the administration of chaulmoogra preparations by injection for two and a half years to children between 10 months of age and five years, as a form of treatment.[59] The children, who had been born in the colony and were mostly still in the early stage of the disease, received intramuscular injections of the mixed chaulmoogra ethyl esters with 50 per cent iodine, either alone or alternatively with other chaulmoogra preparations. The study concluded that the treatment of early or slightly advanced cases of leprosy in children with the newer chaulmoogra preparations was attended by a large percentage of apparent cures.[60] Today we know that administration of chaulmoogra injections were not only horribly painful but also of very little efficacy. The trials were conducted amidst much optimism, yet within a short time they came under criticism, as is evident from a defensive report written two years later.[61]

---

58 The League of Nations Leprosy Commission took advice from Wade and helped him institute the International Leprosy Association. Correspondence between H.W. Wade and Etienne Burnet (5 September 1931) League of Nations Archives, Geneva.

59 Chaulmoogra oil from *Hydnocarpus wightiana* and *Hydnocarpus anthelmintica* was used in traditional Ayurvedic medicine in India for the treatment of leprosy and other skin conditions. It was introduced into Western medicine in the late nineteenth century and became the treatment of choice for a decade between the 1920s and 1930s. Victor Heiser introduced the Mercado method to the Philippines which enabled its administation by hypodermic injection. See John Parascandola, 'Chaulmoogra Oil and the Treatment of Leprosy'. Available at: www.lhncbc.nlm.nih.gov/lhc/docs/published/2003/pub2003048.pdf (accessed 2 February 2010).

60 C. Nicolas and E. Roxas-Pineda, 'Results of Anti-Leprosy Treatment of Children in the Culion Leprosy Colony by C Nicolas and E Roxas-Pineda of the Medical Section, Culion Leprosy Colony', p. 4, unpublished mss, Culion Archives, Culion Island, the Palawan Group, the Philippines.

61 Manuscripts of Investigations prepared in 1929: 'Progress of Leprosy Treatment at the Culion Leper Colony' by C.B. Lara, Chief Physician Culion Leper Colony Philippine Health Service, unpublished mss, Culion Archives, Culion Island, the Palawan Group, the Philippines. In response to criticism, Lara wrote that 'It is probable that such propaganda, together with the above cited authoritative statements, has created a deeply rooted impression that leprosy treatment at Culion has been, is, and will probably, continue to be a failure … Since then, however, the results have been more gratifying, and present indications give us reason to expect further progress in the future, provided that the present conditions will continue to obtain. It would seem, therefore, desirable to retrace the progress of the

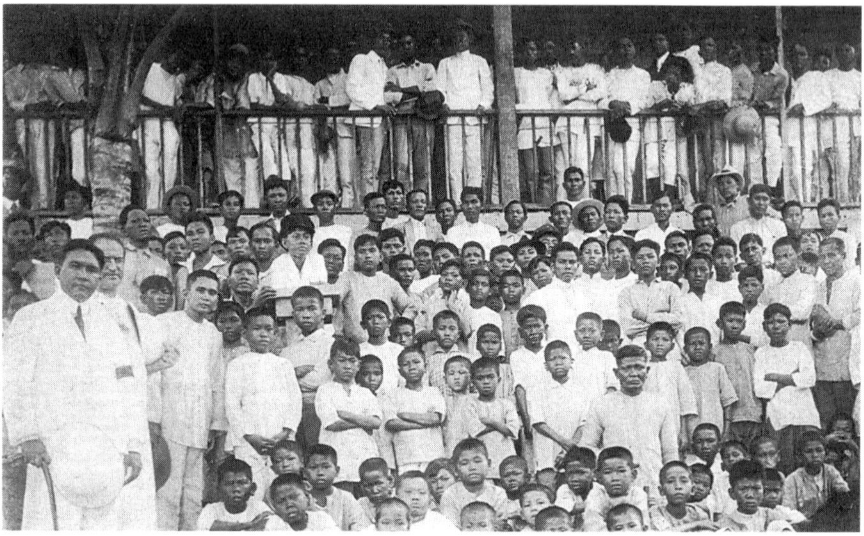

Figure 6.1 Leprosy-affected boys at Culion Leprosarium, the Philippines, 1920
Source: Used by permission.

Such studies received renewed encouragement and justification from international efforts to coordinate medical research against leprosy. In response to a request at the Strasbourg Leprosy Conference in 1923, the League of Nations Health Committee began a worldwide inquiry into leprosy. In 1926, at the Sixth Session of the Health Organization of the League of Nations, Professor Chagas, the Brazilian physician responsible for the discovery of Chagas disease who served as an elected member of the Committee of Hygiene for the League of Nations, described leprosy as a medical and social issue requiring the cooperation of all civilized countries and needing a coherent approach.[62] In a speech to the Leprosy Committee of the League of Nations, he outlined the fundamental questions requiring urgent attention as subjects for international research centres. Close and sustained examination of the children of leprosy-affected people had the potential to shed light on early diagnosis, time of incubation, intrauterine or inherited infection and/or immunity. Implicit within these subjects for research was a narrowing of focus upon the family and in particular the unborn child. No one knew how leprosy was transmitted and how long it took for it to be transmitted: doctors knew that the disease was spread between individuals, but were puzzled that it did not spread more often between

treatment work at Culion and to present the actual situation; to show evidence not only that Culion is not an unsuitable place "for the effective administration of treatment" but also that a large proportion of even advanced cases can be, or has been, successfully treated'.

[62] C. Chagas, *Rapport préliminaire sur le problème de la lèpre, préséntе par le prof.* [C]C [1926], C.252 M 96 1926 pp. 95–7 also CH 466 Vol No 299. League of Nations Archives, Geneva.

spouses and they wondered if there was something in the human organism that either favoured or formed an obstacle to transmission of the disease. They were still unsure of the precise diagnosis of the symptoms of the disease, particularly in the early phases. They were equally in need of information of the time of incubation, which seemed to be very long. Most pertinently there were unanswered questions around the possibility of intrauterine transmission: was the disease transmitted *in utero*, through breast milk, or by skin to skin contact? The provisional report of the Secretary for the specially convened Leprosy Commission, Etienne Burnet, echoed the view that 'the time had come to organize large scale experiments'. Amongst other statements, he suggested that the children of lepers were 'particularly valuable material' and it was 'highly desirable that every country affected by leprosy should have one or several asylums for children separated at birth from their parents and, if need be, another asylum, or special wards, for their children who have remained in contact with lepers for any length of time'.[63]

The medical people on Culion were not slow to appreciate the opportunity that the large number of people in the settlement represented for scientific inquiry. The recommendations of the League of Nations enabled the doctors on Culion to turn a liability into a rich field for research, and the annual reports reveal an appreciation of the children as offering a unique opportunity for understanding leprosy. Most of the medical people who worked in leprosy certainly did not do so for recognition within the medical fraternity. As much as leprosy-affected people have been marginalized, so too have leprosy workers, both medical and paramedical. Wade and Lara and the other doctors on Culion worked in isolated conditions fuelled only by their passion for the work. If they were medically ambitious, their ambition was dedicated to solving the problem of the disease. Nonetheless the problems presented by the disease and the public health policies of the time conspired to create a climate in which people became a medical resource and the disadvantages of the situation were turned to experimental advantage, resulting in a very real impact on the people affected by the disease.

A study in 1938 of the earliest recognizable manifestations and clinical course of the disease undertook observation of 629 children. These children had been in continuous contact with leprosy-affected parents for from a few months to several years. This study concluded that the early development of the disease could be seen in an appreciable portion before the age of three years and the earliest lesions developed on parts of the body that had most frequently and most intimately come into contact with the source of infection. It describes the study group as children

[63] *Commission pour l'étude de la lèpre*, 1928. On 14 May 1928, the Leprosy Commission drew up a programme, and Etienne Burnet, as Secretary for the Commission, embarked on a study tour to the Baltic Countries, the Americas, and the Far East, including India, Malay States, Java, the Philippines, Canton, Shanghai, Japan and Honolulu. His report was published as League of Nations: Health Organisation, *Report on the Study Tour of the Secretary of the Leprosy Commission in Europe, South America and the Far East (January 1929–June 1930)*, CH 887 (Geneva, 1930). League of Nations Archives, Geneva.

under observation for at least one year.[64] Unsurprisingly, the following year, 67 children in the colony were reported as having to be 'dropped to the leper [*sic*] list'. Eighteen children had developed lesions since the previous year and 49 had shown the first recognizable lesions at the beginning of the year. The experiment must have continued because the report for 1939 revealed that 'only children two years of age or older had been transferred from the Colony to the Balala Nursery'.

> Excluding clinical lepers [*sic*] detected in 1938, but including those who became leprous in 1939, the average nonleprous child population (age range from newly born to about four years) for the year was 266. The proportion becoming leprous during the past 12 months was therefore about 18 percent. This figure would be considerably higher if only the children above one year of age (147) are to be considered (i.e. about 33 percent).[65]

But they already knew this. In a study of 398 children of leprous parents living in Culion on 31 December 1924, Rodriguez found 14.8 per cent of the children were bacteriologically positive, 2.8 per cent with distinct clinical manifestations, and 24.4 per cent with suspicious manifestations of the disease. It is difficult not to suspect that the children who had been left with their parents were there for the sake of the study, a study which had been all too successful in demonstrating that children were particularly susceptible to leprosy and if left in contact with affected leprosy sufferers would stand a one-in-three chance of getting it.

Experimental work using children continued until the end of the war. A report in 1945 reveals that all the children born on Culion before 1932 had, for 13 years, served as material for regular observations and special studies concerning early leprosy. Observations of these children began at birth and continued every two months, in some cases more often, for as long as the children remained in the colony.[66] These studies had already yielded new information which could only have been obtained from uninterrupted and continuing observations. It looked forward to further analysis of the existing data for a better understanding of the disease as well as continuing the observations on the same group of children for the duration of their lifetime. It believed that a fresh approach to treatment and prophylaxis of the disease might emerge from the more recent studies. It therefore

64 Casimiro B. Lara, 'Early Leprosy in Children of Lepers: Further Observations on the Early, Definitely, Identifiable Leprosy Lesions, Culion Leprosy Colony' (submitted for publications 27 May 1938), unpublished mss, Culion Archives, Culion Island, the Palawan Group, the Philippines.

65 'Annual Report of the Medical Section Culion Leper Colony for the Calendar Year 1939', unpublished mss, Culion Archives, Culion Island, the Palawan Group, the Philippines.

66 Observations were interrupted between January 1942 and July 1945, because of the war and the subsequent lack of sufficient, specially trained examiners, but after August 1945 observations were resumed as before.

urged 'that this material – the children of lepers' would continue to be observed from birth. At the same time it emphasized that 'all possible care and consideration should be given to the human aspects involved'.[67]

But there was an even greater problem. In a tragic irony, early separation from their mothers increased the likelihood of infant mortality, for in the attempt to save children from leprosy, many died from gastrointestinal diseases which would likely have arisen for lack of access to breast milk. By the 1930s, the death rate per 1,000 children was 348.48. The 1930 report expresses this:

> Of the 28 children who died in 1930, 12 were born in the same year, and 20 were only 1 year old or younger. The infant mortality was about 40 percent. This is surprising since the artificial feeding has undoubtedly given more satisfactory results than in the previous year. A large proportion of the deaths was due to respiratory and digestive tract infections; this may suggest deficient vitamin A in the diet, a condition that is considered to predispose to such affections. During the last quarter of the year, cod liver oil was given systematically to the older children but this could not be done for the nurslings without provoking diarrhea.[68]

The next year showed only a slight improvement and revealed that the attrition rate had risen since artificial feeding had commenced in 1928. In the average population of 5,548, the infant mortality rate was 32.6 per cent. This was slightly lower than the rate for the previous year, 1930, which was 40 per cent, but it was still distinctly higher than for 1929 and 1927 which was 19.4 per cent for each year, and for 1928, which was 26.5 per cent.[69]

The doctors of course were damned if they did and damned if they didn't. When new babies had been removed from their parents, they died like flies. If they were left with their parents, they contracted the disease. The doctors must have been shocked by the success of their studies because they soon expressed the urgent necessity of 'segregating all children of lepers as early as possible after birth, if they are to be protected from the infection and thus prevented, besides from propagating and perpetuating the disease'.[70] Culion had become a nursery for leprosy and the babies were the test tubes.

---

[67] 'Annual Report of the Medical Section, Culion Leper Colony for the Year 1945', unpublished mss, Culion Archives, Culion Island, the Palawan Group, the Philippines.

[68] 'Annual Report of the Medical Section Culion Leper Colony for the Year ending December 31, 1930 by Casimiro B Lara, Chief Physician', p. 46, unpublished mss, Culion Archives, Culion Island, the Palawan Group, the Philippines.

[69] 'Annual Report of the Medical Section Culion Leper Colony for the Year Ending December 31, 1931', p 54, unpublished mss, Culion Archives, Culion Island, the Palawan Group, the Philippines.

[70] 'Annual Report of the Medical Section Culion Leper Colony for the Calendar Year 1939', p. 17, unpublished mss, Culion Archives, Culion Island, the Palawan Group, the Philippines.

Culion was not unique. Children served as an observational resource elsewhere too. As part of their activities, the Leprosy Commission to the League of Nations circulated an 'Enquiry Concerning Leprosy' including one question about the 'Regime and Institutions for the Children of Lepers'. Responses to this question included reports, photographs and plans of institutions throughout the world. On the basis of the responses to the questionnaire, the specifics of practices conducted in leprosy institutions such as Surinam, Fiji, Macao and Malaysia can be identified. Photographs of children receiving prophylactic oral doses of chaulmoogra in Paramaribo, Surinam, can be seen side-by-side with photographs of children taking part in sports days at the Federal Leper Settlement in the Straits Settlements of the Federated Malay Straits.[71] In leprosy colonies throughout the world where people were isolated and segregated, administrators were faced with the same problem. People did not die from leprosy, they lived for decades with the disease and they were usually capable of living, working and reproducing within the context of a lifetime of incarceration. The policy in the Philippines came to represent one possible solution to the problem and the policies in Japan represented another equally valid approach.[72]

Japanese Leprosaria and Birth Control Policies

In the Edo period (1603–1867), in Japan, leprosy was variously attributed to an inherited poison passed through the blood, food poisoning (from eating fish, for example), or the result of living in a certain environment. Some of the people with the disease lived either a semi-religious life or as mendicants, gathering around sacred sites and hot springs.[73] As in most countries throughout the world, the status of a leprosy-affected person depended upon the economic resources at their command.

---

[71] Studies on transmission of leprosy to children were conducted at Culion (Jose Rodriguez, 'Studies on Early Leprosy in Children of Lepers', *Philippine Journal of Science* 31/2 (1929): pp. 115–46, in Dutch Guiana (P.H.J. Lampe, 'Fate of Children Born of Leprous Parents in the Groot-Chatillon Leprosy Asylum', *International Journal of Leprosy* 1/1 (1933): pp. 5–15) and also in India.

[72] 'In the Philippine Islands marriage between patients is also allowed, but the children are separated as soon after birth as possible and brought up in special institutions. The incidence of leprosy in these children is in proportion to the age when separated from their parents. It is sometimes possible to get children whose parents have leprosy adopted by healthy people' and 'It is reported that in Japan marriage of patients in institutions is allowed provided that the male is sterilised. Few children are said to be born in these institutions'. Government of India, Central Advisory Board of Health, *Report on Leprosy and its Control in India*, p. 30.

[73] Burns, 'From "Leper Villages" to Leprosaria', pp. 105–7.

Japanese policy on leprosy in the modern era became tied to its sense of itself as a nation and national pride. The numbers affected by the disease were considered a national disgrace.[74] Dr Kensuke Mitsuda (1876–1964) who was the most influential leprologist in the country lamented the impact of the statistics on the image of Japan abroad: 'Japan, a country proud of the purity of its own pedigree and blood, is now known as the world's leading leprosy nation, far worse than European and American nations.' He was deeply concerned that it would be considered 'barbarous, uncivilized and primitive'.[75] In 1907 the (Old) Leprosy Prevention Law was enacted, having application mainly to vagrants affected by the disease. As part of this initiative, the country was divided into five regions and a public sanatorium was established in each region. After the First World War, the new public health policy moved more strongly towards ensuring absolute segregation by expanding sanatoria and, among other measures, providing abortion 'when requested by a patient'. In addition the 1931 revision of the (Old) Leprosy Prevention Law gave superintendents the authority to discipline inmates, adding a dimension of criminality to leprosy confinement in Japan. This was intensified with the use of cells to imprison recalcitrant inmates or those who had been convicted of a crime.

From 1915 onwards, patients who requested permission to marry had also to consent to sterilization.[76] An expansion programme began with the purpose of establishing a system of state-run sanatoria in 1927 and a mega-colony like Culion, called Oshima Seishoen Sanatorium, was erected on an island in the Inland Sea.[77] In 1931 the (Old) Leprosy Prevention Law was widened in scope to apply to everyone suffering from leprosy, rather than those who were vagrant and this legislation was accompanied by the establishment of a national or state-run system of sanatoria. The 2005 report of the Japan Law Foundation: Verification Committee Concerning Hansen's Disease Problem stated that the 'The Leprosy Prevention Law was established immediately before the fifteen year period of war [1931-1945] in which Japan fought in Asia and the Pacific … In the midst of this prolonged war period, the policy on Hansen's Disease was also placed within the framework of a eugenic policy to create better citizens who were superior physically and psychologically'.[78]

---

[74] In 1900 there were 30,359 leprosy-affected people in Japan and in 1923, there were 100,000 reportedly affected by the disease. Burns discusses the shame that these figures represented as well as the collapse of the distinction between actual sufferers and those who were in the same familial 'lineage' as those with the disease. Ibid., pp. 108–9.

[75] Japan Law Foundation, 'Verification Report', p. 121.

[76] Fujio Ohtani, *The Walls Crumble: The Emancipation of Persons Affected by Hansen's Disease in Japan* (Tokyo, 1998), p. 37.

[77] Ibid., p. 70.

[78] Japan Law Foundation, 'Verification Report', p. 23.

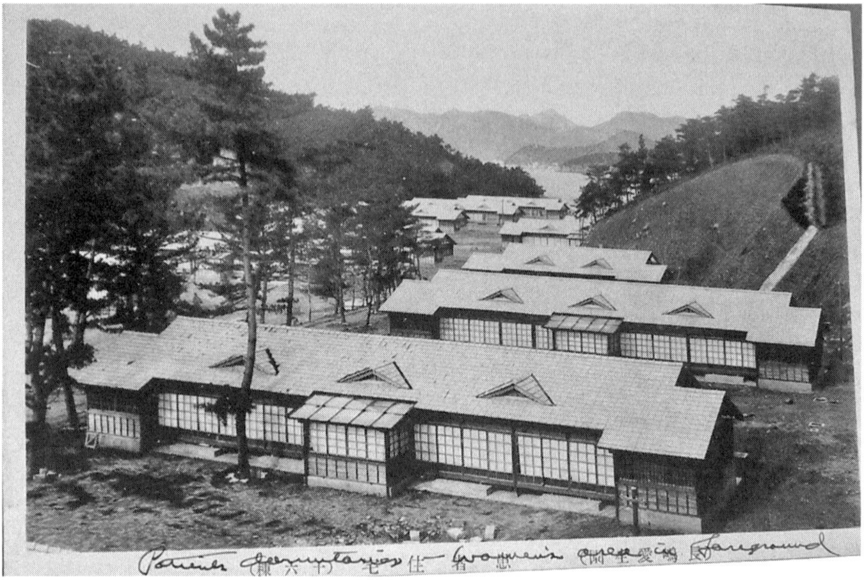

Figure 6.2 Patients' dormitories, women's area in the foreground at Nagashima Leprosarium, Japan, 1931

Source: Used by permission.

The Leprosy Free Prefectures Campaign entailed removal of all leprosy-affected people into sanatoria. Then in 1948 the Eugenic Protection Law legalized sterilization and the termination of pregnancies of people who were at risk of producing defective descendants.[79] This included 'ill and physically weak people, women who had given birth many times, and poor people, whose children would become ill or weak or could become delinquent due to bad surroundings.'[80] The clause including people with leprosy was ambiguous. Optional sterilization could be exercised 'if the person or the person's spouse has leprosy and it may be contagious to the person's descendents', in spite of the well-known fact that leprosy was not hereditary.[81] Doctors reasoned that when a 'mentally competent person gave consent, the illegality of sterilisation, even for medical reasons, could be exempted.' The Verification Report adds that 'Whether or not the 'consent of the patient' in a Hansen's disease sanatorium really meant a free decision of the patient, was never asked'.[82] So 'Sterilisation of Hansen's disease patients continued to be carried out as a fait accompli, even with the possibility that it was

[79] Ohtani states that 'nearly all of those who reside on state-operated sanatoria have been surgically sterilized', *The Walls Crumble*, p. 37.

[80] Japan Law Foundation, 'Verification Report', pp. 53–4.

[81] Ibid., p. 54.

[82] Ibid., p. 52.

in violation of the Penal Law'.[83] It had been the practice since 1915 and became a precondition for marriage for those confined in sanatoria.[84] Even after the war, the government continued its policy of increasing admissions and accommodation within the sanatoria, admitting 4,500 in 1949. The committee found that 'After the war was lost, the idea of enhancing the eugenic policy to build a "civilized nation" was very strong among the population policy makers and doctors at the time'.[85]

The establishment of national leprosaria in Japan coincided with the building of leprosy colonies and the enactment of legislation in other parts of the world.[86] This was the period of the 'model' leprosy colony or settlement influenced by Molokai, Hawaii and the Culion Leper Colony and the hospital and agricultural colony of Fontilles in Spain that had been established in 1907.[87]

Japan's policy on leprosy was continually reported internationally without adverse comment and was in fact considered praiseworthy. *Leprosy in India* in 1935 contained notes from a journey to Japan by Dr Isaac Santra. He reported the standard practice in Japan in which 'every patient on death is autopsied' and there was a 'vast collection of material' at Aiseien Nagashima, Okayama. He also learnt that the married male patients were sterilized on their own consent.[88] He described how at Oshima, since 1909, 600 had died and the viscera of 230 had been preserved in 10 per cent formalin. He was also aware that autopsies were being performed on foetuses, as well, because he stated that *M leprae* had been found in the viscera of foetuses, but that these bacilli were difficult to differentiate from the tubercle bacillus.[89]

From a medical point of view, there was nothing noteworthy about the standard practice of autopsy, even though in this instance, everyone who died was routinely subjected to it. The most offensive aspect of this process of autopsy was the

---

83 Ibid.

84 Ohtani, *The Walls Crumble*, p. 63.

85 Japan Law Foundation, 'Verification Report', p. 54.

86 The (Old) Leprosy Prevention Law of 1907 was in concert with the Berlin and Bergen International Leprosy Conferences of 1897 and 1909 which recommended segregation. In Nigeria, in March 1908, a Lepers' Ordinance was passed for the Colony of Southern Nigeria. In 1905, legislation was put into place authorizing the creation of the Culion Leper Colony Reservation. The United States of America with the provocation of John Early, a leprosy-affected veteran of the American-Spanish war, and the support of William Danner from the American Mission to Lepers, enacted legislation in 1917 to create a national leprosarium.

87 J. Bernabeu-Mestre and T. Ballester-Artigues, 'Disease as a Metaphorical Resource: The Fontilles Philanthropic Initiative in the Fight against Leprosy 1901–1932', *Social History of Medicine*, 17/3 (2004): pp. 409–21.

88 Dr Isaac Santra, 'Notes on Leprosy in Japan', *Leprosy in India* (1953): pp. 26–7.

89 Santra ended his report saying that 'Places of isolation are not isolated places in Japan. The leper [*sic*] is happy and active … All the conveniences of the West are combined with the hospitality of the East'. He reported that the doctors very generously shared their work with him saying that 'Nothing is secret in Japan except the military'. Ibid., p. 28.

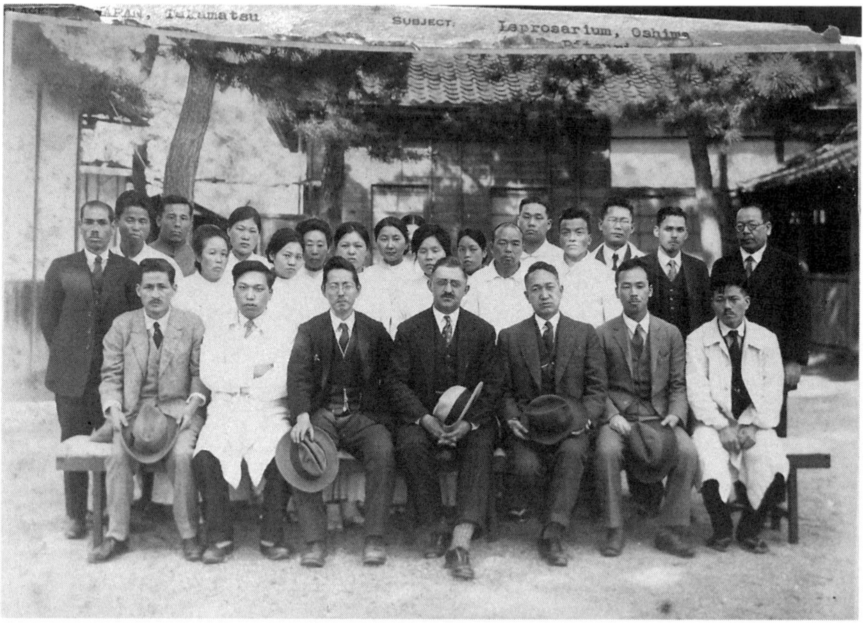

Figure 6.3 Dr H.W. Wade (medical director of Culion) with members of staff from Oshima Leprosarium, Japan, 1931

Source: Used by permission.

discovery that body parts were indiscriminately stored in various leprosaria, rather than receiving a proper burial once they had served their investigatory purpose. In a disease that symbolically implies disembodiment, this treatment seems to be the ultimate insult. Additionally, if consent had been obtained for sterilization, then there can be no objection either. Yet from the subsequent testimonies of survivors, obtaining consent from inmates under sanatorium conditions was to compel them to submit to a procedure within which they had little choice, if they wished to exercise their right to live anything like a normal life. The evidence provided from foetuses, in the light of the discoveries of the Verification Report, begs the question that it may have very possibly included those of neonates killed at birth. Nonetheless in 1935, no one who worked in the leprosy world and who read Santra's report felt compelled to object to what was happening in Japan.

Although Japanese policy was well known internationally, its applicability to places like India was still debated. One of the significant differences between Japan and the rest of the world at this stage was that outside Japan sterilization in the case of leprosy was not carried out for eugenic purposes. At the inaugural 'All India Leprosy Workers Conference' in Wardha, India, in 1948, for example, Dr Dharmendra presented a paper on the place of sterilization and particularly vasectomy in leprosy control, arguing that it could not be considered on eugenic

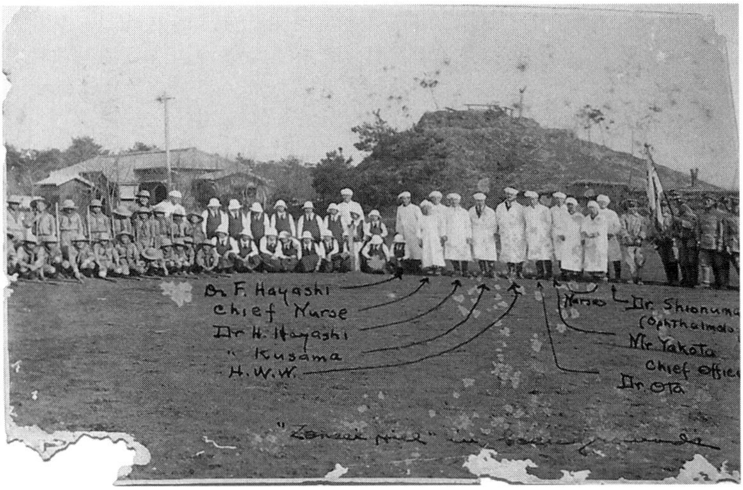

Figure 6.4 Dr H.W. Wade (medical director of Culion), Japan, 1931
Note: This photograph shows him as 'HWW'.
Source: Used by permission.

grounds because there was no evidence that the transmission of the disease had a familial basis. However, he considered that sterilization did have a place principally in infective or suitable cases, provided it was on a voluntary basis, in order to prevent the spread of the disease.[90] He drew heavily on the example of Japan and cited a considerable body of literature from Japanese studies explaining their national policy, the matter of consent, the negligible impact of sterilization on the sex drive as well as its function in preventing pregnancies which were considered to exacerbate the disease. (The Japanese doctors felt that in permitting sterilization they were in fact enabling leprosy-affected people to enjoy normal conjugal relations without the complications of reproduction.) He then outlined a proposal for sterilization in India. This proposal listed likely candidates such as couples in institutions who wished to pursue married life, those who committed crimes of a sexual nature, and those living in informal or self-settled leprosy camps where children may be exposed to the disease.[91] In it, Dharmendra argued that the most common ground for sterilization in cases of leprosy was the prevention of the spread of the disease by preventing the birth of children who would be exposed to leprosy.[92] The discussion which followed was quite divided and was summed up by the Chairman as being about a highly controversial topic, but everyone was in agreement that there should be no

[90] Dr Dharmendra, 'The Place of Vasectomy in Leprosy Control', *Leprosy in India, Special Issue: All India Leprosy Conference, Wardha*, 20/1 (1948): pp. 28–31 and pp. 63–75 respectively.

[91] Dharmendra, 'The Place of Vasectomy in Leprosy Control', p. 69.

[92] 'Social and Economic Aspects of Leprosy', p. 29.

vasectomy on a compulsory basis.[93] The issue of consent made all the difference to the acceptance of sterilization. It became clear long after that although the doctors in Japan seemed to believe that consent had been obtained and in fact assured their overseas medical visitors of this, many, many people who were sterilized would later reveal that they really didn't have a choice.[94]

Finally in 1953, the (New) Leprosy Prevention Law was enacted and by 1955, 91 per cent of all leprosy-affected people in Japan were isolated. Although Robert Hastings, the American editor of the *International Journal of Leprosy*, points out that the (New) Leprosy Prevention Law differed little from laws still operational in various states of the United States at that time, and that similar legislation was still in existence in most parts of the world, this new Japanese legislation was enacted at a time when leprosy institutions throughout the world were beginning to consider opening their doors. The new drugs promin and dapsone were making a dramatic difference to the symptoms of leprosy and people who had been isolated from society for years were struggling to re-enter the outside world. A WHO study on legislation published in 1952 stated that 'At the present time, the compulsory isolation of lepers [*sic*] is still the most commonly employed method of control in use in those countries where leprosy is endemic. Doubt has been thrown on the efficiency of this method by the observation that leprosy has not always diminished where such a policy was vigorously applied … It is for this reason that the Committee recommended that "only infectious cases need to be subjected to some form of isolation"'.[95]

I want to argue that while it was inexcusable, what happened in Japan should be seen within the context of policies throughout the world in which people with the disease were isolated and segregated. What happened in the Philippines was one logical consequence of those policies while what happened in Japan was the other extreme. Cohabitation in leprosy asylums is discussed in the context of sterilization in 1946 by Rogers and Muir in their standard medical textbook on leprosy:

> Owing to difficulties in backward tropical countries in the safe separation of infants from their leper parents early enough to prevent the possibility of their infection, the most effective methods of preventing married patients from begetting children is by sterilization … the marriage of lepers in institutions should only be permitted subject to the same operation being first performed, as has been done by the Americans in Panama. Such expedients are only required when the circumstances do not permit of the strict enforcement of the general rule to isolate the sexes completely in leper settlements.[96]

[93] Ibid., p. 31.

[94] For personal testimonies of people confined in Japan see IDEA website. Available at: www.idealeprosydignity.org/OralHistoryWeb/Japan-Nishimura.html (accessed 5 February 2010)

[95] World Health Organisation, *Leprosy: A Survey of Recent Legislation*, pp. 3–36.

[96] Sir Leonard Rogers and Ernest Muir, *Leprosy*, 3rd edn (Bristol, 1946), p. 130.

Here the 'marriage of lepers in institutions' should only be permitted 'subject to the same operation', that is vasectomy 'being first performed' otherwise the general rule of isolating the sexes should be 'strictly enforced'. Either option would result in preventing newborns from becoming infected with leprosy. While the Verification Committee 2005 report argued that Japan began ignoring international approaches to leprosy control from 1923 after the Strasbourg Conference,[97] I would argue that it was only after the Second World War (and after the impact that the new drugs had on leprosy) that Japanese policies began to be significantly out of step with the rest of the world and instead of loosening their segregation policies, the Japanese tightened them.[98]

In Japan and throughout the world, administrators were caught by an isolation system of their own making. They either had to segregate the sexes for the lifetime of the inhabitants, permit their colonies to become breeding grounds for children who were candidates to be the next generation of leprosy-affected sufferers, or they had to sterilize their inmates, having 'obtained consent'. In some cases, they went to extreme lengths to prevent unwanted births. One Japanese woman's experience gives a harrowing insight into the ambivalent mindset of those entrusted with medical surveillance and the limited choices and painful realities for colony inmates. When she was discovered to be seven months pregnant, she was strongly advised to undergo an abortion: she remembers the child moving its hands and legs on the operating table and the nurse covering the nose and mouth of the baby to stop it from breathing and saying to her 'it is a cute girl and looks very like you'.[99]

Events such as this facilitated the creation of the veritable charnel house that the 2005 Verification Committee's investigation revealed in the sanatoria of Japan:

> The 114 fetus samples, many surgery-extracted materials, and over 2,000 pathological samples, all resting in silence at national sanatoria for Hansen's disease, etc. – what are they saying to us quietly? Are they not powerfully asking us the question 'What have they done?' – to all those who have been involved in the medical treatment of Hansen's disease in this country until now? Even if these corpses are carefully commemorated and respectfully buried, these facts must never be trivialized or forgotten by any means.[100]

The poetry of Haruko Tsuda (1912–1963), who was isolated at 18, expresses in 1961 the grief of the people who were subject to these policies:

---

97 Japan Law Foundation, 'Verification Report', p. 121.

98 Robert Hastings, 'Review of Ohtani, Fujio, *The Walls Crumble*', *International Journal of Leprosy* (September 2000). Available at: http://findarticles.com/p/articles/mi_qa3754/is_200009/ai_n8925248/ (accessed 25 October 2011).

99 Michio Miyasaka, 'Punishing Paternalism: An Ethical Analyses of Japan's Leprosy Control Policy', *Eubios Journal of Asian and International Bioethics*, 19/4 (2009): pp. 103–7, p. 105.

100 Japan Law Foundation, 'Verification Report', p. 68.

> Lying amidst the tattered dark blue bedclothes
> I feel like a convict
> Not permitted to give life
> In the twilight years of life
> No child to muse about
> Time passes slowly
> When waiting for death
> While not one familiar face comes to call.[101]

The segregation of people in Japan continued until 1996, well after leprosy colonies throughout the rest of the world had ceased to function as isolation centres. One of the leprosy-affected residents of Suruga sanotarium, Tokio Nishimura, describes the impact of the 2001 landmark Kumamoto District court ruling that the (New) Leprosy Prevention Law of 1953 was unconstitutional:

> The most painful thing for me was that we couldn't have children. This was the crime of the government. That's why we wanted to fight and regain our human rights in court. When the Leprosy Prevention Law was abolished in 1996, nothing changed. No change in the community's attitude, no change in anything. The change was brought at the time of the Kumamoto District court case. The government apologized officially for their mistake, and it was only then when things started to move forward. Some of us started to think about leaving the sanatoria, and some have done that. Through this court case, we started to become different. We started to feel different. Each one of us started to recover our humanity. We started to change. People started to leave the sanatorium, people started to resume communication with their families, people started to go freely to the local health facilities. None of this was seen before the Kumamoto District lawsuit.[102]

The response to the court action raised the most obvious question as to how these violations of human rights could have taken place and part of the job of the Verification Committee was to answer that question for the sake of the future. With a great deal of frankness and a disarming sense of shared responsibility, the committee analysed the contributing factors. Many of these were unique to Japan, but this instance of the treatment of people affected by leprosy should also be placed within the international context of medical research into the disease from the late nineteenth century onwards. The Japanese experience should also be viewed within the context of the public health policies against leprosy throughout the world and if in fact the rest of the world knew how the Japanese were dealing

[101] Available at: www.idealeprosydignity.org/OralHistoryWeb/Japanese%20Poets.html (accessed 5 February 2010).

[102] Available at: www.idealeprosydignity.org/OralHistoryWeb/Japan-Nishimura.html (accessed 5 February 2010).

with their leprosy-affected and how they cited this approach as a possible option in the raft of measures available to public health administrators. More importantly, the struggles of leprosy-affected people for legal status and respect, as people, rather than as medical resources, span the modern history of the disease and in spite of their seeming helplessness, these people with the disease called leprosy have managed to salvage dignity and recognition.

Bibliography

Manuscript Sources

Culion Museum and Archives, Culion Is., the Palawan Group, the Philippines Annual Reports: 1929–1945.

League of Nations Archives, Geneva Leprosy Commission.

Printed Primary Sources

Armauer Hansen, G.H. and C. Looft, *Leprosy: In its Clinical and Pathological Aspects*, trans. Norman Walker (Bristol: John Wright & Co, 1895).

Blom, K., 'Armauer Hansen and Human Leprosy Transmission: Medical Ethics and Legal Rights', *International Journal of Leprosy*, 41/2 (1973): pp. 199–207.

Burnet, E. *Provisional Report Presented to the Leprosy Commission at its Meeting in Tokyo in April 1930* (CH 836/Leprosy 7).

Burnet, E. *Provisional Report Presented to the Leprosy Commission at its Meeting in Tokyo in April 1930: Consideration of Urgent Matters to which the Commission drew attention at its May Session, 1928* (CH Leprosy 7a), League of Nations Archive, Geneva.

Carter, H.V., *On Leprosy and Elephantiasis with Plates* (London: George Edward Eyre and William Spottiswoode, 1874).

Carter, Henry Vandyke, *Report on Leprosy and Leprosy Asylums in Norway with References to India* (London: George Edward Eyre and William Spottiswoode, 1874).

C. Chagas, *Rapport préliminaire sur le problème de la lèpre, présénte par le prof.* [C]C [1926], C.252 M 96 1926 pp. 95–7 also CH 466 Vol No 299. League of Nations Archives, Geneva.

Cochrane, R.G. *The Epidemiology, Pathology and Diagnosis of Child Leprosy (being the Dr Elizabeth Mathai Endowment Lectures, 1942–43, delivered at the Medical College, University of Madras)* (Madras: Superintendent Government Press, 1943).

Dharmendra, Dr, 'The Place of Vasectomy in Leprosy Control', *Leprosy in India, Special Issue: All India Leprosy Conference, Wardha*, 20/1 (1948): pp. 28–31 and pp. 63–75.

Dyer, Isadore, 'The Berlin Leprosy Conference', *New Orleans Medical and Surgical Journal*, 50/6 (1897): pp. 357–68

Eiglemeier, K., N. Honoré, S.A.Woods, B. Caudron and S.T. Cole, 'Use of an Ordered Cosmid Library to Deduce the Genomic Organization of *Mycobacterium leprae*', *Molecular Microbiology*, 7/2 (1993): pp. 197–206.

Fite, G.L. and H.W. Wade, 'The Contribution of Neisser to the Establishment of the Hansen bacillus as the Etiologic Agent of Leprosy and the So-Called Hansen-Neisser Controversy', *International Journal of Leprosy*, 23/4 (1955): pp. 418–28.

Government of India, Central Advisory Board of Health, *Report on Leprosy and its Control in India* (New Delhi: Government of India, 1942).

Hansen, G. Armauer, *The Memories and Reflections of Dr. G. Armauer Hansen*, trans. G.A. Hansen (Würzburg: Germany Leprosy Relief Association, 1976).

Hastings, Robert C. (ed.), *Leprosy* (New York: Longman, 1985).

IDEA website. Available at: www.idealeprosydignity.org/OralHistoryWeb/Japan-Nishimura.html (accessed 5 February 2010).

Japan Law Foundation: Verification Committee Concerning Hansen's Disease Problem, 'Verification Committee Concerning Hansen's Disease Problem: Final Report' (Summary Version). Available at: www.leprosyhistory.org/english/bulletin.htm.

Lampe, P.H.J. 'Fate of Children Born of Leprous Parents in the Groot-Chatillon Leprosy Asylum', *International Journal of Leprosy* 1/1 (1933): pp. 5–15.

Leprosy in India, Special Issue: All India Leprosy Conference, Wardha, 20/1 (1948).

Pedley, J.C. and J.G. Geater, 'Does Droplet Infection Play a Role in the Transmission of Leprosy?', *Leprosy Review*, 47/2 (1976): pp. 97–102.

Ridley, D.S. and W.H. Jopling, 'Classification of Leprosy According to Immunity: A Five-Group System', *International Journal of Leprosy*, 34 (1966): pp. 255–73.

Rodriguez, J., 'Studies on Early Leprosy in Children of Lepers', *Philippine Journal of Science* 31/2 (1929): pp. 115–46.

Rogers, Sir Leonard and Ernest Muir, *Leprosy*, 3rd edn (Bristol: John Wright and Sons, 1946).

Rokstad, Professor Ingvald, 'Gerhard Henrich Armauer Hansen: Address Delivered at Inauguration of the Armauer Hansen Memorial Room, February 18, 1962', *International Journal of Leprosy*, 32/1 (1964): pp. 64–70.

Santra, Dr Isaac, 'Notes on Leprosy in Japan', *Leprosy in India* (1953): pp. 26–7.

Stanley, Stein, *Alone No Longer* (Carville: The Star, 1963).

Virchow, Rudolf, trans. George L. Fite, 'Virchow's Leprosy from *Die Krankhaften Geschwulste*', *International Journal of Leprosy*, 22/1 (1954): pp. 71–79 [and] 22/2 (1954): pp. 205–17.

World Health Organisation, *Leprosy: A Survey of Recent Legislation* (Geneva: WHO, 1954), reprint from the *International Digest of Health Legislation*, 5 (1954).

Secondary Sources

Anderson, Warwick, 'Leprosy and Citizenship', *Positions: East Asia Cultures Critique*, 6 (1998): pp. 707–30.

Bernabeu-Mestre, J. and Ballester-Artigues, T., 'Disease as a Metaphorical Resource: The Fontilles Philanthropic Initiative in the Fight against Leprosy 1901–1932', *Social History of Medicine*, 17/3 (2004): pp. 409–21.

Burns, Susan L., 'From "Leper Villages" to Leprosaria: Public Health, Nationalism and the Culture of Exclusion in Japan', in Carolyn Strange and Alison Bashford (eds), *Isolation: Places and Practices of Exclusion* (London and New York: Routledge, 2003), pp. 104–18.

Douglas, Mary, 'Witchcraft and Leprosy: Two Strategies of Exclusion', *Man*, New Series 26/4 (1991): pp. 723–36.

Edmond, Rod, *Leprosy and Empire: A Medical and Cultural History* (Cambridge: Cambridge University Press, 2006).

Gould, Tony, *Don't Fence Me In: From Curse to Cure: Leprosy in Modern Times* (London: Bloomsbury, 2005).

Gussow, Zachary, *Leprosy, Racism, and Public Health: Social Policy in Chronic Disease Control* (San Francisco and London: Westview Press, 1989).

Hastings, R. 'Review of Ohtani, Fujio, *The Walls Crumble*', *International Journal of Leprosy* (September 2000). Available at: http://findarticles.com/p/articles/mi_qa3754/is_200009/ai_n8925248/ (accessed 25 October 2011)

Irgens, Lorentz M., 'The Discovery of *Mycobacterium leprae*: A Medical Achievement in the Light of Evolving Scientific Methods', in Lorentz M. Irgens, Yngve Nedrebo, Sigurd Sandmo and Arne Skivenes (eds), *Leprosy* (Bergen: Selja Forlag, 2006), pp. 33–9.

Miyasaka, Michio, 'Punishing Paternalism: An Ethical Analyses of Japan's Leprosy Control Policy', *Eubios Journal of Asian and International Bioethics*, 19/4 (2009): pp. 103–7.

Moblo, Pennie, 'Blessed Damien of Moloka'i: The Critical Analaysis of Contemporary Myth', *Ethnohistory*, 44/4 (1997): pp. 691–726.

Obregon, Diana, 'Building National Medicine: Leprosy and Power in Colombia, 1870–1910', *Social History of Medicine*, 15/1 (2002): pp. 89–108.

Ohtani, Fujio, *The Walls Crumble: The Emancipation of Persons Affected by Hansen's Disease in Japan* (Tokyo: Tofu Kyokai Association, 1998).

Parascandola, John, 'Chaulmoogra Oil and the Treatment of Leprosy'. Available at: www.lhncbc.nlm.nih.gov/lhc/docs/published/2003/pub2003048.pdf (accessed 2 February 2010).

Rawcliffe, Carole, *Leprosy in Medieval England* (Suffolk, UK and Rochester, NY: Boydell P, 2006).

Robertson, Jo, 'Culion, the "Island of the Living Dead": Or Another Look at Leprosy and Citizenship', in Astri Andresen, Kari Tove Elvakken and Tore Gronlie (eds), *Politics of Prevention, Health Propaganda, and the Organisation of Hospitals, 1800–2000* (Bergen: Rokkansenteret, 2005), pp. 81–91.

Robertson, Jo, 'The Leprosy Asylum in India', *Journal of the History of Medicine and Allied Sciences*, 64/4 (2009): pp. 474–517.

Rodriguez, Cristina Verzola (ed.), *Culion Island: A Leper Colony's 100-Year Journey Toward Healing* (Philippines: Culion Foundation and Fundacion ANESVAD, 2003).

Vogelsang, Th. M., 'The Hansen-Neisser Controversy, 1879–1880', *International Journal of Leprosy*, 31/1 (1963): pp. 74–80.

Vogelsang, Th. M., 'Gerhard Henrik Armauer Hansen 1841–1912: The Discoverer of the Leprosy Bacillus: His Life and Work', *International Journal of Leprosy*, 46/3 (1978): pp. 257–332.

Wexler, Nancy, 'Learning to be a Leper: A Case Study in the Social Construction of Illness', in Elliott G. Mishler (ed.), *Social Contexts of Health, Illness, and Patient Care* (New York: Cambridge University Press, 1981), pp. 169–74.

Worboys, Michael, 'Was there a Bacteriological Revolution in Late Nineteenth-Century Medicine?', *Studies in History, Philosophy, Biology and Biomedical Science*, 38 (2007): pp. 20–42.

Chapter 7
Gifts, Commodities and the Demand for Organ Transplants

Sally Wilde

Introduction

Much discussion of organ transplantation has been dominated, whether consciously or not, by two conceptual models. The market model conceptualizes organs for transplantation as commodities that could, at least theoretically, be bought and sold, with supply and demand balanced in the same way as other commodities, by variations in price.[1] The gift model, in contrast, conceptualizes gift-giving as the only ethical and just way of providing organs for transplantation.[2] Underneath both these models there resides a deeper and widely shared assumption, that once the need for an organ transplant is determined by medical authority, this need acquires some of the characteristics of a moral imperative. In other words, medically determined need results in a 'demand' for an organ, in both the economic and the everyday sense of the word. Such medically determined demand is a classic example of a black box.[3] What medicine has to offer is widely regarded as of inherent value, and few outside the field of medicine ever lift the lid and look inside the box at the factors determining demand for medical treatment.

In contrast, what follows is an examination of some of the changes since the 1950s in both demand and supply within the transplantation business. Variations in the availability of body parts are not neglected, but this chapter breaks new ground in also examining a small sample of the factors affecting changes in the

---

[1] Mark J. Cherry, *Kidney for Sale by Owner, Human Organs, Transplantation, and the Market* (Washington, DC, 2005); James S. Taylor, *Stakes and Kidneys, Why Markets in Human Body Parts are Morally Imperative* (Aldershot, 2005).

[2] Renée C. Fox and Judith P. Swazey, *The Courage to Fail, A Social View of Organ Transplants and Dialysis* (Chicago, 1974). For a discussion of the broader issues raised by gift exchange in medicine see: Sally Wilde, 'Surgical Theatre, Gifted Performance: The Moral Economy of Surgical Training', in Christy Collis and Maggie Nolan (eds), *Benevolence, Journal of Australian Studies* 85 (Perth, 2005), pp. 27–36, pp. 194–8; see also: Marcel Mauss, *The Gift, the Form and Reason for Exchange in Archaic Societies* (New York, 1990); James G. Carrier, *Gifts and Commodities, Exchange and Western Capitalism since 1700* (London, 1995).

[3] N. Rosenberg, *Inside the Black Box: Technology and Economics* (Cambridge, 1982).

demand for human organs and tissues. This brief preliminary look inside the black box reveals a wide range of culturally specific influences on the variations in demand over time and from place to place. Principle-driven texts, whatever their perspective, tend to erase the cultural dimension and treat time-bound and culturally specific circumstances as both ongoing and universal. This chapter, in contrast, seeks to move forward from the gift versus commodity debate and the emphasis on problems with the supply of organs. It proposes that cultural and temporal specificity are central rather than tangential aspects of the organ transplant business and provides clear evidence that medically determined demand does not inexorably rise at all times and in all places. This opens up the potential for a wide range of local policy initiatives, especially for those who take it for granted that in medicine, prevention is better than cure.

Preliminary Observations

One of the key problems identified in almost all recent discussion of organ transplantation is that there are more people wanting organs or tissue than people prepared to provide them.[4] A recent volume on organ donation in the United States, for instance, began by arguing that the field of organ transplantation 'faces the challenge of reducing the ever widening gap between the demand for and the supply of transplantable organs'.[5] This is also the starting point for the recent outpouring of works advocating the legal sale of organs, which often also emphasize that the result of the shortage of organs for transplantation is a loss of lives. Mark Cherry, for instance, begins his book *Kidney for Sale by Owner* with statistics on the number of people in the United States who died whilst 'queuing for available organs'.[6] In the parlance of the market, demand exceeds supply. Demand is taken for granted as large, likely to grow fast, and believed to include hidden demand because of supply problems. Even critics of organ donation programmes Renée Fox and Judith Swazey, in *Spare Parts*, their sequel to *The Courage to Fail*, identify 'an escalating shortage of organs due to the increased scale and scope

[4] Rainer W.G. Gruessner and Enrico Benedetti (eds), *Living Donor Organ Transplantation* (New York, 2008); Margaret Lock, *Twice Dead, Organ Transplants and the Reinvention of Death* (Berkeley, 2002); D. Joralemon, 'Shifting Ethics: Debating the Incentive Question in Organ Transplantation', *Journal of Medical Ethics*, 27/1 (2001): pp. 30–35; Stefan Timmermans, 'The Cause of Death vs. the Gift of Life', in Stefan Timmermans and Jonathan Gabe (eds), *Partners in Health, Partners in Crime* (Oxford, 2003), pp. 49–73, p. 56.

[5] Institute of Medicine of the National Academies, *Organ Donation, Opportunities for Action* (Washington, DC, 2006), p. ix.

[6] Cherry, *Kidney for Sale*, p. ix; Taylor, *Stakes and Kidneys*, p. 1; this is also the underlying rationale behind: Stephen Wilkinson, *Bodies for Sale, Ethics and Exploitation in the Human Body Trade* (London, 2003) and Martin Rothblatt, *Your Life or Mine, How Geoethics Can Resolve the Conflict Between Public and Private Interests in Xenotransplantation* (Aldershot, 2004), who argues for using organs from non-human beings.

of the transplantation endeavour' as one of the key issues.[7] This emphasis on the shortage of organs has been particularly marked since the early 1980s, when the introduction of a new generation of immunosuppressive drugs was followed by what Fox and Swazey describe as a 'boom' in the transplant business.[8]

The debate about how to resolve this perceived problem can be summarized as a debate concerning the merits of gifts versus commodities. The pioneers among those who favour the gift conceptualization were first Richard Titmuss in 1970 and in 1974 Renée Fox and Judith Swazey.[9] Titmuss focused on international variations in how medical supplies of blood were provided. He argued that blood donation produces better outcomes than blood as a commodity. His was an ideologically driven defence of the British National Health Service and its ethos of gifts and social rights to health, and he made what became a very influential case for the collectivist view. Fox and Swazey were mainly interested in kidney dialysis and kidney and heart transplants in the United States. Their empirical data allowed them to conclude that gifts in organ transplantation are very weighty objects for both donors and recipients. As a consequence, whilst ultimately preferring gifts to market mechanisms, they nevertheless wrote about the tyranny of the gift.[10]

There is now a considerable body of work that favours the opposing 'commodity' view of organ and tissue transplantation. Virtually all of this literature addresses only one aspect of organ transplantation, that is, how to increase the supply of organs.[11] Members of the pro-commodification camp generally assume that markets are the best way to raise supply to meet ever growing demand, arguing in a more or less nuanced fashion via philosophical reasoning that the sale of body parts is morally warranted on the grounds of individual autonomy.[12] Almost all of these works fail to examine two key

---

[7] Renée C. Fox and Judith P. Swazey, *Spare Parts: Organ Replacement in American Society* (New York, 1992), p. xv; Fox and Swazey, *Courage to Fail.*

[8] Fox and Swazey, *Spare Parts*, p. 7.

[9] Richard Titmuss, *The Gift Relationship* (London, 1970); for a thoughtful discussion of the issues raised by Titmuss' work see: Catherine Waldby and Robert Mitchell, *Tissue Economies, Blood, Organs, and Cell Lines in Late Capitalism* (Durham, NC, 2006).

[10] Fox and Swazey's work remains enormously influential. In particular, two recent collections of papers on the subject either overtly or implicitly pay homage to it: Stuart J. Youngner, Renée C. Fox and Laurence J. O'Connell (eds), *Organ Transplantation, Meanings and Realities* (Madison, 1996); Carla M. Messikomer, Judith P. Swazey and Allen Glicksman (eds), *Society & Medicine, Essays in Honor of Renée C. Fox* (New Brunswick, 2003).

[11] Cherry, *Kidney for Sale*; Taylor, *Stakes and Kidneys*; Wilkinson, *Bodies for Sale*; Michele Goodwin, *Black Markets: The Supply and Demand of Body Parts* (Cambridge, 2006); Rothblatt, *Your Life or Mine*; Cecile Fabre, *Whose Body is it Anyway? Justice and the Integrity of the Person* (Oxford, 2006).

[12] J.S. Taylor, 'Black Markets, Transplant Kidneys and Interpersonal Coercion', *Journal of Medical Ethics*, 32/12 (2006): pp. 698–701; Cherry, *Kidney for Sale*; Taylor, *Stakes and Kidneys*; Wilkinson, *Bodies for Sale.*

assumptions. The first assumption is that the demand for organs and tissue must inexorably grow; the second assumption is that the direct sale of organs would provide better outcomes than the current system. But neither of these assumptions can be taken for granted. The first assumption is actually false, as will be demonstrated by an examination of the recent history of the demand for the two most commonly transplanted human body parts, kidneys and corneas, and the second assumption is yet to be tested widely in practice.

Selling organs may solve some problems in the transplantation business, but it also creates new ones, and remains enormously controversial, as the flood of pronouncements on the issue by ethicists and philosophers attests. Selling kidneys is current practice in a range of countries, including Brazil, China, India and Russia.[13] The sale of kidneys has been particularly well studied in Iran, where it has been legal since 1988. There has been no waiting list for kidney transplants in Iran since 1999, but paid donors, even in legal and well-regulated settings such as this, often feel exploited and resentful after the event, and the transmission of disease with the kidney is not uncommon.[14] In a recent study of 16 Australians who went overseas to try and buy themselves a kidney, only six had a good result. Three did not receive a transplant, despite spending time in an overseas hospital waiting on dialysis, and seven acquired serious infections along with their new kidneys.[15] On current evidence, it would appear that at least some of the organs which are bought and sold are of lower quality than those which are gifted, a finding which supports that of Titmuss nearly 40 years ago.[16]

Within the world of economics, those on the left of the political spectrum have historically been more interested in the demand side of the equations, while conservatives have tended to have more to say about the supply side. However, bioethics debates about organ transplantation are rather more complex than this. Whilst virtually all of the literature advocating markets in organs is concerned with the problems of supply, the debate has become equally bound up with a

---

[13] Clive O. Callender, Micean Johnikin and Patrice Miles, 'Cultural Differences in Living Organ Donation: A Global Perspective', in Gruessner and Benedetti, *Living Donor*, pp. 6–15.

[14] Ahad J. Ghods, 'Incentives in Non-Western Countries: The Iranian Model', in Gruessner and Benedetti, *Living Donor*, pp. 75–80; B. Broumand, 'Living Donors: The Iran Experience', *Nephrology, Dialysis, Transplantation*, 12 (1997): pp. 1830–31; Nancy Scheper-Hughes, 'Illegal Organ Trade: Global Justice and the Traffic in Human Organs', in Gruessner and Benedetti, *Living Donor*, pp. 106–21.

[15] Sean E. Kennedy, Yvonne Shen, John A. Charlesworth, James D. Mackie, John D. Mahony, John J.P. Kelly and Bruce A. Pussell, 'Outcome of Overseas Commercial Kidney Transplantation: An Australian Perspective', *Medical Journal of Australia*, 182/5 (2005): pp. 224–7.

[16] Titmuss, *The Gift Relationship*.

patients' rights rhetoric.[17] In addition, many of the authors who favour a 'gift' approach to the supply of organs also fail to offer a critique of the demand side of the equation. There is a widespread tendency among both those who favour gifts and those who favour the sale of organs to assume that the provision of health care of all kinds, as decided by clinicians, is somehow a 'good thing'. If a treatment is invented and a doctor recommends that a patient should have it/would benefit from it, this decision is seldom questioned. The patient should, it is argued, be able to have it. Although for some time economists have studied what they call the phenomenon of 'supplier-induced demand' for health care, this attitude has not percolated through to the debates over organ transplants.[18] Despite discussions of whether or not there is 'over-servicing' in other areas of health care (providing too many tests and/or unnecessary treatment), this question has seldom been asked about organ transplants. The most important exception to this is still the work of Fox and Swazey, and recent work by Renée Fox has become increasingly critical of the assumption that more is better in health care. But even this work fails to seriously consider the components of demand for transplantable organs and tissue.[19]

Gifts are entangled objects and are about relationships and power, in a way that commodities are not.[20] In particular, unrequited gifts impose a very heavy burden on both donor and recipient. Benign gifts, the sort that cement friendships and family relationships, are about gift exchange, reciprocal obligations and intergenerational transfers. Gifts that cannot be repaid, however, are about power, and in the case of living related kidney donation they may also be entangled in family manipulation or even exploitation, as Farhat Moazam has shown in her very fine and thought-provoking book on kidney transplants in Pakistan.[21] The post-mortem gifts of organs also raise complex and culturally specific issues as Margaret Lock and William La Fleur have both shown in the case of Japan, for

[17] Michelle Goodwin, for instance, has argued that allowing the sale of kidneys would help redress the dramatic inequalities in access to kidney transplants faced by African Americans: Goodwin, *Black Markets*.

[18] J.R. Richardson, 'The Inducement Hypothesis: That Doctors Generate Demand for their Services', in J.R.G. Butler and D.P. Doessal (eds), *Health Economics: Australian Readings* (Sydney, 1989); L.J. Opit, 'The Cost of Health Care and Health Insurance in Australia: Some Problems Associated with the Fee-for-Service System', *Social Science and Medicine*, 18/11 (1984): pp. 967–72.

[19] Renée C. Fox, 'Toward an Ethic of Iatrogenesis', in William R. LaFleur, Gernot Böhme and Susumu Shimazono (eds), *Dark Medicine: Rationalizing Unethical Medical Research* (Bloomington, 2007), pp. 149–64; Fox and Swazey, *Courage to Fail*; Fox and Swazey, *Spare Parts*.

[20] Nicholas Thomas, *Entangled Objects: Exchange, Material Culture and Colonialism in the Pacific* (Cambridge, MA, 1991).

[21] Farhat Moazam, *Bioethics and Organ Transplantation in a Muslim Society; A Study in Culture, Ethnography and Religion* (Bloomington, 2006).

instance.[22] I propose therefore to shift the focus a little from gifts vs. commodities, both of which, I believe, have their pros and cons, to the mechanisms for distributing scarce resources.

Anything that is in short supply can be rationed by queue, or it can be rationed by price, and in fact human body parts have been rationed by both mechanisms since the day that organ and tissue transplants began.[23] When body parts are rationed by price, it is self-evident that the rich go to the front of the queue. In the United States, the government was persuaded to make end stage renal failure (ESRF) a special case, and unlike America's other health services, the costs of treatment, whether dialysis or transplant, are theoretically covered for all citizens.[24] Despite this, there is considerable evidence that the poor, and especially poor African Americans, are far less likely to receive a kidney transplant than rich whites, even though the medically determined demand is significantly higher in the black population.[25] Nevertheless, one of the richest countries in the world can afford to make kidney transplants widely available to its citizens through a combination of government funding and more or less coordinated queues, whilst wealthy citizens waiting in those queues can afford to become medical tourists, travelling to other countries in search of somebody sufficiently badly in need of money to be prepared to sell them a kidney. Elsewhere in the world, the situation is rather different. In countries without government- or charity-funded health care systems, the uninsured never make it on to a queue and only the rich can afford a kidney transplant.[26] In countries such as Kenya or Ecuador, the same poverty that means there are very few trained transplant surgeons affects the availability of dialysis, thus the standard debate on demand which posits the value of transplant

---

22 Lock, *Twice Dead*; W.R. LaFleur, 'Transplanting the Transplant: Japanese Sensitivity to American Medicine as an American Mission', in Messikomer, Swazey and Glicksman, *Society and Medicine*, pp. 87–107.

23 Fox and Swazey, *Spare Parts*.

24 G.E. Schreiner, 'How End-Stage Renal Disease-Medicare Developed', *Seminars in Nephrology*, 17/3 (1997): pp. 152–9; A.R. Hull, 'The Legislative and Regulatory Process in the End Stage Renal Disease Program', *Seminars in Nephrology*, 17/3 (1997): pp. 160–69; J.S. Cameron, *History of the Treatment of Renal Failure by Dialysis* (Oxford, 2002), especially ch. 21, 'The Growth of Long-Term Dialysis for Long-Term Renal Failure in its Fiscal and Sociopolitical Context', pp. 309–27.

25 Goodwin, *Black Markets*; Arnold M. Epstein, John Z. Ayanian, Joseph H. Keogh, Susan J. Noonan, Nancy Armistead, Paul D. Cleary, Joel S. Weissman, Jo Ann David-Kasdan, Diane Carlson, Jerry Fuller, Douglas Marsh and Rena M. Conti, 'Racial Disparities in Access to Renal Transplantation, Clinically Appropriate or Due to Underuse or Overuse?', *New England Journal of Medicine*, 343/21 (2000): pp. 1537–45.

26 Roberto S. Kalil and Lawrence G. Hunsicker, 'Kidney Transplantation: Geographical Differences', in Gruessner and Benedetti, *Living Donor*, pp. 139–43; Scheper-Hughes, 'Illegal Organ Trade'; W.H. Hörl, F. de Alvaro and P.F. Williams, 'Healthcare Systems and End-Stage Renal Disease Therapies – An International Review: Access to ESRD Treatments', *Nephrology, Dialysis, Transplantation*, 14/supp6 (1999): pp. 10–15.

over ongoing dialysis is meaningless, as ESRF is normally followed by death. This is one of the reasons why the gift/commodity dichotomy does not, actually, make a lot of sense. So much of the organ transplant business is already driven by market forces, before the question is even asked about who should be first in line.

While it is reasonable to assume that most recipients of donated organs will value such an opportunity for extended or enhanced life, it is also important to recognize the extent to which the demand for human body parts is doctor-driven as well as culturally shaped. Demand is heavily influenced by the people who make their living supplying the services surrounding transplants, taking organs out of one body and putting them in another. It is driven by medical understandings of the body and techno-scientific considerations. If doctors determine that somebody would benefit from a transplant, the argument goes, then they 'should' be able to have access to somebody else's body part. Organ transplantation is a part of both wealthy health care systems and the medical dominance paradigm and patients are only indirectly the source of demand for organs. But medical professionals are by no means the only influence on the demand for transplantable organs, and the story is actually quite complex. Generally, there has been a dearth of work on the factors which impact directly on the demand for organs or tissue. It is therefore time to lift the lid of the black box and briefly examine a few of the cultural and temporal factors affecting the demand for (as well as the supply of) two of the most common transplants, corneas and kidneys.

Corneas

Corneal transplantation – technically called penetrating keratoplasty – is the most commonly performed and successful of all tissue transplants. In 1990, for instance, 36,037 corneas were transplanted in the United States compared to 8,886 kidneys, 2,160 livers, 1,673 hearts and 412 pancreases.[27] As a treatment for corneal blindness, transplants are effective, can be performed as day surgery and the grafts typically have a fairly long survival compared to transplants of other organs. Studies from centres as diverse as Texas and Hyderabad indicate that corneal transplants are routinely performed without tissue typing or systemic immunosuppressive drugs, but despite this, only about 10 per cent of first-time corneal grafts suffer rejection within a year, and of these, well over half can generally be rescued with the administration of steroids and other immunosuppressants.[28] Consequently, around the world high 10-year survival rates are common. Since

[27] Patricia Aiken-O'Neill and Mark J. Mannis, 'Summary of Corneal Transplant Activity', *Cornea*, 21/1 (2002): pp. 1–3; Fox and Swazey, *Spare Parts*, p. 7. While the cornea figures are for 1990, the figures for other organs relate to 1989.

[28] Jerry Y. Niederkorn, 'The Immune Privilege of Corneal Grafts', *Journal of Leukocyte Biology*, 74 (2003): pp. 167–71; Virender S. Sangwan, Balasubramanya Ramamurthy, Urmi Shah, Prashant Garg, Mitthanamalli S. Sridhar and Gullapalli N. Rao,

the 1980s, the median survival of corneal grafts in Australia, for instance, has been about 15 years.[29] By almost any measure, penetrating keratoplasties are one of the big success stories of post-Second World War transplantation, and hundreds of thousands of people around the world have had their sight restored by this procedure. However, contrary to the common perception of transplant surgery, in many major developed countries the demand for corneas does not exceed supply. Despite the fact that penetrating keratoplasty is a relatively common and successful operation, there is no inexorable growth in the demand for corneas. On the contrary, the number of corneal transplants performed in the United States has been falling for about 15 years, while the numbers in countries such as Australia and New Zealand are fairly stable. In those countries which have well-developed eye-banking systems, the supply of corneas regularly meets demand, and waiting lists for corneal transplants are typically short, dependent as much on surgeon time and operating theatre availability as the availability of corneas. Indeed, the United States exports thousands of corneas every year. Whilst the number of transplants in the United States fell from 36,037 in 1990 to 33,260 in 2000, the number of corneas donated rose. As a result, the number of corneas exported increased from 7 per cent of the total in 1990 to 29 per cent of the total 10 years later.[30] Some eye banks elsewhere, including in Italy and Australia, also frequently have more corneas than are needed locally. These are either sent inter-state, used for research, or exported. There are a number of countries, including Israel and Japan, that have a shortage of corneas, while others, including the United States and Australia, do not. The reasons for this are complex, affecting both demand and supply, and each side of this equation will be considered in turn.

Factors Affecting the Demand for Corneas

There have been a number of studies of the indications for corneal transplant, and they demonstrate both wide geographic variations and significant changes over time.[31] Some of the geographic variations are naturally occurring. Keratoconus,

---

'Outcome of Corneal Transplant Rejection: A 10-Year Study', *Clinical and Experimental Ophthalmology*, 33/6 (2005): pp. 623–7.

29 K.A. Williams, N.B. Hornsby, C.M. Bartlett, H.K. Holland, A. Esterman and D.J. Coster (eds), *Australian Corneal Graft Registry Report 2004* (Adelaide, 2004), p. 12.

30 Aiken-O'Neill and Mannis, 'Summary of Corneal Transplant Activity'.

31 S. Louise Moffatt, Victoria A. Cartwright and Thomas H. Stumpf, 'Centennial Review of Corneal Transplantation', *Clinical and Experimental Ophthalmology*, 33/6 (2005): pp. 642–57; N. Al-Yousuf, I. Mavrikakis, E Marvrikakis and S.M. Daya, 'Penetrating Keratoplasty: Indications Over a 10 Year Period', *British Journal of Ophthalmology*, 88/8 (2004): pp. 998–1001; C. Banu Cosar, M.S. Sridhar, Elisabeth J. Cohen, Evan L. Held, Paulo de Tarso, S. Alvim, Christopher J. Rapuano, Irving M. Raber and Peter R. Laibson, 'Indications for Penetrating Keratoplasty and Associated Procedures, 1996–2000', *Cornea*, 21/2 (2002): pp. 148–51; Kendall Dobbins, Francis W. Price and William E. Whitson, 'Trends

for instance (a progressive distortion and thinning of the corneal surface), is one of the leading causes of corneal blindness in a wide range of countries, but it is particularly common among Maori and Pacific Islanders. While it was responsible for only about 15 per cent of corneal transplants in the United States in 2002, it was the indication for nearly half of the corneal transplants in New Zealand in the same year.[32] But another of the common indications for corneal transplant that showed particularly wide geographic variation results from iatrogenic injury. At the end of the twentieth century, the leading indication for corneal transplant in the United States, Canada, France and Singapore was a condition called pseudophakic bullous keratopathy or PBK.[33] This form of iatrogenic injury is not well known, even among doctors, but in the 1980s and 1990s there was an epidemic of PBK in the United States, and a number of other countries.[34] PBK is a swelling of the cornea caused by a thinning of the endothelial layer on the inside surface of the cornea. Sometimes it is linked to naturally occurring problems, but the cause of the late twentieth-century epidemic of PBK was damage to the endothelial layer during or after cataract surgery. One study from the American midwest found that between 1982 and 1996, PBK was the most common indication for corneal transplant, accounting for 31.5 per cent of all cases, although it was generally falling in incidence.[35] Another study from the east coast found that PBK was still the leading indication for corneal graft in the period 1996–2000, accounting for 27.2 per cent of cases.[36]

Cataracts were once a leading cause of blindness, but are now routinely removed in most Westernized countries by an operation which can take as little as 15 minutes. A small incision is made in the eye, the cataract is destroyed and removed, and a synthetic lens is inserted through the incision. The results are generally very good and complications are relatively infrequent. However, cataract surgery is an incredibly common operation. Indeed, in the year 2000 an article in the *British Medical Journal* claimed that it was the most commonly performed operation in the world, although no figures were provided to support this claim.[37]

---

in the Indications for Penetrating Keratoplasty in the Midwestern United States', *Cornea*, 19/6 (2000): pp. 813–16.

32 Moffatt et al., 'Centennial Review'.

33 Banu Cosar et al., 'Indications for Penetrating Keratoplasty'; Al-Yousuf et al., 'Penetrating Keratoplasty'; Dobbins et al., 'Trends in the Indications'.

34 Alan Sugar, 'An Analysis of Corneal Endothelial and Graft Survival in Pseudophakic Bullous Keratopathy', *Transactions of the American Ophthalmological Society*, 87 (1989): pp. 762–801; Emile J. Farge, 'Eye Banking: 1944 to the Present', *Survey of Ophthalmology*, 33/4 (1989): pp. 260–63.

35 Dobbins et al., 'Trends in the Indications'.

36 Banu Cosar et al., 'Indications for Penetrating Keratoplasty'.

37 David Spalton and Doug Koch, 'The Constant Evolution of Cataract Surgery', *British Medical Journal*, 321/7272 (2000): p. 1304. It is certainly not the most commonly performed operation everywhere. In Australia, for instance, in 2006 cataract removal was

As a complication of cataract surgery, PBK is now occurring less frequently than in the 1980s, because of changes in surgical technique and the type and location of the replacement lenses.[38] However, given that about two million cataracts are removed every year in the United States alone, even a complication rate of 0.3 per cent would result in 6,000 cases of PBK a year, or somewhere between one in five and one in six of all corneal transplants in the United States. During the 1990s, intra-ocular lenses in front of the iris (and hence just behind the cornea where they may damage the endothelial layer) were largely supplanted by foldable lenses inserted directly into the capsule behind the iris from which the cataract is removed. These changes have been associated with a falling incidence of PBK. This in turn has been directly linked to falls in the number of corneal transplants in the United States, from just over 36,000 in 1990 to just over 33,000 in 2000.[39] However, it might be noted that levels of PBK remain relatively high in those places, including some parts of India, that continue to use the older and less expensive cataract surgery technology. In the United Kingdom, where ophthalmologists were slower to adopt the use of intra-ocular lenses for cataract surgery, much of this epidemic was avoided. However, PBK still accounted for between 7 and 8 per cent of all corneal transplants in the UK in the 1990s.[40]

The indication for a further large proportion of corneal transplants is also directly linked to medical intervention in the eye. This is because however good they are, corneal transplants don't last forever. Those provided for older patients may see them out, so to speak, but transplants in younger people, for conditions such as keratoconus, eventually fail and need to be replaced. At the end of the twentieth century, 22 per cent of corneal transplants in Canada, 21 per cent in Taiwan, 15 per cent in Germany, 13 per cent in Israel, 19 per cent in Australia, 14 per cent in the UK and 18 per cent in the United States were second or third transplants because of a failed graft.[41] But while these numbers may rise as people live longer (and their eyes outlive the transplant), they are just as likely to fall, if ways are found to improve graft survival.

However, demand for corneas is not only driven by clinical indications. It is also driven by wealth, including by the availability of doctors trained to perform corneal transplants, patients able to pay for the surgery and/or a government-funded health system which covers the procedure. Much of the literature calling for the sale of organs and tissue has focused on ways to legally and ethically

about the seventh most common surgical procedure. But nevertheless, it is an exceedingly common operation almost everywhere from India to Indiana.

[38] Marvin L. Kwitko and Charles D. Kelman (eds), *The History of Modern Cataract Surgery* (The Hague, 1998).

[39] Aiken-O'Neill and Mannis, 'Summary of Corneal Transplant Activity'; Banu Cosar et al., 'Indications for Penetrating Keratoplasty'; Dobbins et al., 'Trends in the Indications'.

[40] Al-Yousuf et al., 'Penetrating Keratoplasty'.

[41] Moffatt et al., 'Centennial Review'; Williams et al., *Australian Corneal Graft Registry*, table 3.1, p. 53.

justify the movement of human body parts from places where, because of poverty, the supply potentially exceeds the demand, to places where, because of wealth, the demand exceeds the supply. But the corneal transplant story is very different. While the demand for corneas *exceeds* the supply in many areas of Africa, Asia and the Middle East, there is no shortage of corneas in a wide range of wealthy countries with well-organized eye-banking systems, including the United States, the United Kingdom, Italy, Australia and New Zealand. The next section of this chapter therefore briefly examines some of the factors affecting the supply of corneas.

Factors Affecting the Supply of Corneas

Eye-banking is not without its problems, but it is very much easier to organize the collection and distribution of corneas than of organs such as kidneys. First, the cornea does not have to be removed from a beating-heart donor and may safely be removed up to 24 hours after death. The ethical, legal and emotional problems of redefining death to enable the donation of organs such as kidneys or hearts do not, therefore, apply to corneas. Relatives may be left in peace to grieve, and whilst approaching bereaved family members is never easy, raising the subject of donation after death is less stressful and intrusive for all concerned. Second, corneas can be stored for significant periods of time – 2–3 days under refrigeration and for three or four weeks under the more expensive system using an organ culture medium.[42] Third, there are relatively few problems associated with rejection and potential incompatibility between donor and recipient.[43] Corneas are checked to ensure that they are disease-free and in good condition and, if so, they can be stored for several days, or flown inter-state or overseas. In most places with well-established eye-banking systems, including the United States, the United Kingdom, Italy, Australia, New Zealand and parts of India, corneal transplant surgery is routinely scheduled in advance, to suit the convenience of the surgeon and the patient, with a high degree of confidence that a cornea will be available when required.[44]

---

42 Wing Chu, 'The Past Twenty-Five Years in Eye Banking', *Cornea*, 19/5 (2000): pp. 754–65; K.A. Williams, L.M. Noack, S.J. Alfrich, R. Danz, S.A. Erickson and D.J. Coster, 'Assessment of the Dutch Organ-Culture System of Corneal Preservation within the Eye Bank of South Australia', *Australian and New Zealand Journal of Ophthalmology*, 16/1 (1988): pp. 21–5.

43 Niederkorn, 'The Immune Privilege of Corneal Grafts'; Sangwan et al., 'Outcome of Corneal Transplant Rejection'.

44 Chu, 'The Past Twenty-Five Years in Eye Banking'; John Armitage and David Easty, 'Bankable Assets', *Nursing Times*, 89/25 (1993): pp. 36–7; K.A. Williams et al., 'Donor Cornea Procurement: Six-Year Review of the Role of the Eye Bank of South Australia', *Australian and New Zealand Journal of Ophthalmology*, 18/1 (1990): pp. 77–89; G.K. Chopra, F. De Vincentis, D. Kaufman and D. Collie, 'Effective Corneal Retrieval in a General Hospital: The Royal Melbourne Hospital Eye Bank', *Australian and New*

In Nepal, ophthalmologist Sanduk Ruit originally set up an eye bank in a hospital in Kathmandu.[45] However, there were few donors because most Nepalese deaths do not take place in hospital and many Hindus and Buddhists fear that those whose corneas are removed will be blind when they are re-incarnated. Realizing that a large proportion of those who died at home were taken to a temple on the Bagmati River for cremation, Dr Ruit discussed the issues with both Buddhist monks and Hindu priests. In 1997, following agreement that restoring the sight of a blind person would increase the good karma of the family, collection of corneas was moved from the hospital to the temple. Within two years there was a five-fold increase in the number of corneas collected and the effective removal of waiting lists for corneas in Nepal. In France, in contrast, a lack of coordination in requesting consent for corneal donation has been associated with a persistent shortage of corneas for transplant.[46] In one study of a hospital in Rouen, more than 70 per cent of those relatives who were asked agreed to the donation of corneas, but fewer than 40 per cent of the relatives of those who died in the hospital were ever approached in the first place. These contrasting stories illustrate how well-organized legally and culturally specific eye banks are crucial to the supply side of the corneal transplant business. Almost all effective eye banks were set up by, or under pressure from, ophthalmologists, that is to say: demand from surgeons for corneas created the supply.

Key features of the history of eye-banking include:

1. Improved methods of corneal storage: in the 1970s and early 1980s, whole eyes were stored in wet pots. In the early 1980s most eye banks changed to a system of only removing the cornea, rather than the whole eye, from cadavers and keeping them in solution in cool storage for 2–3 days. Current solutions for cold storage enable corneas to be kept viable for about 10 days. There is also now a system in use in some centres, where corneas are stored in a culture medium at higher temperatures, and remain viable for 3–4 weeks.[47]
2. Improved methods of death notification: in their early years, many eye banks were based at a single hospital and set up arrangements with the hospital staff to be notified of deaths, so that they could then approach the relatives and request the donation of corneas. Some eye banks in the United

Zealand Journal of Ophthalmology, 21/4 (1993): pp. 251–5; Gullapalli Rao, 'Eye Banking – are we really up to it in India?', *Indian Journal of Ophthalmology*, 52/3 (2004): p. 183.

45 David Heiden, 'Dr Sanduk Ruit and Corneal Transplantation in Nepal', *The Western Journal of Medicine*, 176/1 (2002): pp. 71–2. Dr Ruit is best known internationally for his high-volume, low-cost cataract treatment, that can be carried out in poor and remote areas with minimal equipment.

46 M. Muraine, D. Toubeau, E. Menguy and G. Brasseur, 'Analysing the Various Obstacles to Cornea Postmortem Procurement', *British Journal of Ophthalmology*, 86/8 (2002): pp. 864–9.

47 Chu, 'The Past Twenty-Five Years in Eye Banking'.

States also had good relationships with their local coroner, and received a large proportion of corneas from that source. However, the most successful eye banks are those which have managed to set up arrangements for automatic death notifications from a wide range of sources, thus providing the largest possible pool of donor relatives who can be approached with a request for corneas.

3. Improved methods of distribution: in the past, many eye banks regularly had corneas which passed their expiry date because no local ophthalmologist had a patient waiting for a transplant. However, corneas can be (and are) safely flown from place to place and administrative arrangements to match waiting patients and available corneas have generally reduced this problem in most developed countries.
4. Improved safety: in many developed countries, including the United States and the European Union, the corneal transplant business is increasingly heavily government-regulated, with strict safety standards for storage and handling, as well as for screening the donor, to make sure that disease is not transmitted to the patient with the cornea.

In areas with well-developed eye-banking systems, patients do not generally have to wait very long for a cornea. The interval between diagnosis and surgery is as likely to be a function of a shortage of operating theatre time, or the surgeon's time, as any shortage of corneas. In Queensland in Australia, for instance, where a single eye bank serves the state, patients are scheduled for surgery some weeks ahead as an elective procedure, the surgeon books a request for a cornea with the eye bank, and a cornea is generally available on the day.[48] Indeed, in Queensland offering surplus corneas to the neighbouring state of New South Wales is possibly more common than cancelling surgery because no cornea is available. In general terms, removing tissue from dead eyes and transplanting it into living eyes some days later is now a routine procedure. Corneas and other parts of the eye such as sclera are laid out on operating theatre trolleys in their little containers in as matter-of-fact a fashion as swabs and forceps.

In some parts of the world, however, corneas are not so readily available as in North America, Western Europe and Australasia. Generally, mismatches between the supply of and the demand for corneas are the result of organizational failures or cultural resistance, or both. In many countries, including Japan, Israel and Syria, there are cultural reasons why people are reluctant to donate corneas.[49] The

---

48 Sally Wilde, 'Obtaining Permission to Save Sight: A History of the Queensland Eye Bank', unpublished paper, Queensland Eye Bank, 1999.

49 Anon, 'U.S. Eye Bank Sends Transplant Tissue to Israel', *Ophthalmology Times*, 31/23 (2006): p. 43; Jennifer A. Webb, 'Eye Bank to Provide Tissue for Worldwide Research, Transplants', *Ophthalmology Times*, 31/11 (2006): p. 8; Bina Venkataraman, 'Countries Make Push to Increase Eye Donors', *New York Times*, 15 July 2008. Available at: www.nytimes.com/2008/07/15/health/15corn (accessed 15 September 2008).

Grand Mufti of Syria was recently reported as publicly announcing his intention to donate his corneas after death, as part of a move to make the removal of corneas acceptable, whilst maintaining traditional Muslim respect for the integrity of the dead body.[50] Eye banking is not currently well developed in these countries, and ophthalmologists who wish to perform transplants often have to obtain corneas from other areas with a surplus, particularly the United States.

Summary

The moral of the corneal transplant surgery story, therefore, would seem to be that there are no inexorable forces leading to an increasing demand for corneas. On the contrary, demand has varied both up and down in the recent past, in association with changes in technology and increasing success in treating a leading cause of blindness: cataracts. Further, increases in the supply of corneas have been associated with the provision of well-organized eye banks and the increasingly efficient storage and distribution of corneas. Obtaining consent for donation from relatives, and overcoming cultural resistance to donation, has not generally been accomplished by paying donors, but rather by sustained, difficult, detailed, culturally sensitive work by trained specialists in this stressful, but rewarding, field of work.

The complexities of this story are an important alternative to the simplicities of the calls for markets in body parts. The balance between the supply of and the demand for corneas is the result of multiple factors. Neither demand nor supply are subject to inexorable forces beyond the reach of human intervention. On the contrary, both vary up and down as a result of a mix of social, cultural, economic, scientific, political, administrative and professional forces. But is corneal transplant surgery an isolated example, or is the pattern of demand for other sorts of transplants also subject to variation?

Kidneys

Factors Affecting the Demand for Kidneys

The most common causes of renal failure actually seem to have been more subject to variation than the indications for corneal transplants. In the United States in 2006, more than 50 per cent of all patients presenting with renal failure were diabetics, but in the early years of renal dialysis in the 1950s, diabetes was scarcely recognized as a cause of renal failure.[51] However, diabetes as a cause of

50 For a more detailed discussion of the variation in Muslim attitudes to organ and tissue donation see: Moazam, *Bioethics and Organ Transplantation in a Muslim Society*.

51 Phillip M. Hall, 'Prevention of Progression in Diabetic Nephropathy', *Diabetes Spectrum*, 19/1 (2006): pp. 18–24; Cameron, *A History of the Treatment of Renal Failure by Dialysis*, pp. 293–9.

renal failure rose rapidly during the 1970s and, by 1982, 27 per cent of patients receiving renal replacement therapy in the United States (dialysis or kidney transplant) were diabetics, rising to 36 per cent by 1992 and 40 per cent by 1995.[52] In Western Europe, the prevalence of diabetes has tended to be lower and as late as 1976, only 3 per cent of patients treated for renal failure there had diabetes.[53] However, the incidence of renal failure associated with diabetes in Europe has since risen significantly, to 11 per cent of renal replacement therapy patients in 1982 and 17 per cent in 1992.[54] Diabetic nephropathy has also been responsible for a rapidly rising proportion of cases of renal failure elsewhere in the world, including in Japan, Taiwan, Australia and New Zealand.[55] Partly, this is the result of improvements in the treatment of diabetes, so that sufferers live long enough to develop renal failure. Before the introduction of insulin in 1923, no type I autoimmune diabetics lived long enough for the disease to inflict much damage on their kidneys. It has been estimated that renal failure from diabetic nephropathy takes 20–30 years to develop, so that the first generation of patients with this condition would not have emerged before the 1950s. The story for type II (adult-onset) diabetes is slightly different, but again, improvements in treatment have meant that since the 1950s, more of these patients have survived long enough to suffer from kidney failure. People with diabetes are living longer, more of them are surviving vascular disease and more of them are being accepted onto renal replacement therapy programmes.[56]

A further important factor in the growth in the number of patients suffering from ESRF is that the incidence of type II diabetes has increased around the world since the 1960s, in association with the 'obesity epidemic'. This epidemic first became apparent in the United States and, as is well known, the associated incidence of type II diabetes is particularly high among African Americans, Asians and Native Americans.[57] Elsewhere, the incidence of type II diabetes is also high in Taiwan and Japan, among Pacific Islanders and in New Zealand.[58] In some countries,

52 Eberhard Ritz, Ivan Rychlik, Francesco Locatelli and Serge Halimi, 'End Stage Renal Failure in Type 2 Diabetes: A Medical Catastrophe of Worldwide Dimensions', *American Journal of Kidney Diseases*, 34/5 (1999): pp. 795–808, p. 797.

53 Cameron, *A History of the Treatment of Renal Failure*, p. 296.

54 Ritz et al., 'End Stage Renal Failure', p. 797.

55 I. Rychlik, G. Miltenberger-Miltenyi and E. Ritz, 'The Drama of the Continuous Increase in End-Stage Renal Failure in Patients with Type II Diabetes Mellitus', *Nephrology, Dialysis, Transplantation*, 13/supp8 (1998): pp. 6–10; Cameron, *A History of the Treatment of Renal Failure*; Ritz et al., 'End Stage Renal Failure'.

56 Domenico Di Landro and Gian Franco Romagnoli, 'Foreword', Type II diabetes issue, *Nephrology, Dialysis, Transplantation*, 13/supp8 (1998): p. 1.

57 Ritz et al., 'End Stage Renal Failure'; Epstein et al., 'Racial Disparities in Access to Renal Transplantation'; Goodwin, *Black Markets*.

58 R. Trevisan, M. Vedovato and A. Tiengo, 'The Epidemiology of Diabetes Mellitus', *Nephrology, Dialysis, Transplantation*, 13/supp8 (1998): pp. 2–5; Ritz et al., 'End Stage Renal Failure', p. 798.

including the United States, Australia and New Zealand, ethnic variations in the susceptibility to type II diabetes are compounded by the association between onset of the disease and deprivation.[59] Atherosclerosis as a contributor to kidney disease has also been strongly associated with socio-economic factors.[60]

These causes of renal failure are currently being attacked on two fronts. The first is a set of major public health campaigns advocating healthier diet and lifestyle, and the second is better medical management of diabetes (of both kinds), so that it does not go on to cause renal failure. Blood pressure management using ACE inhibitors appears to be particularly effective.[61] The outcomes of these initiatives currently remain uncertain, but meanwhile, in countries such as the United States and Australia, renal failure is increasingly a problem associated with stigmatized lifestyles, and, in Australia, particularly with Aboriginal communities.

Diabetic nephropathy is not the only cause of renal failure whose incidence has changed since the 1950s. The current most common causes of renal failure in Australia and New Zealand are diabetes and hypertension, together accounting for about half of all new cases.[62] But when kidney transplants began in Australia in the 1960s, two of the major causes of renal failure were congenital abnormalities leading to reflux, and renal failure associated with taking phenacetin and other analgesics in combination, a condition known as analgesic nephropathy.[63] The congenital abnormalities and reflux still occur, but they are now generally better managed, so that they do not go on to lead to renal failure. Phenacetin was banned

---

[59] Matthew Cox, Paul J. Boyle, Peter Davey and Andrew Morris, 'Does Health-selective Migration following Diagnosis Strengthen the Relationship between Type 2 Diabetes and Deprivation?', *Social Science and Medicine*, 65/1 (2007): pp. 32–42.

[60] David A. Shoham et al., 'Kidney Disease and the Cumulative Burden of Life Course Socioeconomic Conditions: The Atherosclerosis Risk in Communities Study', *Social Science and Medicine*, 67/8 (2008): pp. 1311–20.

[61] Hall, 'Prevention of Progression in Diabetic Nephropathy'; Giovanni F.M. Strippoli, Maria Craig, Francesco P. Schena and Jonathan C. Craig, 'Antihypertensive Agents for Primary Prevention of Diabetic Nephropathy', *Journal of the American Society of Nephrology*, 16/10 (2005): pp. 3081–91; Jorge L. Gross, Mirela J. de Azevedo, Sandra P. Silveiro, Luís Henrique Canani, Maria Luiza Caramori and Themis Zelmanovitz, 'Diabetic Nephropathy: Diagnosis, Prevention, and Treatment', *Diabetes Care*, 28/1 (2005): pp. 164–76.

[62] Stephen McDonald, Sean Chang and Leonie Excell, 'New Patients Commencing Treatment in 2005', *Australia and New Zealand Dialysis and Transplant Registry Report 2006* (Adelaide, 2006), p. 44. Glomerulonephritis was also important, accounting for 24 per cent and 22 per cent of new cases in Australia and New Zealand respectively in 2005.

[63] Rates of analgesic nephropathy were far higher in Australia than elsewhere, associated with heavy use of the products 'Vincents' and 'Bex', but the problem was widely recognized in the 1970s. J. Rodney Cove-Smith, 'Analgesic Nephropathy in the United Kingdom: Incidence, Clinical Features and Pathogenesis', *Journal of Clinical Pathology*, 34/11 (1981): pp. 1255–60; in the United States, analgesics of the aspirin/phenacetin/caffeine type (APCs) were re-formulated without phenacetin after it was banned as dangerous in 1983. Brand names include Saridon and Coricidin.

in Australia and some other countries in the 1970s, although other analgesics have subsequently been associated with renal failure, especially when taken in combination.[64] There has been a marked decrease in the incidence of analgesic nephropathy as a cause of renal failure in both Europe and Australia, and in 2005, for instance, just 3 per cent of new patients with renal failure had analgesic nephropathy.[65]

Overall, these shifts represent a major epidemiological change from the 1960s, and raise many complex issues of fairness and equity. In the United States, for instance, a study published in the *NEJM* in 2000 found that African Americans in renal failure were less likely to be put on the waiting list for a kidney transplant than whites.[66] Mainly, this was because they were less likely to meet the requisite health conditions because of other health problems. But it also seems that whites who did not meet the requisite health conditions for a kidney transplant were more likely to manage to get onto a waiting list anyway. In Australia, a 1997 NHMRC discussion paper on the issues raised by the allocation of transplant resources noted that Aboriginal people may be less likely to receive a kidney transplant because there are insufficient histocompatible donors.[67]

Clearly, the demand for kidney transplants is the result of a complex set of factors and has been the subject of very considerable change over the last 40 years, with some causes of renal failure falling, and others rising. Currently, major causes of renal failure are linked to at least theoretically preventible disease. As a group of European nephrologists put it in 1999:

> [End stage renal disease] in patients with type 2 diabetes is a problem of dramatically increasing importance worldwide. It constitutes a medical catastrophe, not only because of the heavy strains it puts on health budgets and logistics of medical care, but also because of the immense human suffering that is hidden behind these dry figures. This is all the more deplorable because

---

64 Thomas V. Perneger, Paul K. Whelton and Michael J. Klag, 'Risk of Kidney Failure Associated with the Use of Acetaminophen, Aspirin, and Non-Steroidal Anti-Inflammatory Drugs', *New England Journal of Medicine*, 331/25 (1994): pp. 1675–9; Marc E. De Broe and Monique Elseviers, 'Analgesic Nephropathy', *New England Journal of Medicine*, 338/7 (1998): pp. 446–52.

65 McDonald et al., 'New Patients', p. 44; this finding has, however, been challenged: Paul Michielsen and Paul de Schepper, 'Trends of Analgesic Nephropathy in Two High-Endemic Regions with Different Legislation', *Journal of the American Society of Nephrology*, 12 (2001): pp. 550–56; see also: Joseph K. McLaughlin, Loren Lipworth, Wong-Ho Chow and William J. Blot, 'Analgesic Use and Chronic Renal Failure: A Critical Review of the Epidemiological Literature', *Kidney International*, 54/3 (1998): pp. 679–86.

66 Epstein et al., 'Racial Disparities in Access'.

67 National Health & Medical Research Council, *Ethical Issues Raised by Allocation of Transplant Resources, Ethical Issues in Organ Donation Discussion Paper No. 3* (Canberra, 1997).

impressive evidence suggests that renal disease in these patients is preventable, if not completely, at least to a large extent.[68]

Factors Affecting the Supply of Kidneys

Some of the enormous body of work dealing with the issues raised by the supply of kidneys has already been discussed, and this section will not go over that same well-worn ground.[69] However, it is worth highlighting two key elements of the story that sometimes get lost in the detailed (and often polemical) discussions. Firstly, just as the demand for kidney transplants varies geographically, so does the supply, and while the buying and selling of kidneys is against the law in many countries, in others, including South Africa, China, India, Iran, Iraq, Lebanon, Pakistan, Philippines, Turkey, Bulgaria, Estonia, Georgia, Romania, Russia and Brazil it is current practice. Different countries have introduced different legislative frameworks and whether paid or unpaid, people are more willing to donate in some areas than in others.[70] In this context, it is pertinent to remember that this is not a problem to which there are ever likely to be universally acceptable solutions. Whilst there may be widespread consensus over the clinical considerations when removing a kidney from one body and implanting it in another, the same does not apply to public attitudes to this process. Secondly, despite the recent spate of philosophical arguments in favour of allowing the living to sell one of their kidneys, it is not just the supply of kidneys from the living that is controversial. The supply of kidneys from the dead can be controversial too.

In the United States and many other Western countries, consensus around new definitions of death emerged in the 1970s.[71] Partly, these new definitions of so-called 'brain death' were required because developments in intensive care and life support systems meant that patients who would once have unequivocally died now could be, and were, connected to machines that breathed for them and kept their hearts beating for prolonged periods of time. But the concept of brain death also enabled the removal of organs, including kidneys, from 'beating-heart donors'. As many people have pointed out, although dead, these patients look as if they are asleep, a state of affairs that may cause distress and makes approaching relatives about organ donation a particularly stressful and skilled task. While the

---

68 Ritz et al., 'End Stage Renal Failure', p. 805.

69 For a convenient survey of many of the issues raised by living donor kidney transplantations see the first 11 chapters of: Gruessner and Benedetti, *Living Donor*.

70 Callender et al., 'Cultural Differences in Living Organ Donation'.

71 Many US state legislatures introduced relevant legislation in the 1970s, and brain death was a practical working concept for most US physicians and surgeons by the time of the President's Commission report on the subject in 1981. See Martin S. Pernick, 'Brain Death in a Cultural Context: The Reconstruction of Death, 1967–1981', in Stuart J. Youngner, Robert M. Arnold and Renie Schapiro (eds), *The Definition Of Death, Contemporary Controversies* (Baltimore, 1999), pp. 3–33.

new medical definition of death was accepted in many countries with little debate, this was not the case in Japan, Denmark or Germany.[72] In Japan, although the concept of brain death received legal backing in 1997, it does not have widespread community support and remains as controversial as euthanasia or abortion in some other cultures.[73] In Denmark, legislative support for the concept was passed in 1990 following considerable public debate, while in Germany there was no definitive legislative support for brain death until 1997, despite many years of de facto acceptance of the concept from both the public and clinicians.[74] China has also resisted pressure from clinicians to introduce legislation permitting the removal of organs from those who are brain dead (but some of whose bodily functions are maintained by mechanical means), while providing a framework within which organs have been removed for sale from executed criminals.[75]

Conclusion

This chapter has considered variations in demand, as well as supply, in the organ transplant business. In the process, a number of key points have emerged. Firstly, and most importantly, the demand for both kidneys and corneas has varied down, as well as up, over the last 50 years. Secondly, demand has not always exceeded supply, especially in the case of corneas. The reasons why this is so are a complex mix of cultural, social, administrative and technological factors that affect both demand and supply. In the case of corneas, for instance, demand fell in the 1990s, because of improved technology in a related area of medicine: cataract removal, while improved supply was associated with interlinked eye-banking systems and the organization of the sustained, difficult and culturally specific work of obtaining consent to donation from relatives. The story of the supply of and demand for kidneys is equally complex. Demand is currently rising steeply, at least partly in association with an international epidemic of type II diabetes. This is a field where policies targeted at prevention seem to offer many attractions. But both the supply of and demand for kidneys vary geographically, as does the legislative framework regulating transplants, and whether paid or unpaid, people are more willing to

---

72 Bo Andreassen Rix, 'Brain Death, Ethics, and Politics in Denmark', in Youngner et al., *The Definition of Death*, pp. 227–38; Bettina Schöne-Seifert, 'Defining Death in Germany: Brain Death and its Discontents', in Youngner et al., *The Definition of Death*, pp. 257–72.

73 Tetsuo Yamaori, 'Strategies for Survival versus Accepting Impermanence: Rationalizing Brain Death and Organ Transplantation Today', in Lafleur et al., *Dark Medicine*, pp. 165–79; Lock, *Twice Dead.*

74 Rix, 'Brain Death'; Schöne-Seifert, 'Defining Death in Germany'.

75 Charlotte Ikels, 'Kidney Failure and Transplantation in China', *Social Science and Medicine*, 44/9 (1997): pp. 1271–83.

donate in some areas than in others.[76] The overall conclusion to be drawn from this evidence is that the problems thrown up by the organ transplant business are never likely to be susceptible to universally acceptable solutions. Localized, culturally specific solutions have had far more success.

Over the last half century, assumptions of altruism from both doctors and patients have been replaced by assumptions of self-interest, and the current pressure for markets in organs should be understood in the context of the far broader trend towards markets and commodification in health care.[77] Market forces and charitable provision used to exist side-by-side in a symbiotic relationship, but even in Western countries, gifts to strangers are no longer taken for granted as normative behaviour. Whilst altruistic giving is deeply embedded in the intellectual and spiritual tradition of a number of cultures, including those influenced by Buddhism and Christianity, deep suspicion of altruism (there's no such thing as a free lunch) is a salient characteristic of twenty-first century free-market ideology. But as the current outpouring of works attests, the buying and selling of human body parts is regarded as deeply problematic by many people in many cultures.

The evidence presented here suggests that the debate about gifts versus commodities in organ transplantation has been associated with a simplistic view of what is actually involved in the business of taking organs out of one body and putting them in another. In contrast, this necessarily brief examination of variations in time and space of just a few of the factors affecting demand (as well as supply), has opened up many new possibilities for consideration by policy-makers. Reflection which is more aware of cultural diversity and changes over time can complicate debate in fruitful ways and point to nuanced decision-making which reflects local circumstances. In addition, attention to the factors affecting demand, rather than supply, has the potential to provide enormous benefits in reducing human suffering. As the old adage has it: prevention is far better than cure.

Bibliography

Primary Sources

Al-Yousuf, N., I. Mavrikakis, E. Marvrikakis and S.M. Daya, 'Penetrating Keratoplasty: Indications Over a 10 Year Period', *British Journal of Ophthalmology*, 88/8 (2004): pp. 998–1001.

[76] Callender et al., 'Cultural Differences in Living Organ Donation'.

[77] R.H. Sprinkle, 'A Moral Economy of American Medicine in the Managed-Care Era', *Theoretical Medicine and Bioethics*, 22/3 (2001): pp. 247–68; Kim Hopper, 'Commentary: On the Transformation of the Moral Economy of Care', *Culture, Medicine and Psychiatry*, 25/4 (2001): pp. 473–84; L. Gilson, 'Trust and the Development of Health Care as a Social Institution', *Social Science and Medicine*, 56/7 (2003): pp. 1453–68.

Banu Cosar, C., M.S. Sridhar, Elisabeth J. Cohen, Evan L. Held, Paulo de Tarso, S. Alvim, Christopher J. Rapuano, Irving M. Raber and Peter R. Laibson, 'Indications for Penetrating Keratoplasty and Associated Procedures, 1996–2000', *Cornea*, 21/2 (2002): pp. 148–51.

Cove-Smith, J. Rodney, 'Analgesic Nephropathy in the United Kingdom: Incidence, Clinical Features and Pathogenesis', *Journal of Clinical Pathology*, 34/11 (1981): pp. 1255–60.

Cox, Matthew, Paul J. Boyle, Peter Davey and Andrew Morris, 'Does Health-selective Migration following Diagnosis Strengthen the Relationship between Type 2 Diabetes and Deprivation?', *Social Science and Medicine*, 65/1 (2007): pp. 32–42.

De Broe, Marc E. and Monique Elseviers, 'Analgesic Nephropathy', *New England Journal of Medicine*, 338/7 (1998): pp. 446–52.

Dobbins, Kendall, Francis W. Price and William E. Whitson, 'Trends in the Indications for Penetrating Keratoplasty in the Midwestern United States', *Cornea*, 19/6 (2000): pp. 813–16.

Epstein, Arnold M., John Z. Ayanian, Joseph H. Keogh, Susan J. Noonan, Nancy Armistead, Paul D. Cleary, Joel S. Weissman, Jo Ann David-Kasdan, Diane Carlson, Jerry Fuller, Douglas Marsh and Rena M. Conti, 'Racial Disparities in Access to Renal Transplantation, Clinically Appropriate or Due to Underuse or Overuse?', *New England Journal of Medicine*, 343/21 (2000): pp. 1537–45.

Gross, Jorge L., Mirela J. de Azevedo, Sandra P. Silveiro, Luís Henrique Canani, Maria Luiza Caramori and Themis Zelmanovitz, 'Diabetic Nephropathy: Diagnosis, Prevention, and Treatment', *Diabetes Care*, 28/1 (2005): pp. 164–76.

Hall, Phillip M., 'Prevention of Progression in Diabetic Nephropathy', *Diabetes Spectrum*, 19/1 (2006): pp. 18–24.

Michielsen, Paul and Paul de Schepper, 'Trends of Analgesic Nephropathy in Two High-endemic Regions with Different Legislation', *Journal of the American Society of Nephrology*, 12/3 (2001): pp. 550–56.

Niederkorn, Jerry Y., 'The Immune Privilege of Corneal Grafts', *Journal of Leukocyte Biology*, 74/2 (2003): pp. 167–71.

Perneger, Thomas V., Paul K. Whelton and Michael J. Klag, 'Risk of Kidney Failure Associated with the Use of Acetaminophen, Aspirin, and Non-Steroidal Anti-Inflammatory Drugs', *New England Journal of Medicine*, 331/25 (1994): pp. 1675–9.

Strippoli, Giovanni F.M., Maria Craig, Francesco P. Schena and Jonathan C. Craig, 'Antihypertensive Agents for Primary Prevention of Diabetic Nephropathy', *Journal of the American Society of Nephrology*, 16/10 (2005): pp. 3081–91.

Sugar, Alan, 'An Analysis of Corneal Endothelial and Graft Survival in Pseudophakic Bullous Keratopathy', *Transactions of the American Ophthalmological Society*, 87 (1989): pp. 762–801.

Trevisan, R., M. Vedovato and A. Tiengo, 'The Epidemiology of Diabetes Mellitus', *Nephrology, Dialysis, Transplantation*, 13/supp8 (1998): pp. 2–5.

Williams, Keryn Anne, Ngaere B. Hornsby, Christine Mary Bartlett, Helene K. Holland, Adrian Esterman and Douglas John Coster (eds), *Australian Corneal Graft Registry Report 2004* (Adelaide: Department of Ophthalmology Flinders Medical Centre, 2004).

Williams, K.A., L.M. Noack, S.J. Alfrich, R. Danz, S.A. Erickson and D.J. Coster, 'Assessment of the Dutch Organ-Culture System of Corneal Preservation within the Eye Bank of South Australia', *Australian and New Zealand Journal of Ophthalmology*, 16/1 (1988): pp. 21–5.

Secondary Sources

Broumand, B., 'Living Donors: The Iran Experience', *Nephrology, Dialysis, Transplantation*, 12/9 (1997): 1830–1.

Cameron, J. Stewart, *A History of the Treatment of Renal Failure by Dialysis* (Oxford: Oxford University Press, 2002).

Carrier, James G., *Gifts and Commodities, Exchange and Western Capitalism since 1700* (London: Routledge, 1995).

Cherry, Mark J., *Kidney for Sale by Owner, Human Organs, Transplantation, and the Market* (Washington, DC: Georgetown University Press, 2005).

Chopra, G.K., F. De Vincentis, D. Kaufman and D. Collie, 'Effective Corneal Retrieval in a General Hospital: The Royal Melbourne Hospital Eye Bank', *Australian and New Zealand Journal of Ophthalmology*, 21/4 (1993): pp. 251–5.

Chu, Wing, 'The Past Twenty-Five Years in Eye Banking', *Cornea*, 19/5 (2000): pp. 754–65.

Fabre, Cecile, *Whose Body is it Anyway? Justice and the Integrity of the Person* (Oxford: Clarendon Press, 2006).

Farge, Emile J., 'Eye Banking: 1944 to the Present', *Survey of Ophthalmology*, 33/4 (1989): pp. 260–63.

Fox, Renée C., 'Toward an Ethic of Iatrogenesis', in William R. LaFleur, Gernot Böhme and Susumu Shimazono (eds), *Dark Medicine: Rationalizing Unethical Medical Research* (Bloomington: Indiana University Press, 2007), pp. 149–64.

Fox, Renée C. and Judith P. Swazey, *The Courage to Fail, A Social View of Organ Transplants and Dialysis* (Chicago: University of Chicago Press, 1974).

Fox, Renée C. and Judith P. Swazey, *Spare Parts: Organ Replacement in American Society* (New York: Oxford University Press, 1992).

Gilson, Lucy, 'Trust and the Development of Health Care as a Social Institution', *Social Science and Medicine*, 56/7 (2003): pp. 1453–68.

Goodwin, Michele, *Black Markets: The Supply and Demand of Body Parts* (Cambridge: Cambridge University Press, 2006).

Gruessner, Rainer W.G. and Enrico Benedetti (eds), *Living Donor Organ Transplantation* (New York: McGraw Hill Medical, 2008).

Heiden, David, 'Dr Sanduk Ruit and Corneal Transplantation in Nepal', *The Western Journal of Medicine*, 176/1 (2002): pp. 71–2.

Hopper, Kim, 'Commentary: On the Transformation of the Moral Economy of Care', *Culture, Medicine and Psychiatry*, 25/4 (2001): pp. 473–84.

Hörl, W.H., F. de Alvaro and P.F. Williams, 'Healthcare Systems and End-Stage Renal Disease Therapies – an International Review: Access to ESRD Treatments', *Nephrology, Dialysis, Transplantation*, 14/supp6 (1999): pp. 10–15.

Hull, A.R., 'The Legislative and Regulatory Process in the End Stage Renal Disease Program', *Seminars in Nephrology*, 17/3 (1997): 160–69.

Ikels, Charlotte, 'Kidney Failure and Transplantation in China', *Social Science and Medicine*, 44/9 (1997): pp. 1271–83.

Joralemon, D., 'Shifting Ethics: Debating the Incentive Question in Organ Transplantation', *Journal of Medical Ethics*, 27/1 (2001): pp. 30–35.

Kennedy, Sean E., Yvonne Shen, John A. Charlesworth, James D. Mackie, John D. Mahony, John J.P. Kelly and Bruce A. Pussell, 'Outcome of Overseas Commercial Kidney Transplantation: An Australian Perspective', *Medical Journal of Australia*, 182/5 (2005): pp. 224–7.

Kwitko, Marvin L. and Charles D. Kelman (eds), *The History of Modern Cataract Surgery* (The Hague: Kugler Publications, 1998).

LaFleur, William R., Gernot Böhme and Susumu Shimazono (eds), *Dark Medicine: Rationalizing Unethical Medical Research* (Bloomington: Indiana University Press, 2007).

Lock, Margaret, *Twice Dead, Organ Transplants and the Reinvention of Death* (Berkeley: University of California Press, 2002).

McLaughlin, Joseph K., Loren Lipworth, Wong-Ho Chow and William J. Blot, 'Analgesic Use and Chronic Renal Failure: A Critical Review of the Epidemiological Literature', *Kidney International*, 54/3 (1998): pp. 679–86.

Mauss, Marcel, *The Gift, the Form and Reason for Exchange in Archaic Societies* (New York: W.W. Norton, 1990).

Messikomer, Carla M., Judith P. Swazey and Allen Glicksman (eds), *Society & Medicine, Essays in Honor of Renée C. Fox* (New Brunswick: Transaction Publishers, 2003).

Moazam, Farhat, *Bioethics and Organ Transplantation in a Muslim Society; A Study in Culture, Ethnography and Religion* (Bloomington: Indiana University Press, 2006).

Moffatt, S. Louise, Victoria A. Cartwright and Thomas H. Stumpf, 'Centennial Review of Corneal Transplantation', *Clinical and Experimental Ophthalmology*, 33/6 (2005): pp. 642–57.

Muraine, M., D. Toubeau, E. Menguy and G. Brasseur, 'Analysing the Various Obstacles to Cornea Postmortem Procurement', *British Journal of Ophthalmology*, 86/8 (2002): pp. 864–9.

National Health & Medical Research Council, *Ethical Issues Raised by Allocation of Transplant Resources, Ethical Issues in Organ Donation Discussion Paper No. 3* (Canberra: Australian Government Publishing Service, 1997).

Opit, L.J., 'The Cost of Health Care and Health Insurance in Australia: Some Problems Associated with the Fee-for-Service System', *Social Science and Medicine*, 18/11 (1984): 967–72.

Rao, Gullapalli, 'Eye Banking – are we really up to it in India?', *Indian Journal of Ophthalmology*, 52/3 (2004): p. 183.

Richardson, J.R., 'The Inducement Hypothesis: That Doctors Generate Demand for their Own Services', in J.R.G. Butler and D.P. Doessal (eds), *Health Economics: Australian Readings* (Sydney: Australian Professional Publications, 1989), pp. 215–37.

Ritz, Eberhard, Ivan Rychlik, Francesco Locatelli and Serge Halimi, 'End Stage Renal Failure in Type 2 Diabetes: A Medical Catastrophe of Worldwide Dimensions', *American Journal of Kidney Diseases*, 34/5 (1999): pp. 795–808.

Rosenberg, N., *Inside the Black Box: Technology and Economics* (Cambridge: Cambridge University Press, 1982).

Rothblatt, Martin, *Your Life or Mine, How Geoethics Can Resolve the Conflict Between Public and Private Interests in Xenotransplantation* (Aldershot: Ashgate, 2004).

Rychlik, I., G. Miltenberger-Miltenyi and E. Ritz, 'The Drama of the Continuous Increase in End-Stage Renal Failure in Patients with Type II Diabetes Mellitus', *Nephrology, Dialysis, Transplantation*, 13/supp8 (1998): pp. 6–10.

Sangwan, Virender S., Balasubramanya Ramamurthy, Urmi Shah, Prashant Garg, Mitthanamalli S. Sridhar and Gullapalli N. Rao, 'Outcome of Corneal Transplant Rejection: A 10-Year Study', *Clinical and Experimental Ophthalmology*, 33/6 (2005): pp. 623–7.

Schreiner, G.E., 'How End-Stage Renal Disease-Medicare Developed', *Seminars in Nephrology*, 17 (1997): pp. 152–9.

Shoham, David A., Suma Vupputuri, Jay S. Kaufman, Abhijit V. Kshirsagar, Ana V. Diez Roux, Joseph Koresh and Gerado Heiss, 'Kidney Disease and the Cumulative Burden of Life Course Socioeconomic Conditions: The Atherosclerosis Risk in Communities Study', *Social Science and Medicine*, 67/8 (2008): pp. 1311–20.

Spalton, David and Doug Koch, 'The Constant Evolution of Cataract Surgery', *British Medical Journal*, 321/7272 (2000): p. 1304.

Sprinkle, R.H., 'A Moral Economy of American Medicine in the Managed-Care Era', *Theoretical Medicine and Bioethics*, 22/3 (2001): pp. 247–68.

Taylor, J.S., *Stakes and Kidneys, Why Markets in Human Body Parts are Morally Imperative* (Aldershot: Ashgate, 2005).

Taylor, J.S., 'Black Markets, Transplant Kidneys and Interpersonal Coercion', *Journal of Medical Ethics*, 32/12 (2006): pp. 698–701.

Thomas, Nicholas, *Entangled Objects: Exchange, Material Culture and Colonialism in the Pacific* (Cambridge, MA: Harvard University Press, 1991).

Timmermans, Stefan, 'The Cause of Death vs. the Gift of Life', in Stefan Timmermans and Jonathan Gabe (eds), *Partners in Health, Partners in Crime* (Oxford: Blackwell, 2003), pp. 49–73.

Titmuss, Richard, *The Gift Relationship* (London: George Allen & Unwin, 1970).

Waldby, Catherine and Robert Mitchell, *Tissue Economies, Blood, Organs, and Cell Lines in Late Capitalism* (Durham, NC: Duke University Press, 2006).

Wilde, Sally, 'Surgical Theatre, Gifted Performance: The Moral Economy of Surgical Training', in Christy Collis and Maggie Nolan (eds), *Benevolence*, *Journal of Australian Studies* 85 (Perth: API Network, 2005), pp. 27–36.

Wilkinson, Stephen, *Bodies for Sale, Ethics and Exploitation in the Human Body Trade* (London: Routledge, 2003).

Williams, K.A., M.A. White, P.R. Badenoch, T.R. Wedding, S.J. Alfrich, M.A. Sawyer, L.M. Noack, E.W. Johnstone, G. Zilm and D.J. Coster, 'Donor Cornea Procurement: Six-Year Review of the Role of the Eye Bank of South Australia', *Australian and New Zealand Journal of Ophthalmology*, 18/1 (1990): pp. 77–89.

Youngner, Stuart J., Robert M. Arnold and Renie Schapiro (eds), *The Definition of Death, Contemporary Controversies* (Baltimore: Johns Hopkins University Press, 1999).

Youngner, Stuart J., Renée C. Fox and Laurence J. O'Connell (eds), *Organ Transplantation, Meanings and Realities* (Madison: University of Wisconsin Press, 1996).

Chapter 8

Science Fiction, Cultural Knowledge and Rationality: How Stem Cell Researchers Talk About Reproductive Cloning

Nicola J. Marks

Introduction

In 1996, a sheep code-named 6LL3 was born in Roslin, just outside Edinburgh, UK. She was later named Dolly and became possibly the most famous sheep in the world. She was the first mammal created from an adult cell – not from the union of a sperm and an egg, not from an embryonic cell; she was created through reproductive cloning.[1]

Dolly grabbed the headlines for a number of reasons. Firstly, she shattered an important biological dogma according to which cells, once fully differentiated, can only ever be that one kind of cell. Indeed, Dolly was generated from an udder cell from a fully grown ewe; the nucleus of this cell was put into an enucleated egg (a technique called somatic cell nuclear transfer or SCNT) and tricked into thinking it was a fertilized egg. It started dividing, until an embryo was formed, implanted into a surrogate ewe and brought to term. So the cells in Dolly's body have the same nuclear DNA as the original udder cell and that one original udder cell contains all the necessary information to give rise to a whole new sheep.

Secondly, Dolly was seen as newsworthy because people at once drew the connection with potential human reproductive cloning, despite Ian Wilmut, her creator, downplaying this.[2] Human cloning, or at least the creation of human-like beings without the need for sexual intercourse, had been foreshadowed in

[1] Ian Wilmut et al., 'Viable Offspring Derived from Fetal and Adult Mammalian Cells', *Nature*, 385/6619 (1997): pp. 810–13.

[2] Alan Petersen, 'Replicating Our Bodies, Losing Our Selves: News Media Portrayals of Human Cloning in the Wake of Dolly', *Body and Society*, 8/4 (2002): pp. 72–3, p. 79; Gina Kolata, *Clone: The Road to Dolly and the Path Ahead* (London, 1997), pp. 21–35.

science fiction for decades.[3] It was mentioned indirectly in *Brave New World*[4] and *Frankenstein or, The Modern Prometheus*,[5] and more directly in *The Boys from Brazil*[6] and Woody Allen's film *Sleeper*.[7] With Dolly, human reproductive cloning was leaving the realm of fiction and entering that of scientific possibility.

Thirdly, Dolly opened up the possibility of 'therapeutic cloning', potentially an extremely powerful medical technology. This involves taking a cell from a patient, transferring its nucleus into an enucleated egg (again using somatic cell nuclear transfer), starting the process of cell division until a two- to three-day-old embryo is obtained. Then, instead of implanting the embryo into a surrogate, as was the case with Dolly, it would be transformed into a cell line (an embryonic stem cell line) with the potential to give rise to all cells in the body. Since these cells would contain the same nuclear DNA as the patient, they would be immunologically compatible with him or her, thus theoretically providing an endless supply of cells for therapy. Supporters of stem cell research and cloning have been keen to highlight this exciting medical possibility. However, many tried to distance 'therapeutic cloning' from the less palatable 'reproductive cloning'; this was not easy given their similar technical origins.[8]

Immediately after the announcement of Dolly's birth, scientists, journalists, politicians, intellectuals of all sorts and members of the public started voicing their opinions. A mixture of awe and fear was evident.[9] Clones (including human ones) were imagined and discussed in multiple ways. For some, Dolly was 'one of the most significant scientific breakthroughs of the decade'[10] but for others she conjured up images of '"photocopied" individuals and automated production lines or artificial incubators producing multiple adult clones'.[11] Calls were made for

---

[3] See Jon Turney, *Frankenstein's Footsteps: Science, Genetics and Popular Culture* (New Haven and London, 1998), p. 214; Brigitte Nerlich et al., 'Fictions, Fantasies, and Fears: The Literary Foundation of the Cloning Debate', *Journal of Literary Semantics*, 30/1 (2001): pp. 37–52.

[4] Aldous Huxley, *Brave New World* (London, 1950 [1932]).

[5] Mary Shelley, *Frankenstein or, the Modern Prometheus* (Oxford and New York, 1980 [1818]).

[6] Ira Levin, *The Boys from Brazil* (London, 1976).

[7] *Sleeper*, directed by Woody Allen (1973).

[8] E.g. Sarah Parry, 'The Politics of Cloning: Mapping the Rhetorical Convergence of Embryos and Stem Cells in Parliamentary Debates', *New Genetics and Society*, 22/2 (2003): pp. 145–68; Joan Haran et al., *Human Cloning in the Media: From Science Fiction to Science Practice* (London, 2007), pp. 31–4.

[9] Dorothee Nelkin and M. Susan Lindee, 'Cloning in the Popular Imagination', *Cambridge Quarterly of Healthcare Ethics*, 7/2 (1998): pp. 145–9.

[10] BBC News, *1997: Dolly the Sheep Is Cloned* (22 February 1997).

[11] Wellcome Trust, *Public Perspectives on Human Cloning. A Social Research Study* (London, 1998), p. 13.

rationality and calm,[12] but also for emergency legislation banning reproductive cloning.[13] The public and the media were accused of being misguided by absurd fears that were blamed on science fiction.[14]

Although many expressed concerns about lay people confusing science 'fiction' and science 'fact', this chapter will show that this distinction is not as simple as it may appear. Indeed, when talking about these cutting-edge areas of research, people – including scientists – imagine particular futures for these areas in order to make sense of them in the present. They draw on existing cultural tropes to do so, including those from the science fictional genre. Some imagined futures will be described as fact, others as fantasy; some will come into being, others will not. Importantly though, these future-oriented discourses are not neutral. They may *enable* particular futures to come into being – they are 'performative'. They may also shore up the authority of particular groups, individuals or types of intellectual inquiry – they can be strategic.

The aim of this chapter then is to explore reproductive cloning by examining the futures that scientists imagine for this technology. I analyse whether they attempt to locate these imagined futures within the realms of fact or fantasy, and what discursive strategies they employ to do this. The chapter opens with a brief overview of the scholarship showing that science is not simply fact or (science) fiction simply fantasy. After describing the data collection, it discusses the literature that shows scientists use science fiction-derived imagery to discredit those who criticize embryo research and cloning. Drawing on interview data, it then focuses on stem cell researchers' discourses about reproductive cloning. These scientists express multiple views about the area; this contrasts with the dominant discourse of 'reproductive cloning bad, therapeutic cloning good' found by others.[15] In addition, stem cell researchers here not only attempt to discredit people's fears about stem cell research and cloning by associating these with science fiction, but also draw on science fiction to express their own concerns. The chapter examines scientists' focus on appearing 'rational'; therefore the ways in which fiction-based accounts and 'gut reactions' are elided in favour of 'technical' explanations are also highlighted. In conclusion, I argue that fears and concerns, be they expressed by scientists or members of the public, should not be dismissed simply because they draw on fictional cultural tropes. Instead fiction – including science fiction and speculative fiction, utopian and dystopian visions – should be seen as an important vehicle to express our

---

12 THES Editorial, *Dolly Is Just Cloning Around* (Times Higher Education Supplement, 28 February 1997).

13 Such legislation was implemented in the UK shortly after the announcement of Dolly's birth, *Human Reproductive Cloning Act* (London, 2001).

14 Ayala Ochert, *Fear and Cloning* (Times Higher Education Supplement, 30 January 1998). See also a comment by one of Wilmut's colleagues, Harry D. Griffin, *Dolly: The Science Behind the World's Most Famous Sheep* (n.d.).

15 Haran et al., *Human Cloning in the Media*, p. 31.

unease and excitement about the future of science and medicine. In particular, it highlights a common concern about the integrity of human bodies and what should/not be done to them

Science, Literature and Struggles for Authority

A rich scholarship in science studies has shown that the 'facts' of science are not simple reflections of nature or reality. What scientists consider to be the problem at hand (the one that is worth investigating and that is 'investigatable') depends on the material world, but also on scientists' particular interests and on the theories that they have already accepted.[16] When a hypothesis is tested experimentally, there are always multiple potential ways of interpreting the results. The matter is not settled solely by further reference to nature or further experimentation, but also by social factors.[17] The kinds of hypotheses that are put forward and accepted will reflect the material world, but also the local culture.[18] They may serve the purpose of those with the most political power.[19] So science and scientific facts do not exist outside of society, even though they rely heavily on the materiality of the objects of study: 'science matters, culture matters'.[20]

---

16 David Bloor, *Knowledge and Social Imagery* (London, 1991 [1976]); see also Susan Merrill Squier, *Liminal Lives: Imagining the Future at the Frontiers of Biomedicine* (Durham, NC and London, 2004), pp. 28–32.

17 If an experiment seems to contradict someone's theory, this person may not necessarily be convinced to throw their theory out, instead they might critique the way in which the experiment has been conducted or the equipment and skill of the experimenter. This is the 'experimenter's regress' according to Harry M. Collins, *Changing Order: Replication and Induction in Scientific Practice* (London and Beverly Hills, 1985), pp. 83–4. It is through social negotiations that the validity of knowledge claims are accepted, Harry M. Collins and Trevor J. Pinch, *The Golem: What Everyone Should Know About Science* (Cambridge, 1993). For instance, negotiations determine who might be the right kind of person, or 'modest witness', to make particular claims, see Steven Shapin and Simon Schaffer, *Leviathan and the Air-Pump: Hobbes, Boyle, and the Experimental Life* (Princeton, 1985), Donna J. Haraway, *Modest_Witness@Second_Millenium.FemaleMan©Meets_OncoMouse™: Feminism and Technoscience* (New York, 1997).

18 Barry Barnes, 'On the Conventional Character of Knowledge and Cognition', in Karin D. Knorr-Cetina and Michael Mulkay (eds), *Science Observed: Perspectives on the Social Study of Science* (London, 1983), pp. 19–51.

19 See for instance Donna J. Haraway, 'A Cyborg Manifesto: Science, Technology, and Socialist-Feminism in the Late Twentieth Century', in *Simians, Cyborgs and Women: The Reinvention of Nature* (London, 1991), pp. 243–51.

20 Anne Fausto-Sterling, 'Science Matters, Culture Matters', *Perspectives in Biology and Medicine*, 46/1 (2003): pp. 109–24.

Similarly, discourses found in literary texts and popular culture are not 'just fiction'. Dominant images in the media, films or books provide us with ways of seeing and interpreting the world, and with language to express our concerns.[21] Fictional accounts can help make sense of, normalize or, on the contrary, problematize behaviours, technologies and objects; they have 'epistemological power'.[22] Literature for instance, because it is 'between knowledge and unawareness' opens a unique location for scholarly inquiry.[23] Therefore 'popular culture matters' too.[24]

Science fiction, or speculative fiction,[25] is particularly important given that science and medicine are so embedded in our everyday lives: how we see ourselves and our bodies is increasingly shaped by biomedical research.[26] Our genetic makeup – our DNA – in particular has come to be synonymous with who we are; genetic determinism and essentialism abound in discourses about our identity.[27] Science fiction enables us to explore, explicitly and 'in graphic ways', the different futures (both utopian and dystopian) that science opens for us.[28]

Fiction provides a set of culture tropes, especially metaphors, which we draw on. These metaphors 'structure our understanding of events, convey emotions and attitudes, and allow us to place public issues and events in a shared context of

---

21 Dorothee Nelkin and M. Susan Lindee, *The DNA Mystique: The Gene as a Cultural Icon* (New York, 1995), especially pp. 11–14, see also José Van Dijck, *Imagenation: Popular Images of Genetics* (Basingstoke, 1998), pp. 12–17, Haran et al., *Human Cloning in the Media*, pp. 6–8.

22 Squier, *Liminal Lives*, p. 5.

23 Ibid., p. 22.

24 Nelkin and Lindee, *The DNA Mystique*, p. 11.

25 Margaret Atwood makes a distinction between 'science fiction proper', concerned with technologies and ideas that are not yet in the realms of possibility, and 'speculative fiction', which 'employs the means already more or less to hand, and takes place on Planet Earth', 'The Handmaid's Tale and Oryx and Crake "In Context"', *PMLA*, 119/3 (2004): pp. 513–17, p. 513. However, although she prefers the label 'speculative fiction', some of Atwood's work can arguably be called science fiction, and here this latter label will include both genres.

26 For instance see Sarah Franklin, 'Life Itself: Global Nature and the Genetic Imaginary', in Sarah Franklin, Celia Lury, and Jackie Stacey (eds), *Global Nature, Global Culture* (London, 2000), pp. 188–227, especially pp. 188–98, Nikolas Rose, 'The Politics of Life Itself', *Theory, Culture & Society*, 18/6 (2001): pp. 1–30.

27 Genetic essentialism indicates that our essence can be found in our genes, genetic determinism indicates that who we are, who we will become and how we will act are all written in our DNA, see Nelkin and Lindee, *The DNA Mystique*, especially pp. 2–3 and pp. 149–68.

28 Atwood, 'The Handmaid's Tale and Oryx and Crake "In Context"', pp. 515–16.

common belief'.[29] Gamson and Modigliani introduce the concept of 'interpretive packages' which are clusters of elements such as 'metaphors, catchphrases, visual images, moral appeals and other symbolic devices' that characterize a temporarily dynamic discourse which provides people with 'interpretation and meaning for relevant events'.[30] There are a variety of competing packages available for people to draw upon in order to make sense of the world, but these packages are also themselves shaped by shared cultural meanings. These packages are signalled by 'condensing symbols'[31] which often correspond to strong images from particular works of fiction.

So science and (science) fiction cannot simply be set up in contrast to each other. Instead, they both are shaped by and shape the culture in which they are embedded. However, scientists are often at great pains to distance what they do from science fiction; they contrast science as provider of objective facts with fiction as provider of subjective fantasies.[32] They set up a 'hierarchy of genres': they exclude events and people (such as maverick scientists or concerned publics) from the realms of good science by describing them with terms indicative of the fictional genre.[33] Scientists paint themselves as rational and objective whilst others are dismissed as irrational, subjective and emotional.

Nevertheless, scientists do not only deal in 'facts'. They regularly project themselves into the future where they imagine their hypotheses confirmed by others' work or possible cures becoming widely used. These projections are very important in showing policy-makers, funders and members of the public the potential of particular areas of research.[34] They may even be vital in creating a

---

[29] Nelkin and Lindee, *The DNA Mystique*, p. 16.

[30] William A. Gamson and Andre Modigliani, 'Media Discourse and Public Opinion on Nuclear Power: A Constructionist Approach', *The American Journal of Sociology*, 95/1 (1989): pp. 1–37, p. 2. They discuss for example the interpretative package 'Progress' which frames nuclear power as an issue relating to 'technological development and economic growth' which resonates with cultural myths about technological fixes and technological heroes.

[31] Ibid., p. 3.

[32] Squier, *Liminal Lives*, pp. 14–16. Scientists need to carefully patrol the boundary between science and the rest of society when they wish to step into the policy arena and play the role of 'neutral' advice providers; see Sheila Jasanoff, *The Fifth Branch: Science Advisers as Policymakers* (Cambridge, MA and London, 1990), Anne Kerr et al., 'The New Genetics: Professionals' Discursive Boundaries', *The Sociological Review*, 45/2 (1997): pp. 279–303.

[33] Haran et al., *Human Cloning in the Media*, pp. 131–5.

[34] Mads Borup et al., 'The Sociology of Expectations in Science and Technology', *Technology Analysis & Strategic Management*, 18/3/4 (2006): pp. 285–98; Nik Brown, 'Hope against Hype – Accountability in Biopasts, Presents and Futures', *Science Studies*, 16/2 (2003): pp. 3–21; Nik Brown and Mike Michael, 'A Sociology of Expectations: Retrospecting Prospects and Prospecting Retrospects', *Technology Analysis and Strategic*

future for particular technologies and areas of research; as such these expectations are 'performative'.[35]

Scientists draw on what Waldby has called the 'biomedical imaginary', the cultural references and mythologies (like the genesis story) which guide and shape biomedical thought and interpretations but often remain unacknowledged.[36] As Squier, drawing on Waldby, argues:

> The very fact that imagery and metaphor are thought to be sites extraneous to science suggests *the investment science has in the marginality and obscurity enabled by those discursive modes*. Thus we can look to imagery and metaphor for the *expressions of excess fantasy and desire*, finding therein those sites of unresolved tension, cultural paradox, and stubborn ambiguity that are crucial, if generally overlooked, aspects of biomedicine.[37] (emphasis added)

There are therefore a number of factors that shape how scientists make sense of science; these need further examination. Members of the public draw on four different types of knowledge to make sense of science: 'technical' knowledge; 'methodological' knowledge, such as knowledge of the limitations of genetic testing; 'institutional' knowledge, such as the links between research and funding or commercialization; and 'cultural' knowledge, about the social and cultural contexts in which knowledge is produced.[38] It seems likely that scientists do the same.

In summary then, science and fiction are not easily disentangled, and the study of how scientists deploy fictional references (either to promote particular futures or to criticize others' concerns) is an important location for sociological analysis. In particular, it may highlight how science maintains its authority, as well as reveal some of the 'excess fantasy and desire' or fears scientists have in relation to human clones.

Management, 15/1 (2003): pp. 3–18; Cynthia Selin, 'Expectations and the Emergence of Nanotechnology', *Science, Technology, & Human Values*, 32/2 (2007): pp. 196–220.

[35] Speech Act Theory argues that discourses can bring about changes in the material world. For example see Bronislaw Szerszynski, 'Risk and Trust: The Performative Dimension', *Environmental Values*, 8 (1999): pp. 239–52; Maja Horst, 'Public Expectations of Gene Therapy: Scientific Futures and Their Performative Effects on Scientific Citizenship', *Science, Technology, & Human Values*, 32/2 (2007): pp. 150–71.

[36] Catherine Waldby, *The Visible Human Project: Informatic Bodies and Posthuman Medicine* (London, 2000), pp. 136–7. For example, scientists draw on 'genesis iconography' to make sense of their work, ibid., pp. 131–5.

[37] Squier, *Liminal Lives*, p. 15.

[38] Anne Kerr et al., 'The New Genetics and Health: Mobilising Lay-Expertise', *Public Understanding of Science*, 7/1 (1998): pp. 41–60.

Data Collection in Context

Interview Data and Discourse Analysis

Research for this chapter was part of a broader project examining stem cell scientists' discourses about their work and about public engagement. The data here are from interviews with scientists from either the UK or Australia. These two countries were chosen as they both are English-speaking, have heavily invested in stem cell research and have similar systems of governance. Interviews lasted between 40 and 105 minutes (most lasting 60 minutes). To access a range of voices, I spoke to junior and senior, academic and commercial scientists working with adult and/or embryonic stem cells (in humans and/or animals) or in areas relating to stem cell science (such as immunology). I conducted 37 one-to-one in-depth semi-structured interviews and three group interviews, interviewing a total of 48 scientists.[39] The focus here is on how they talked about 'reproductive' rather than 'therapeutic' cloning and 28 scientists specifically talked about this technology. Qualitative methods were used since the aim was to explore scientists' accounts to gain an in-depth understanding of, for example, discursive strategies, not obtain the percentage of scientists strongly opposed to cloning.

These discourses were analysed following Gilbert and Mulkay's approach,[40] and Potter and Wetherell's development of this work.[41] That is the analysis of discourse as a 'topic' – for instance the study of interpretative regularities or of discursive repertoires – is seen as 'methodologically prior' to that of discourse as a 'resource' – where what interviewees say is taken to reflect how things 'really are'.[42] Discourse is not restricted to particular utterances, and discourse analysis:

---

[39] In addition, I organized two multi-disciplinary discussions bringing together stem cell researchers, social scientists, lawyers and ethicists. In total, the discourses of 54 stem cell researchers were accessed. These data were complemented by attending conferences and by an examination of publicly available material including media coverage and parliamentary transcripts; these will not be discussed here.

[40] Nigel G. Gilbert and Michael Mulkay, *Opening Pandora's Box: A Sociological Analysis of Scientists' Discourse* (London, 1984).

[41] Jonathan Potter, 'Discourse Analysis and Constructionist Approaches: Theoretical Background', in John T.E. Richardson (ed.), *Handbook of Qualitative Research Methods for Psychology and the Social Sciences* (Leicester, 1996), pp. 125–56; Jonathan Potter and Margaret Wetherell, 'Analyzing Discourse', in Alan Bryman and Robert G. Burgess (eds), *Analyzing Qualitative Data* (London and New York, 1994); *Discourse and Social Psychology: Beyond Attitudes and Behaviour* (London, 1987); Margaret Wetherell, 'Racism and the Analysis of Cultural Resources in Interviews', in Harry van den Berg, Margaret Wetherell and Hanneke Houtkoop-Steenstra (eds), *Analyzing Race Talk: Multidisciplinary Perspectives on the Research Interview* (Cambridge and New York, 2003), pp. 11–30.

[42] Gilbert and Mulkay, *Opening Pandora's Box*, p. 8 and pp. 13–17.

> is concerned with talk and texts as social practices … has a triple concern with action, construction and variability … [and has a] concern with the rhetorical or argumentative organization of talks and texts.[43]

So the analysis also investigates how authority is given to particular truth claims and examines discourse in its institutional, cultural and historical settings.[44]

Although interviews are not the same as naturally occurring talk, they are not 'culturally unique'[45] and provide an interesting insight into what scientists say in this context which is perhaps less confrontational than parliamentary debates. Here, respondents were given pseudonyms to help protect their anonymity. All emphases in quotes were added by the author. In places, long interview excerpts are reproduced to highlight some of the complexities and intricacies of respondents' discourses.

Discursive Contexts

The interview data were collected in 2004–2005, which corresponds to a unique set of circumstances. Shortly after Dolly's birth, the first human embryonic stem cell line was created.[46] It was this combination of cloning and stem cell technologies that made therapeutic cloning seem an exciting possibility.

In 1998 and then in 2001, some scientists claimed to be working on reproductive cloning; these were Richard Seed (a physicist), Panos Michael Zavos, Severino Antinori (two fertility specialists) and Brigitte Boiselier (a biochemist, head of a human cloning company and member of the Raelian Sect).[47] No evidence ever surfaced to confirm any success in their endeavours. Nevertheless, clear legislative and regulatory frameworks were called for in many countries to address cloning as well as stem cell-based developments in embryo research.

In the UK, research on embryos for improving infertility treatments was already regulated under the 1990 *Human Fertilisation and Embryology Act*.[48]

---

43 Potter and Wetherell, 'Analyzing Discourse', p. 48.

44 Wetherell, 'Racism and the Analysis of Cultural Resources in Interviews', pp. 14 and 24.

45 Kerr et al., 'The New Genetics: Professionals' Discursive Boundaries', see also Wetherell, 'Racism and the Analysis of Cultural Resources in Interviews', p. 13.

46 James A. Thomson et al., 'Embryonic Stem Cell Lines Derived from Human Blastocysts', *Science*, 282/5391 (1998): pp. 1145–7.

47 Maja Horst, 'Cloning Sensations: Mass Mediated Articulation of Social Responses to Controversial Biotechnology', *Public Understanding of Science*, 14/2 (2005): pp. 185–200; Brigitte Nerlich and David D. Clarke, 'Anatomy of a Media Event: How Arguments Clashed in the 2001 Human Cloning Debate', *New Genetics and Society*, 22/1 (2003): pp. 43–59; Mary C. Ingram-Waters, 'Public Fiction as Knowledge Production: The Case of the Raelians' Cloning Claims', *Public Understanding of Science*, 18/3 (2009): pp. 292–308.

48 *Human Fertilisation and Embryology Act* (London, 1990).

This was extended in 2002 to allow the creation (whether by cloning – SCNT – or fertilization)[49] and use of embryos for research into 'serious conditions' under licence from the Human Fertilisation and Embryology Authority.[50] In parallel, as mentioned in the introduction, reproductive cloning was banned through emergency legislation the same year.

In Australia the use (not the creation) of embryos was legalized and regulated in a nationally consistent manner from 2002[51] but cloning, both reproductive and therapeutic, had been put under moratorium the same year.[52] In 2006, Australian legislation was updated to allow the creation of embryos through cloning technologies for research.

In 2004, during my data collection, a ground-breaking paper was published by Korean scientists led by Woo Suk Hwang and collaborating with American colleagues; they claimed to have created a human stem cell line through cloning (SCNT).[53] This demonstrated that therapeutic cloning was possible. Then in 2005, another paper was published by the same group, this time claiming to have produced over 10 patient-specific cloned stem cell lines, signalling that therapeutic cloning could be efficient enough to be used in a clinical setting.[54] However, after some ethical concerns were raised, both papers were eventually shown to be deliberate frauds.[55]

So when my interviews took place, therapeutic cloning was legal in the UK but its moratorium was about to be reviewed in Australia. In addition, the claims by reproductive cloners had not led to any evidence of human reproductive cloning. Therapeutic cloning still seemed promising as one of the Korean papers had come out, but the fraud had not yet been brought to light. However, Dolly's premature death in early 2003[56] indicated the potential limitations of cloning technologies.[57]

---

49 The Prolife Alliance had argued that cloned embryos did not come under the auspices of the HFEA, thus leaving a legal loophole, *R* v. *Secretary of State for Health, Ex Parte Bruno Quintavalle on Behalf of Pro-Life Alliance* (2001). The case was successful in the High Court but overturned on appeal.

50 *Human Fertilisation and Embryology (Research Purposes) Regulations* (London, 2001).

51 *Research Involving Human Embryos Act* (Canberra, 2002).

52 *Prohibition of Human Cloning Act* (Canberra, 2002).

53 Woo Suk Hwang et al., 'Evidence of a Pluripotent Human Embryonic Stem Cell Line Derived from a Cloned Blastocyst', *Science*, 303/5664 (2004, retracted): 1669–74.

54 'Patient-Specific Embryonic Stem Cells Derived from Human SCNT Blastocysts', *Science*, 308/5729 (2005, retracted): pp. 1777–83.

55 David Cyranoski, 'Verdict: Hwang's Human Stem Cells Were All Fakes', *Nature*, 439/7073 (2006): pp. 122–3.

56 John Whitfield, *Obituary: Dolly the Sheep* (Nature News Online, 18 February 2003).

57 To date, no stem cell lines have been successfully created from cloned human embryos.

Findings: Stem Cell Researchers, Cultural Tropes and Boundary Maintenance

Both in the UK[58] and Australia,[59] public discussions in the media and parliament were important locations where embryo research and cloning were discussed and their future decided. During these, particular discursive strategies were used in order to promote/demote different areas of research. Of interest here are three main themes: the separation of therapeutic from reproductive cloning, the exclusion of 'maverick' scientists from the realms of good science and the use of fictional imagery.

A dominant discourse emerged after the announcement of Dolly's birth and the creation of human embryonic stem cell lines: the majority of supporters of embryo research and therapeutic cloning sought to distance themselves from a minority of scientists engaged in what was described as inappropriate behaviour: reproductive cloning. The distancing was done at two levels. Firstly, scientists, the media and some politicians drew rhetorical boundaries separating therapeutic cloning and reproductive cloning, describing the former as essential research – leading to therapies for multiple diseases – which needed to be legalized, and the latter as bad science that needed to be prohibited.[60] Secondly, would-be reproductive cloners

---

[58] Michael Mulkay, 'Rhetorics of Hope and Fear in the Great Embryo Debate', *Social Studies of Science*, 23/4 (1993); Michael Mulkay, 'The Triumph of the Pre-Embryo: Interpretations of the Human Embryo in Parliamentary Debate over Embryo Research', *Social Studies of Science*, 24/4 (1994); Michael Mulkay, 'Frankenstein and the Debate over Embryo Research', *Science, Technology, & Human Values*, 21/2 (1996); Michael Mulkay, *The Embryo Research Debate: Science and the Politics of Reproduction* (Cambridge, 1997); Parry, 'The Politics of Cloning'; Clare Williams et al., 'Envisaging the Embryo in Stem Cell Research: Rhetorical Strategies and Media Reporting of the Ethical Debates', *Sociology of Health & Illness*, 25/7 (2003): pp. 793–814; Jenny Kitzinger and Clare Williams, 'Forecasting Science Futures: Legitimising Hope and Calming Fears in the Embryo Stem Cell Debate', *Social Science & Medicine*, 61/3 (2005): pp.731–40.

[59] Katherine I. Morley and Wayne Hall, 'Regulation of Embryonic Stem Cell Research and Therapeutic Cloning: The Australian Debate', *Plaintiff*, 55 (2003): pp. 20–23; Olivia Harvey, 'Regulating Stem-Cell Research and Human Cloning in an Australian Context: An Exercise in Protecting the Status of the Human Subject', *New Genetics & Society*, 24/2 (2005): pp. 125–36; Olivia Harvey, 'Regulating Stem Cell Research and Human Cloning in an Australian Context: The Lockhart Review', *New Genetics and Society*, 27/1 (2008): 125–36; Susan Dodds and Rachel A. Ankeny, 'Regulation of hESC Research in Australia: Promises and Pitfalls for Deliberative Democratic Approaches', *Journal of Bioethical Inquiry*, 3/1–2 (2006): pp. 95–107; Rachel Ankeny and Susan Dodds, 'Hearing Community Voices: Public Engagement in Australian Human Embryo Research Policy, 2005–2007', *New Genetics and Society*, 27/3 (2008): pp. 217–32.

[60] Parry, 'The Politics of Cloning', p. 179; Haran et al., *Human Cloning in the Media*, pp. 31–4; Eric Jensen, 'The Dao of Human Cloning: Utopian/Dystopian Hype in the British Press and Popular Films', *Public Understanding of Science*, 17/2 (2008): pp. 123–43, pp. 129–34.

were 'expelled' by other scientists from bona fide science.[61] They were also criticized in the media, which is rather unusual since medical scientists normally enjoy public support there.[62]

A variety of science fiction stories and characters were drawn upon to talk about cloning, including *The Boys from Brazil*, *Frankenstein* and *Brave New World*. Soon after Dolly's birth, they were utilized by the public[63] and in the media[64] to express concerns about reproductive cloning and the 'imminent threat' of mass-produced clones lacking proper human identity. This makes sense, since this area of research was in its infancy. The same was true of IVF in the 1990s when embryo research was discussed at length in the lead-up to the legislation being voted on in the UK and when similar discourses inspired by science fiction were used: 'What could be more natural than to fill the missing parts of the test-tube story along Frankenstein lines?'.[65] In addition, anyone who claimed to want to clone humans was labelled 'mad scientist' or 'Dr Frankenstein'[66] by the media.

However, fictional characters and references to irrationality were more commonly used by those in favour of stem cell research and cloning: they projected fictional accounts onto their opponents (those who disagreed with destroying embryos for instance).[67] Again, as in the 1990 debates over IVF:

> When Frankenstein appeared within the context of pro-research discourse, he was made to speak, not of the dangers of science, but of the credulity, ignorance, and dogmatism of those who were unwilling to endorse the advance of science knowledge.[68]

[61] Sarah Parry, 'Stem Cell Scientists' Discursive Strategies for Cognitive Authority', *Science as Culture*, 18/1 (2009): pp. 89–114, pp. 103–4; Petersen, 'Replicating Our Bodies, Losing Our Selves', p. 82.

[62] Ibid., pp. 83–4.

[63] Wellcome Trust, *Public Perspectives on Human Cloning*, p. 14.

[64] Petersen, 'Replicating Our Bodies, Losing Our Selves', pp. 76–82, pp. 85–6; Brigitte Nerlich et al., 'Clones and Crops: The Use of Stock Characters and Word Play in Two Debates About Bioengineering', *Metaphor and Symbol*, 15/4 (2000): pp. 223–39, pp. 230–33; Iina Hellsten, 'Dolly: Scientific Breakthrough or Frankenstein's Monster? Journalistic and Scientific Metaphors of Cloning', *Metaphor and Symbol*, 15/4 (2000): pp. 213–21, pp. 216–18.

[65] Mulkay, 'Frankenstein and the Debate over Embryo Research', p. 158.

[66] Petersen, 'Replicating Our Bodies, Losing Our Selves', pp. 82–4; Joan Haran, 'Managing the Boundaries between Maverick Cloners and Mainstream Scientists: The Life Cycle of a News Event in a Contested Field', *New Genetics & Society*, 26/2 (2007): 203–19; Haran et al., *Human Cloning in the Media*, pp. 76–8.

[67] For instance, Mulkay, 'Frankenstein and the Debate over Embryo Research'; Williams et al., 'Envisaging the Embryo in Stem Cell Research'; Haran et al., *Human Cloning in the Media*, p. 61.

[68] Mulkay, 'Frankenstein and the Debate over Embryo Research', p. 169.

So supporters of stem cell research and therapeutic cloning used science fiction as a 'rhetorical weapon'.[69] Drawing on Gamson and Modigliani, the condensing symbol here is 'Frankenstein' which has 'cultural resonance'[70] with shared popular culture and can convey a dystopian image of science. However, by being projected onto opponents of embryo research, it indicates these people are silly to believe in science fiction and that their fears are unfounded.

Proponents of IVF and embryo research in the 1990s had also drawn on fictional narratives to support this research. Indeed they needed to project themselves into the future and imagine the possibilities of IVF. However, these projections were always utopian and, as there were no well-known and readily available utopian fictions with which to associate these imaginings, these were never labelled as fantasies. Therefore, the people articulating them could maintain their cognitive authority by not being associated with science fiction.[71]

I now turn to my data which confirms some of the above findings but contrasts with others. In particular, scientists not only project fictional imagery onto others to dismiss their fears, but also themselves draw on fictional cultural tropes (including science fiction like *The Boys from Brazil*) to express their own concerns.

Multiple Views on Reproductive Cloning

I found more variety in my informants' discourses about reproductive cloning than those discussed above – this could be due to the larger sample size and to the private setting compared to those of the media and parliament. Approximately half expressed some level of concern for human reproductive cloning, whilst half expressed some level of support for it, especially as an infertility treatment (only eight respondents totally rejected it). Most respondents had not considered this latter use, so their initial reaction was often interesting. They then thought through this during the interview, sometimes ending up rejecting this idea more, sometimes less, as I will discuss below.

Another difference with the above discourses is that my informants did not mention any of the 'mad scientists' attempting human reproductive cloning. This is most likely due to the timing of my research: when the above data were collected, reproductive cloners had the attention of the media. However, by the time I was interviewing, these claims had been dismissed and stem cell research had retained its aura of 'good science'.

The discourse of some scientists reflected the dominant discourse above: reproductive cloning was described as unacceptable, but therapeutic cloning as useful. For instance a stem cell scientist from Australia states:

---

69 Kitzinger and Williams, 'Forecasting Science Futures', p. 737.

70 Gamson and Modigliani, 'Media Discourse and Public Opinion on Nuclear Power', p. 5.

71 Mulkay, 'Rhetorics of Hope and Fear in the Great Embryo Debate'; Mulkay, 'Frankenstein and the Debate over Embryo Research'.

Martin: If you can imagine using my own cells and creating a zygote and so the cells would be exactly the same genetic material as myself, so if I graft these cells in myself there won't be a graft rejection, and so this is the original idea, *this is a very interesting means of regenerating organs*.

...

Martin: So as I said for me, therapeutical [*sic*] cloning is not really a big ethical issue. Concerning the other, *reproductive cloning*, I think this is something *completely* [hesitation] *freaky*? So it just has to be completely forbidden.

Martin imagines a possible future in which SCNT can help organ regeneration, but advocates a ban on reproductive cloning which he describes in pejorative terms as 'freaky'. Not all scientists however were as enthusiastic about the future promise of therapeutic cloning. This is discussed elsewhere.[72]

Some stem cell researchers said they felt uncomfortable about the idea of reproductive cloning, but were not sure why. The following was the response by an Australian PhD student working on adult stem cells to a question about the acceptability of reproductive cloning for treating infertility:

Caroline: [shakes head] Yeah, no, I would, I mean it's hard because you're dealing with people that really want children. Yeah, I would tend to not agree with that.

Interviewer: Can you understand why you don't agree with that?

Caroline: Um [hesitation] No! [hesitation] It might simply be because you're using the term reproductive cloning.

Caroline was one of the scientists who had not already thought in depth about her view on reproductive cloning as a treatment for infertility

Many scientists raised safety issues as the reason not to let reproductive cloning go forward: 'It's quite clear that it's completely unsafe and you shouldn't think of doing it.' Others put forward another hurdle: the need for DNA mixing, which happens in fertilization, but would be by-passed by cloning:

Philip: I think I'll give you an even better argument against it that's strictly a biological argument: evolution has gone to a lot of trouble to make sexual reproduction, we waste an awful lot of energy on it, it must be there for good reason.

[72] Nicola J. Marks, 'Localities and Temporalities in Stem Cell Research: Dynamics of Expectation in the UK and Australia' (paper presented at the Society for Social Studies of Science Annual Meeting, Tokyo, Japan, 27 August 2010).

This requirement for mixing and the related need for human uniqueness came up frequently in both the UK and Australia.

Several scientists stated they did not have a particular problem with reproductive cloning, especially if it could be used as an infertility treatment and if the safety issues could be solved. An Australian embryonic stem cell researcher stated:

> Heidi: So, at this point I would never say that one should start developing cloning technology for infertility treatment in a clinical setting at this point, because it's not safe. But if you took that argument out and people found that cloning was a safe technology, or it became a safe technology, then I don't see what the argument against it is.

Another argued:

> Danielle: I guess personally I don't have a personal ethical or moral conflict with reproductive cloning, I don't know why that is, I don't know if that's because I'm a scientist or that's because you know I personally know someone that's struggled with infertility, I'm not sure why that is, or, but I think that if it was safe … I don't see the future as being everyone's going to be cloned or anything like that, I don't really see a problem with it, I have a realistic I think view of what it could be applied for.

Danielle was suggesting that her accepting view of reproductive cloning could be due to her being a scientist; this implies that she is not swayed by unfounded fears and has an educated opinion based on 'technical' knowledge. Alternately, her view could be shaped by her personal experience with friends who are infertile, suggesting a role for 'cultural knowledge' in shaping her views.

This diversity of views shows that the same science 'facts' lead to scientists expressing different opinions about what areas of research can and should go forward. Their views then seem to be shaped by something beyond the detail of the science.

Science Fiction as a 'Rhetorical Weapon'

Despite the variety of views just discussed, many scientists expressed their personal view as if it were the obvious one to hold. As did many of the scientists investigated by others, they attempted to discredit people's concerns by placing these in the realm of fiction. Some informants criticized members of the public for drawing on science fiction to make sense of cloning. In the following quote, an

Australian adult stem cell researcher condemns both the media and the press for associating scientists with Dr Frankenstein:

> Clara: There's lot of [hesitation] bad press you know, *Dr Frankensteins*, so that's the other thing, I find that really annoying, this whole, like with the cloning debate, and the public issue was because you know a scientist is going to go away and clone something just because they can … We all have better things to do!

Here, Clara is implying that scientists are responsible people who would not waste their time on something as unsavoury as human reproductive cloning. Similarly, a British embryonic stem cell scientist bemoans science fiction's perceived influence on the low public opinion of scientists:

> Anthony: But once something starts becoming a bit controversial … you've got you know *all this Frankenstein cloning*, then people start to get suspicious, 'this is scientists just playing around'.

Neither Clara nor Anthony portrayed these imagined uses of Dr Frankenstein as ways of expressing concerns over the potential of science to run away and lead to unintended consequences. They steeped criticisms of scientists in science fiction, and could thus dismiss them as irrational. Neither of these respondents suggested that some of their (well-respected) colleagues may not oppose reproductive cloning in such unequivocal terms.

Another informant from Australia downplayed concerns about scientists attempting human reproductive cloning. To do this he drew on science fiction imagery but also highlighted that if scientists had wanted to clone humans, they already could have done this by using technologies other than somatic cell nuclear transfer:

> Victor: If you really set your mind to actually doing something destructive, you could, *The Boys from Brazil, that's something that comes up all the time*, you know in the field, but the fact is that embryo splitting has been around for a long time, so if you wanted to, you can split an embryo … I'm sure it would work, although I don't know if anyone's tried it … since the 1980s, embryos splitting's been around, no one's done it, the whole point is, OK fine you might just want to do it for the hell of it, if you don't have a reason, people won't do it, *there's a lot of the stuff you can do in different ways, but no-one's ever bothered to do it.*

In *The Boys from Brazil* Joseph Mengele survives the end of the war and flees to Sao Paulo where he produces clones out of tissue he took from the late Adolf

Hitler.[73] Victor indicates that the image fiction projects of scientists is distorted as these people are not megalomaniacs bent on world destruction or re-creating Hitler. Evidence for this is the fact that scientists have not 'bothered' to use another available technology to create clones (embryo splitting). So concerns about reproductive cloning are not well founded according to Victor.

A different stem cell researcher, this time from the UK, also criticized members of the public for basing their views on science fiction, after I mentioned that some people may fear clones would not have their own identity:

> Ted: I think [clones] would have their own identity, because, I come back to identical twins, in practice, *I think we're being kind of skewed by ... The Boys from Brazil kind of scenario, of creating mini-Hitl*ers, you're probably too young to remember *a film by Woody Allen, called Sleeper*, have you seen that? It's probably worth watching that, because [the] grandmaster's nose [is] to be cloned to form a new one. *It's ridiculous obviously* but in practice, when we have identical twins, we might say, oh, they look very similar, but we don't somehow think they are the same person, or they have the same identity, we treat them as separate people, so *we are completely capable of distinguishing between genetic identity and psycho-social identity.*

Ted is highlighting the idea that a person's genetic makeup does not determine their 'psycho-social' identity. In other words, he condemns genetic determinism and highlights the role of nurture as well as nature in identity formation. According to Ted, clones would be unique individuals. Ted is partly blaming science fiction such as *The Boys from Brazil* or *Sleeper* for this focus on genetic determinism. For him these scenarios are 'ridiculous obviously': they will not occur in practice and only serve to worry and confuse people. However, as will be shown below, not everyone disbelieves these scenarios which also do not clearly rest on genetic deterministic understandings of human identity.

Scientists here project science fiction imagery onto publics, whose fears then no longer have to be taken seriously and can be dismissed.

Science Fiction as a Means of Expression

Some of my informants expressed their own concerns using science fiction images, rather than projecting these onto others. For instance, I had asked a UK adult stem cell researcher what he thought about his country being one of the only ones to have legalized human SCNT (the first steps towards therapeutic and reproductive cloning). In the following quotes, he answers by criticizing other countries' bans

[73] Levin, *The Boys from Brazil*; José Van Dijck, 'Cloning Humans, Cloning Literature: Genetics and the Imagination Deficit', *New Genetics and Society*, 18/1 (1999): pp. 9–22.

for being based on emotions rather than facts. He then describes his own concerns about reproductive cloning, and draws on imagined futures derived from science fiction to express them:

John: Yes, I think, well you have to ask why the other countries have made it illegal, you know, and *it's mostly these sorts of semi-religious or emotional things* about, about them being human embryos or human cells … I don't really see that you know we should take a different view about these cells to any other cells, unless people are proposing to grow them up into, into live human beings, where there's a whole set of different issues that come up, but, so no, I think our legislation is sensible.

Interviewer: So what issues concern you about reproductive cloning then? Is it the safety issues?

John: … I mean I think *the first thing is safety*, and unless it's absolutely safe, you shouldn't do it. There are issues of more sort of widespread issues of public health … Sexual reproduction actually has a function of mixing up the gene pool and if reproductive cloning became common place *you could end up with a really rather restricted gene pool*. Um, *I don't terribly like the idea of having one hundred copies of some of the world's dictators*, [laugh] [hesitation] *which could easily happen.*

Interviewer: Do you think that? That that could happen? I mean in terms of environmental factors being important, for example, I mean I don't necessarily, I mean Dolly was different to her mum for example …

John: Well we don't know actually. Um, but I think it's quite possible that a dear leader would make one hundred copies of himself [laugh].

By highlighting his approval of UK legislation, John indicates that 'semi-religious or emotional things' should not guide science policy, thus presumably suggesting instead a role for scientific facts. He expresses his approval for the banning of reproductive cloning and gives three reasons. The first relates to safety and, as mentioned above, is often used as grounds not to reproductively clone human beings. The second was also given by several informants and highlights the importance of having a varied gene pool for species adaptation in case of environmental changes. The third is the most remarkable here. John suggests that allowing reproductive cloning could lead to the creation of 'one hundred copies of some of the world's dictators'.

This last scenario is, in my view, clearly inspired by *The Boys from Brazil* in which 94 clones are produced from Hitler's tissue. John does not see this as fantasy, and argues that it is quite possible and 'could easily happen'. When I quiz him about the role of nurture in shaping identity, he indicates that there is no clear evidence that environment would play a large role: 'Well we don't know actually'. Although John may acknowledge the cultural reference to science fiction, he does not portray his concerns about reproductive cloning as based on irrational fears; rather the idea that a leader would want to use cloning to make 100 copies of himself is presented as quite reasonable. However his laugh may indicate he realizes other people may not take these concerns seriously.

Thus, John contrasts unsatisfactory legislation or decision-making around science, which he describes as based on emotions and religion, with sound decisions based on evidence and risk assessments – even if these risks are re-interpretations of science fiction scenarios. He avoids sounding contradictory by portraying the storyline of politicians wanting to clone themselves as realistic. He bases these claims on the evaluation of available data (such as the status of current scientific knowledge or the character of current leaders) and by implication, then, is not displaying emotion-based judgements. So being able to present one's views as 'rational' is important. I will come back to this in the next section.

John's is a very genetically deterministic view. He imagines clones as 'copies' with the same characteristics as the original dictator. This contrasts with Ted's view above. Other informants, this time from Australia, also expressed a belief in determinism:

> Barry: In terms of reproduction I see no real merit in having a cloned individual because it's really only a facsimile of, genetically, of someone who's already there.

By using the label 'facsimile', Barry is using 'metaphors' of clones as 'photocopies'[74] to dismiss reproductive cloning. Thus, similarly to publics and media,[75] he is drawing on cultural imagery and projects an image of clones as mere copies of the original.

One scientist working in immunology in Australia was unusual in that he expressed the following very specific concern about therapeutic cloning sliding into reproductive cloning:

> David: *There's only one way to make a complex organ: that is do reproductive cloning and abort the foetus and take the organs*, that's the only way to do it. So people haven't thought that next step through. That's the real reason that I'm against cloning, reproductive cloning … So you could say I need a kidney to live,

[74] Nerlich and Clarke, 'Anatomy of a Media Event', pp. 51, 53.

[75] Wellcome Trust, *Public Perspectives on Human Cloning*; Nerlich et al., 'Fictions, Fantasies, and Fears'; Nerlich and Clarke, 'Anatomy of a Media Event'; Haran et al., *Human Cloning in the Media*.

> I'll make a clone of myself, get a woman to bear that child until the third trimester, pay her to have an abortion, take the baby and take his two kidneys. They'd be exactly the same tissue type as mine, implant them in me, I've got perfect kidney function. *So that's really Frankenstein stuff, but that's totally and utterly doable.*

David is imagining an undesirable future in which human clones (foetuses that are aborted) are created for immunologically compatible body parts. This contrasts with more common utopian futures found in the media and described by other scientists (see above) in which therapeutic cloning is used to create compatible body parts from cell lines. Similar to John above, David invokes a specific cultural trope from science fiction (Frankenstein), but does not indicate that this association is irrational or that his views are therefore mere fantasies. He describes a very detailed scenario in which complex organs are found to be impossible to make from cell lines and in which the initial promises of therapeutic cloning are not realized, leading to a reproductive cloning/organ harvesting dystopian situation.

This storyline is in fact very similar to that of *The Island*,[76] which came out several months later. In this film, organs for rich people were initially going to come from cell cultures, but greed and technical problems led to the need to create full (adult) human clones. Although describing an imagined future that could easily be a science fiction plot, David does not portray his views as unrealistic. In fact, his use of the Frankenstein trope could be a way of signalling his awareness that his scenario may *seem* fantastical, and his rejection of this point of view; he is pre-empting criticisms of his imagined future. David here expresses concern about the commodification of clones' bodies and their use as spare parts. Although these cloned foetuses are genetically identical to the donors, they should still be afforded some kind of dignity.

Scientists do not only draw on science fiction to express dystopian futures for reproductive cloning. For example, an Australian adult stem cell scientist discusses a friend's experiment:

> Pierce: I've just had a mate of mine who cloned a mouse from an olfactory receptor in the nose … it's what Woody Allen did in *Sleeper*.

Pierce directly associates his friend's work with the storyline of a fictional movie. The plot of *Sleeper* was raised by another scientist above and labelled as unrealistic ('ridiculous obviously'). Here however, an experiment that has taken place is described by analogy with fiction. In fact, Pierce then goes on to explain that his friend contacted Allen to tell him about his experiment. This indicates the friend knew of this fictional storyline and highlights the 'biological imaginaries' that shape the experiments that scientists undertake. Of course, here, the clone in question is that of a mouse; it is not clear that the same sort of language would be

[76] *The Island*, directed by Michael Bay (2005).

used if the cloning was of a human. It is quite possible that human bodies are seen as more special, or sacred, than that of animals.

I have argued that fictional scenarios created in the entertainment industry and scientists' imagined futures are not so distant. Scientists do not only draw on fictional imagery to discredit others, but also to express their visions of future scientific developments, which make sense of their current positions on cloning. These imagined futures however are not portrayed as irrational or fictional, but as realistic.

Reconstructing 'Rational' Reasoning

In this section, I explore how scientists make sense of the views they express about reproductive cloning, stem cell research and regulation. Some researchers are happy to paint their views as grounded in values and other cultural factors. Others work hard to 'rationalize' them and present them as objective and factual.

In the following quotes, I discuss stem cell regulation with a researcher in Australia:

> Peter: … But to ban [embryonic stem cell research], *because a certain sub-population of the community has a strong feeling* that no one should have access to this because they don't believe in it themselves, *I think that's wrong*, I think that's ethically wrong …
>
> Interviewer: If say embryonic stem cell research went forward and somatic cell nuclear transfer was, became more safe and reproductive cloning became safe, what would you say to that? …
>
> Peter: I don't think that's acceptable.
>
> Interviewer: OK. Why do you not think that's acceptable?
>
> Peter: […] [hesitation] Because you're making, well because, even though we think it's safe, if something. There's a couple of reasons. First of all, I can't see any point in making a new human for the sake of you know making a new person that's going to grow up as a person, you know, I don't see any medical, necessarily any medical benefit that couldn't be achieved in another way. There's something, *maybe I have some religion in there somewhere deep down*, there's something wrong about that, *it just doesn't feel right to me*, I don't see the need for it and it doesn't feel right.
>
> Interviewer: So do you then think it should be banned?

Peter: But I don't … so it comes back to where, where do you think human life begins. I don't have a problem with, dealing with cells in the dish all the time, I don't think a few cells in the dish are, have a soul basically. I guess if they're used for a therapeutic reason, that's fine, but to make a whole new living organism that can also then pass it's genetic material on, even, mistake or no mistake, to the next generation, and then throughout the rest of mankind, and there's a potential for a tiny mistake to be passed on forever. And you know, possibilities are horrendous ethically, you know, *I can think of disaster scenarios* where you have a cloned person that has some, that you think is fine but has some terrible disease, some new disease, some early ageing disease like Dolly or something that gets to twenty and wants, like everyone else, to have their family, all of a sudden, I know I'm talking about, maybe talking eugenics here but, you don't really want, there's no need to have that situation happen … *we shouldn't allow you know reproductive cloning.*

Peter presents concerns based on religious or emotive grounds as inappropriate reasons to put breaks on science. Then he expresses concerns about reproductive cloning. I ask him if it should therefore be banned. His initial 'gut-reaction'[77] against reproductive cloning is not used as a justification to ban this technology either. Peter finally says that reproductive cloning should not be allowed, but only after he has found and voiced concerns which relate to public health – he imagines a dystopian scenario in which people with unknowable and undetected mutations are created. So concerns about the health and safety of potential clones and future populations are put forward as better (more appropriate and convincing) reasons to ban a practice than ones based on the perceived inherent wrongness of this practice.

According to Gilbert and Mulkay, scientists draw on different repertoires in different contexts in order to present particular versions of events. Specifically, the 'contingent repertoire' is deployed when actions are depicted 'as the activities and judgements of specific individuals acting on the basis of their personal inclinations and particular social positions'.[78] This contrasts to the 'empiricist repertoire' which 'portrays scientists' actions and beliefs as following unproblematically and inescapably from the empirical characteristics of an impersonal natural world'.[79] The former is usually drawn on to explain why people (including scientists) make erroneous judgements, whilst the latter is used to explain the correctness of one's

[77] Later in the interview Peter agrees this label describes his concerns about reproductive cloning.

[78] Gilbert and Mulkay, *Opening Pandora's Box*, p. 57.

[79] Ibid., p. 56.

own decisions, which flowed inevitably from the 'proper' interpretation of nature. This is called the 'asymmetrical' 'accounting for error'.[80]

Utilizing these analytical tools, it can be argued that Peter is attempting to explain the error in others' views that stem cell research should be banned by drawing on the contingent repertoire – the 'personal inclinations' of these others is that they are religious. At the same time he uses the empiricist repertoire to explain his position on reproductive cloning – he portrays the need to ban it as following from safety concerns based on Dolly's early ageing and the risk of passing diseases to future generations. Peter's own personal inclinations are mentioned ('maybe I have some religion in there somewhere deep down') but not put forward as reasons for a ban. A similar analysis of John's discourse above can be done. He describes others' views using the contingent repertoire – 'these sorts of semi-religious or emotional things' – and challenges their role in guiding policy, whilst describing his view using a more empiricist repertoire – for instance talking about the 'really rather restricted gene pool'. Similarly Philip was keen to give me 'strictly a biological argument' to explain his stance on reproductive cloning. So many scientists describe the reasons for their views using the empiricist repertoire, even if they are describing imagined futures that may or may not eventuate.

Other researchers by contrast are more comfortable discussing their views using the contingent repertoire. For example, Zach working on adult stem cells in Australia says the following:

> Zach: I can't see any productive reason for [reproductive cloning] and I, I suppose I'm sort of contradicting myself in saying that if there's no obvious benefit why should you do it, when I've said there's other things that have been banned that shouldn't have been banned because of the possibility of stuff. For that one, I just can't, I can't understand why you would need that sort of an aspect, it seems, and in that case, it's not actually for research, it's for people to have children along other pathways so, I don't know if it needs to be banned I suppose. I'm not really big on banning stuff, so [laugh] I just can't see the necessity for it … It seems a very extreme way, you know, *I'm just not really comfortable with the idea of people basically raising themselves*, and I know it's not the same and nurture comes into it but *I probably just see too much science-fi to* [laugh] *to separate from my way of thinking.*

Zach is commenting on the contradiction between his criticism expressed earlier (data not shown) of stopping therapeutic cloning because of people's concerns about potential abuses and his own concerns about reproductive cloning. He is willing to state that his views are shaped by his socio-cultural environment, in particular science fiction. Like John above, his laugh indicates his realization that others may not therefore take his view seriously. As a PhD student with little experience of speaking in public, Zach appears to be more prepared than other informants to

80 Ibid., pp. 79–82.

acknowledge his views as being contradictory and socially located. He reflects on the difficulty in separating one's views from broader cultural influences. In particular, although he can draw on 'technical' knowledge[81] to highlight the role of nurture, he retains a view of human clones as photocopies of the original cell donors, with the same identity ('raising themselves'). His 'biological imaginary'[82] is here, rather unusually, acknowledged and shown to shape his thinking and explain his concern about genetic determinism.

Many scientists draw mainly on the empiricist repertoire and 'technical' knowledge to express their views and put them forward as rational facts untainted by culture. However, there is space for explicitly contingent and cultural knowledge to be expressed too.

Discussion and Conclusions: Rhetorical Strategies, Cloned Bodies and the 'Imagination Deficit'

This chapter has examined scientists' discourses about reproductive cloning. It has shown that fact and fiction merge and separate in interesting ways. Scientists present different futures for cloning and imagine clones and their bodies in different ways.

Reproductive cloning is at the cutting edge of research. Although the birth of Dolly is an indication that the creation of cloned humans may be possible, there is still much work to be done if this is ever to happen. This 'work' includes 'imaginative work', whereby future-oriented discourses imagine, promote and construct a future in which cloning is a possibility, as well as material work for instance to refine the technology. It is of course possible that the creation of human clones may not occur. This latter future will be facilitated if the materiality of human cells prevents their successful cloning, or if imaginative work that casts a negative image of cloning is successful enough to end interest in this area.

There were various ways in which scientists interviewed here talked about human cloning. Some imagined a future in which it was a treatment for infertility. Others described it as 'freaky' or imagined a future in which genetic diversity was under threat due to too many people using it. For many, there were hurdles to overcome before human cloning should be considered; these often related to the health and safety of future clones. In addition, several scientists expressed some form of 'gut reaction' against this technology (e.g. Peter or Caroline) which may also prevent it from being developed.

Because human reproductive cloning has not been achieved in practice, the imaginative work that refers to it (whether to promote or demote it) is heavily influenced by popular culture, especially science fiction in which reproductive cloning has existed for a long time. Fictional imagery was here utilized in two

81 Kerr et al., 'The New Genetics and Health'.

82 Waldby, *The Visible Human Project*.

key ways. Firstly it was used as a 'rhetorical weapon'[83] to discredit others' views. Stem cell researchers projected science fiction-based accounts into the mouths of members of the public for instance. In this way, concerns raised by these others were placed in the domain of fiction and did not merit careful consideration. This rhetorical strategy, which draws on a 'hierarchy of genres',[84] is commonly adopted by those in favour of a controversial area of research in order to displace criticisms. This projects and imagines members of the public and others as credulous and irrational.

Secondly science fiction and other cultural tropes are part of scientists' 'biological imaginary';[85] they shape, implicitly or explicitly, how scientists speculate about their (proposed) research and that of others. For instance, Zach explicitly drew on science fiction to explain his concern about reproductive cloning, and Pierce's colleague articulated his project about creating a mouse from nose cells by drawing a parallel with *Sleeper*. Similarly, John expressed his concerns about reproductive cloning by referring implicitly to the scenario of *The Boys from Brazil*. So science fiction here, in contrast to others' findings [86], can be used by stem cell researchers overtly to express their views, not simply to dismiss what critics may argue.

These scientists however seem aware that links with fiction could make their views seem merely fantastical. They tried to pre-empt this by laughing or stating something along the lines of 'this may seems crazy, but it is true, and I have plausible evidence' (e.g. 'So that's really Frankenstein stuff, but that's totally and utterly doable'). Extending on this, although some scientists explicitly draw on fictional imagery, they are usually keen to highlight that their views are shaped by rational thought and experimentation. However, this contrast between those who are rational and those who are not needs to be 'constructed'; it is not simply given in nature. As Haraway argues, '[t]he struggle is over who gets to count as a rational actor, as well as an author of knowledge, in the dramas and courts of technoscience'.[87] Here we saw how scientists like John and Peter had difficulty during interviews to make sense of their 'gut reactions' and how they attempted to downplay the 'cultural' components of knowledge in favour of 'technical' ones.[88] One strategy for this was to draw flexibly on the 'contingent' and 'empiricist repertoires'.[89]

When scientists draw on cultural tropes, these achieve specific effects (like displacing criticism or highlighting concerns) by signalling particular 'interpretive

---

83 Kitzinger and Williams, 'Forecasting Science Futures'.

84 Haran et al., *Human Cloning in the Media*.

85 Waldby, *The Visible Human Project*.

86 For instance, Mulkay, 'Frankenstein and the Debate over Embryo Research'; Parry, 'The Politics of Cloning'.

87 Haraway, *Modest_Witness*, p. 89.

88 Kerr et al., 'The New Genetics and Health'.

89 Gilbert and Mulkay, *Opening Pandora's Box*.

packages'.[90] One of these packages is 'the unacceptability of reproductive cloning'. In John's case, 'one hundred dictators' is a 'condensing symbol' which has a particular cultural resonance, through its association with the storyline of *The Boys from Brazil* and is thus likely to suggest similar meanings to various people who might hear it. Drawing on metaphors from *The Boys from Brazil* can be a short-cut way of projecting an image of reproductive cloning as unacceptable.

So stem cell researchers draw on science fiction imagery and particular interpretative packages to project visions of reproductive cloning or of members of the public. However, these reinterpretations of film or book storylines do not always do the originals justice. For example, there can be many ways of reading *The Boys from Brazil*. Here it was deployed as an example of genetic determinism, whereby armies of Hitler clones were generated (this interpretation was either accepted by the likes of John, or projected onto publics and dismissed by Victor). However, Levin's novel highlights the role of nurture in addition to that of genes in determining people's character.[91] There seems to be an 'imagination deficit' as Van Dijck calls it: 'Relevant and interesting literary works were systematically reduced to their seemingly unequivocal or unambiguous plots, without acknowledgement of their rich, multi-interpretable and educational content'.[92]

Some of these impoverished re-deployments of cultural products lead to 'conventional, flattened concepts of the human body, its identity and individuality'.[93] That is, clones are imagined as 'photocopies' of the original, pale imitations. Genes are given an all important role in the generation of psychological identity. These conceptions highlight the angst displayed by stem cell researchers like John or Barry towards the idea of creating clones that would not be 'proper' human beings. This indicates that for them genetics determine what cloned bodies will look like but also *who* clones will be, and human uniqueness should not be diluted or troubled by the creation of clones. In addition, the narcissistic idea of people 'raising themselves' becomes a concern if individuality comes solely from genes.

By contrast, conceptions of potential clones as unique individuals and reproductive cloning as part of tools for assisted reproductive technology reveals an understanding of identity stemming from a combination of nature and nurture. This more complex understanding is reproduced not only in *The Boys from Brazil*, but also in other multi-layered science fiction narratives such as *Blueprint* or *Joshua, Son of None*.[94] For scientists who imagine clones in this way (such as Heidi or Ted), clones would be 'proper' people who deserve respect. Their well-

[90] Gamson and Modigliani, 'Media Discourse and Public Opinion on Nuclear Power'.

[91] Van Dijck, 'Cloning Humans, Cloning Literature', pp. 14–15.

[92] Ibid., p. 9.

[93] Ibid.

[94] Ibid., pp. 15–17; Haran et al., *Human Cloning in the Media*, pp. 58–9; Kate O'Riordan, 'Human Cloning in Film: Horror, Ambivalence, Hope', *Science as Culture* 17 (2008): pp. 145–62, p. 150.

being is of concern if cloning technologies do not improve. This understanding of clones as full human beings, despite their genetic identity (as in sameness) with donors, is also visible in David's concern about the commodification of clones' bodies (including that of foetuses) for use in stem cell treatments. Again, this complex issue is dealt with in a film, *The Island*.[95]

All these scientists imagine clones and their bodies in different ways, sometimes utopian, sometimes dystopian. Despite the rejection by many of science fiction as a means of making sense of human reproductive cloning, I think the richness and diversity of fictional narratives may be very useful in unpicking exactly what it is that we fear or embrace in this technology.

Bibliography

Ankeny, Rachel and Susan Dodds, 'Hearing Community Voices: Public Engagement in Australian Human Embryo Research Policy, 2005–2007', *New Genetics and Society*, 27/3 (2008): pp. 217–32.

Atwood, Margaret, 'The Handmaid's Tale and Oryx and Crake "In Context"', *PMLA*, 119/3 (2004): pp. 513–17.

Barnes, Barry, 'On the Conventional Character of Knowledge and Cognition', in Karin D. Knorr-Cetina and Michael Mulkay (eds), *Science Observed: Perspectives on the Social Study of Science* (London: Sage, 1983), pp. 19–51.

BBC News. *1997: Dolly the Sheep Is Cloned.* 22 February 1997 [cited 5 November 2010]. Available at: http://news.bbc.co.uk/onthisday/hi/dates/stories/february/22/newsid_4245000/4245877.stm.

Bloor, David, *Knowledge and Social Imagery*, 2nd edn (London: Routledge and Kegan Paul, 1991 [1976]).

Borup, Mads, Nik Brown, Kornella Konrad and Harro Van Lente, 'The Sociology of Expectations in Science and Technology', *Technology Analysis & Strategic Management*, 18/3/4 (2006): pp. 285–98.

Brown, Nik, 'Hope against Hype – Accountability in Biopasts, Presents and Futures', *Science Studies*, 16/2 (2003): pp. 3–21.

Brown, Nik, and Mike Michael, 'A Sociology of Expectations: Retrospecting Prospects and Prospecting Retrospects', *Technology Analysis and Strategic Management*, 15/1 (2003): pp. 3–18.

Collins, Harry M., *Changing Order: Replication and Induction in Scientific Practice* (London and Beverly Hills: Sage, 1985).

Collins, Harry M. and Trevor J. Pinch, *The Golem: What Everyone Should Know About Science* (Cambridge: Cambridge University Press, 1993).

Cyranoski, David, 'Verdict: Hwang's Human Stem Cells Were All Fakes', *Nature*, 439/7073 (2006): pp. 122–3.

95 Ibid., pp. 153–6.

Dodds, Susan and Rachel A. Ankeny, 'Regulation of hESC Research in Australia: Promises and Pitfalls for Deliberative Democratic Approaches', *Journal of Bioethical Inquiry*, 3/1–2 (2006): pp. 95–107.

Fausto-Sterling, Anne, 'Science Matters, Culture Matters', *Perspectives in Biology and Medicine*, 46/1 (2003): pp. 109–24.

Franklin, Sarah, 'Life Itself: Global Nature and the Genetic Imaginary', in Sarah Franklin, Celia Lury and Jackie Stacey (eds), *Global Nature, Global Culture* (London: Sage, 2000), pp. 188–227.

Gamson, William A. and Andre Modigliani, 'Media Discourse and Public Opinion on Nuclear Power: A Constructionist Approach', *The American Journal of Sociology*, 95/1 (1989): pp. 1–37.

Gilbert, Nigel G. and Michael Mulkay, *Opening Pandora's Box: A Sociological Analysis of Scientists' Discourse* (London: Cambridge University Press, 1984).

Griffin, Harry D. *Dolly: The Science Behind the World's Most Famous Sheep*. n.d. [cited 18 November 2010]. Available at: http://cdsweb.cern.ch/record/454177/files/p443.pdf.

Haran, Joan, 'Managing the Boundaries between Maverick Cloners and Mainstream Scientists: The Life Cycle of a News Event in a Contested Field', *New Genetics & Society*, 26/2 (2007): pp. 203–19.

Haran, Joan, Jenny Kitzinger, Maureen McNeil and Kate O'Riordan, *Human Cloning in the Media: From Science Fiction to Science Practice* (London: Routledge, 2007).

Haraway, Donna J., 'A Cyborg Manifesto: Science, Technology, and Socialist-Feminism in the Late Twentieth Century', in *Simians, Cyborgs and Women: The Reinvention of Nature* (London: Free Association, 1991), pp. 243–51.

Haraway, Donna J., *Modest_Witness@Second_Millenium.FemaleMan©Meets_OncoMouse™: Feminism and Technoscience* (New York: Routledge, 1997).

Harvey, Olivia, 'Regulating Stem-Cell Research and Human Cloning in an Australian Context: An Exercise in Protecting the Status of the Human Subject', *New Genetics & Society*, 24/2 (2005): pp. 125–36.

Harvey, Olivia, 'Regulating Stem Cell Research and Human Cloning in an Australian Context: The Lockhart Review', *New Genetics and Society*, 27/1 (2008): pp. 33–42.

Hellsten, Iina, 'Dolly: Scientific Breakthrough or Frankenstein's Monster? Journalistic and Scientific Metaphors of Cloning', *Metaphor and Symbol*, 15/4 (2000): pp. 213–21.

Horst, Maja, 'Cloning Sensations: Mass Mediated Articulation of Social Responses to Controversial Biotechnology', *Public Understanding of Science*, 14/2 (2005): pp. 185–200.

Horst, Maja, 'Public Expectations of Gene Therapy: Scientific Futures and Their Performative Effects on Scientific Citizenship', *Science, Technology, & Human Values*, 32/2 (2007): pp. 150–71.

Human Fertilisation and Embryology Act (London: HMSO, 1990).

Human Fertilisation and Embryology (Research Purposes) Regulations (London: HMSO, 2001).

Human Reproductive Cloning Act (London: HMSO, 2001).

Huxley, Aldous, *Brave New World* (London: Chatto & Windus, 1950 [1932]).

Hwang, Woo Suk, Sung Il Roh, Byeong Chun Lee, Sung Keun Kang, Dae Kee Kwon, Sue Kim, Sun Jong Kim, Sun Woo Park, Hee Sun Kwon, Chang Kyu Lee, Jung Bok Lee, Jin Mee Kim, Curie Ahn, Sun Ha Paek, Sang Sik Chang, Jung Jin Koo, Hyun Soo Yoon, Jung Hye Hwang, Youn Young Hwang, Ye Soo Park, Sun Kyung Oh, Hee Sun Kim, Jong Hyuk Park, Shin Yong Moon, and Gerald Schatten, 'Patient-Specific Embryonic Stem Cells Derived from Human SCNT Blastocysts', *Science*, 308/5729 (2005, retracted): pp. 1777–83.

Hwang, Woo Suk, Young June Ryu, Jong Hyuk Park, Eul Soon Park, Eu Gene Lee, Ja Min Koo, Hyun Yong Jeon, Byeong Chun Lee, Sung Keun Kang, Sun Jong Kim, Curie Ahn, Jung Hye Hwang, Ky Young Park, Jose B. Cibelli, and Shin Yong Moon, 'Evidence of a Pluripotent Human Embryonic Stem Cell Line Derived from a Cloned Blastocyst', *Science*, 303/5664 (2004, retracted): pp. 1669–74.

Ingram-Waters, Mary C., 'Public Fiction as Knowledge Production: The Case of the Raelians' Cloning Claims', *Public Understanding of Science*, 18/3 (2009): pp. 292–308.

The Island, directed by Michael Bay (DreamWorks SKG, Warner Bros. Pictures and Parkes/MacDonald Productions, 2005).

Jasanoff, Sheila, *The Fifth Branch: Science Advisers as Policymakers* (Cambridge, MA; London: Harvard University Press, 1990).

Jensen, Eric, 'The Dao of Human Cloning: Utopian/Dystopian Hype in the British Press and Popular Films', *Public Understanding of Science*, 17/2 (2008): pp. 123–43.

Kerr, Anne, Sarah Cunningham-Burley and Amanda Amos, 'The New Genetics: Professionals' Discursive Boundaries', *The Sociological Review*, 45/2 (1997): pp. 279–303.

Kerr, Anne, Sarah Cunningham-Burley and Amanda Amos, 'The New Genetics and Health: Mobilising Lay-Expertise', *Public Understanding of Science*, 7/1 (1998): pp. 41–60.

Kitzinger, Jenny and Clare Williams, 'Forecasting Science Futures: Legitimising Hope and Calming Fears in the Embryo Stem Cell Debate', *Social Science & Medicine*, 61/3 (2005): pp. 731–40.

Kolata, Gina, *Clone: The Road to Dolly and the Path Ahead* (London: Allen Lane, 1997).

Levin, Ira, *The Boys from Brazil* (London: Pan, 1976).

Marks, Nicola J. 'Localities and Temporalities in Stem Cell Research: Dynamics of Expectation in the UK and Australia'. Paper presented at the *Society for Social Studies of Science Annual Meeting*, Tokyo, Japan, 27 August 2010.

Morley, Katherine I. and Wayne Hall, 'Regulation of Embryonic Stem Cell Research and Therapeutic Cloning: The Australian Debate', *Plaintiff*, 55 (2003): pp. 20–23.

Mulkay, Michael, 'Rhetorics of Hope and Fear in the Great Embryo Debate', *Social Studies of Science*, 23/4 (1993): pp. 721–42.

Mulkay, Michael, 'The Triumph of the Pre-Embryo: Interpretations of the Human Embryo in Parliamentary Debate over Embryo Research', *Social Studies of Science*, 24/4 (1994): pp. 611–39.

Mulkay, Michael, 'Frankenstein and the Debate over Embryo Research', *Science, Technology, & Human Values*, 21/2 (1996): pp. 157–76.

Mulkay, Michael, *The Embryo Research Debate: Science and the Politics of Reproduction* (Cambridge: Cambridge University Press, 1997).

Nelkin, Dorothee and M. Susan Lindee, *The DNA Mystique: The Gene as a Cultural Icon* (New York: W.H. Freeman and Company, 1995).

Nelkin, Dorothee and M. Susan Lindee, 'Cloning in the Popular Imagination', *Cambridge Quarterly of Healthcare Ethics*, 7/2 (1998): pp. 145–9.

Nerlich, Brigitte and David D. Clarke, 'Anatomy of a Media Event: How Arguments Clashed in the 2001 Human Cloning Debate', *New Genetics and Society*, 22/1 (2003): pp. 43–59.

Nerlich, Brigitte, David D. Clarke and Robert Dingwall, 'Clones and Crops: The Use of Stock Characters and Word Play in Two Debates About Bioengineering', *Metaphor and Symbol*, 15/4 (2000): pp. 223–39.

Nerlich, Brigitte, David D. Clarke and Robert Dingwall, 'Fictions, Fantasies, and Fears: The Literary Foundation of the Cloning Debate', *Journal of Literary Semantics*, 30/1 (2001): pp. 37–52.

Ochert, Ayala. *Fear and Cloning*. Times Higher Education Supplement, 30 January 1998 [cited 18 November 2010]. Available at: www.timeshighereducation.co.uk/story.asp?storyCode=105707&sectioncode=26.

O'Riordan, Kate, 'Human Cloning in Film: Horror, Ambivalence, Hope', *Science as Culture*, 17 (2008): pp. 145–62.

Parry, Sarah, 'The Politics of Cloning: Mapping the Rhetorical Convergence of Embryos and Stem Cells in Parliamentary Debates', *New Genetics and Society*, 22/2 (2003): pp. 145–68.

Parry, Sarah, 'Stem Cell Scientists' Discursive Strategies for Cognitive Authority', *Science as Culture*, 18/1 (2009): pp. 89–114.

Petersen, Alan, 'Replicating Our Bodies, Losing Our Selves: News Media Portrayals of Human Cloning in the Wake of Dolly', *Body and Society*, 8/4 (2002): pp. 71–90.

Potter, Jonathan, 'Discourse Analysis and Constructionist Approaches: Theoretical Background', in John T.E. Richardson (ed.) *Handbook of Qualitative Research Methods for Psychology and the Social Sciences* (Leicester: BPS Books, 1996), pp. 125–56.

Potter, Jonathan and Margaret Wetherell, *Discourse and Social Psychology: Beyond Attitudes and Behaviour* (London: Sage, 1987).

Potter, Jonathan and Margaret Wetherell, 'Analyzing Discourse', in Alan Bryman and Robert G. Burgess (eds), *Analyzing Qualitative Data* (London and New York: Routledge, 1994), pp. 47–66.

Prohibition of Human Cloning Act (Canberra: The Parliament of the Commonwealth of Australia, 2002).

R v. *Secretary of State for Health, Ex Parte Bruno Quintavalle on Behalf of Pro-Life Alliance* (2001).

Research Involving Human Embryos Act (Canberra: The Parliament of the Commonwealth of Australia, 2002).

Rose, Nikolas, 'The Politics of Life Itself', *Theory, Culture & Society*, 18/6 (2001): pp. 1–30.

Selin, Cynthia, 'Expectations and the Emergence of Nanotechnology', *Science, Technology, & Human Values*, 32/2 (2007): pp. 196–220.

Shapin, Steven and Simon Schaffer, *Leviathan and the Air-Pump: Hobbes, Boyle, and the Experimental Life* (Princeton: Princeton University Press, 1985).

Shelley, Mary, *Frankenstein or, the Modern Prometheus* (Oxford and New York: Oxford University Press, 1980 [1818]).

Sleeper, directed by Woody Allen (Rollins-Joffe Productions, 1973).

Squier, Susan Merrill, *Liminal Lives: Imagining the Future at the Frontiers of Biomedicine* (Durham, NC and London: Duke University Press, 2004).

Szerszynski, Bronislaw, 'Risk and Trust: The Performative Dimension', *Environmental Values*, 8 (1999): pp. 239–52.

THES Editorial. *Dolly Is Just Cloning Around.* Times Higher Education Supplement, 28 February 1997 [cited 18 November 2010]. Available at: www.timeshighereducation.co.uk/story.asp?storyCode=101838&sectioncode=26.

Thomson, James A., Joseph Itskovitz-Eldor, Sander S. Shapiro, Michelle A. Waknitz, Jennifer J. Swiergiel, Vivienne S. Marshall and Jeffrey M. Jones, 'Embryonic Stem Cell Lines Derived from Human Blastocysts', *Science*, 282/5391 (1998): pp. 1145–7.

Turney, Jon, *Frankenstein's Footsteps: Science, Genetics and Popular Culture* (New Haven, CT and London: Yale University Press, 1998).

Van Dijck, José, *Imagenation: Popular Images of Genetics* (Basingstoke: Macmillan Press, 1998).

Van Dijck, José, 'Cloning Humans, Cloning Literature: Genetics and the Imagination Deficit', *New Genetics and Society*, 18/1 (1999): pp. 9–22.

Waldby, Catherine, *The Visible Human Project: Informatic Bodies and Posthuman Medicine* (London: Routledge, 2000).

Wellcome Trust, *Public Perspectives on Human Cloning. A Social Research Study* (London: The Wellcome Trust, 1998).

Wetherell, Margaret, 'Racism and the Analysis of Cultural Resources in Interviews', in Harry van den Berg, Margaret Wetherell and Hanneke Houtkoop-Steenstra (eds), *Analyzing Race Talk: Multidisciplinary Perspectives on the Research Interview* (Cambridge and New York: Cambridge University Press, 2003), pp. 11–30.

Whitfield, John. *Obituary: Dolly the Sheep*. Nature News Online, 18 February 2003 [cited 30 May 2007]. Available at: www.nature.com/news/2003/030217/full/030217-6.html.

Williams, Clare, Jenny Kitzinger and Lesley Henderson, 'Envisaging the Embryo in Stem Cell Research: Rhetorical Strategies and Media Reporting of the Ethical Debates', *Sociology of Health & Illness*, 25/7 (2003): pp. 793–814.

Wilmut, Ian, Angelika Schnieke, Jim McWhir, Alexamder Kind and Keith Campbell, 'Viable Offspring Derived from Fetal and Adult Mammalian Cells', *Nature*, 385/6619 (1997): pp. 810–13.

Chapter 9
Inventing the Healthy Body: The Use of Popular Medical Discourses in Public Anatomical Exhibitions

Elizabeth Stephens

Over the last decade, a large number of popular anatomical exhibitions – *Body Worlds*, *The Amazing Human Body*, *Bodies: The Exhibition*, *Bodies Revealed*, *Our Body, à corps ouvert*, *Our Body: The Universe Within*, *Body Exploration* and *Mysteries of the Human Body* – have toured across the UK, United States, Europe, Australia and Asia to great popular success. Advertised as 'the anatomical display of real human bodies', these exhibitions feature *écorché* figures (that is, bodies whose skin has been removed to reveal the internal anatomy), preserved through a process of plastination (in which the organic fluids are replaced with a clear synthetic polymer). Displays include whole bodies and dissected figures, as well as single organs, parts of the skeleton, the vascular system, and so on. All of these exhibitions owe their exhibitory styles and the availability of plastinated bodies on which they depend to the foundational work of Gunther von Hagens, the German anatomist who invented the process of plastination, and whose *Body Worlds* was both the first of these anatomical exhibitions and remains the best known.[1] (*Body Worlds* claims to have received over 26 million visitors since its first show, in Tokyo, in 1995.)

The Amazing Human Body exhibition, which toured Australia in 2006 and 2007, exemplifies the curatorial style of these exhibitions. Designed, according to its organizer Dr Wayne Castle, to look 'like a medical textbook', each of the exhibits was surrounded by explanatory text intended to direct the viewers' gaze to a particular part of the body and to provide an account of its function.[2] At the Sydney show, Castle, dressed in a white coat that signified his status as a medical professional, delivered lectures on various aspects of human anatomy, using the exhibits as demonstration models. Publicity material reinforced the show's

---

[1] Although none of these other exhibitions is formally affiliated with *Body Worlds*, they all use von Hagens' patented plastination technology and may well source their exhibits from the same processing facilities. (Given the limited number of facilities, it is likely they are all associated with von Hagens to some degree, although von Hagens has also taken steps to distance himself from his competitors' work.)

[2] Claire Doble, 'What Lies Beneath', *Sydney Morning Herald* (2 February 2006): p. 15.

emphasis on the exhibits' medical significance, stating that its purpose was 'to provide audiences with a unique and educational perspective on the inner working of the human body by viewing real human specimens', thereby enabling visitors 'to make more informed decisions about [the body's] care and keeping' (exhibition pamphlet). Through a series of comparative displays that juxtaposed, for instance, a smoker's lung or alcoholic's liver with healthy specimens of these organs, the exhibition claimed to 'encourage healthy lifestyle choices by serving as a wake-up call that demonstrates how our own choices directly affect our health' (exhibition pamphlet). By its own account, then, the central aim of *The Amazing Human Body* was to encourage its audiences to recognize the importance of educating themselves about anatomy, primarily by representing this as an index of bodily health, thereby attesting to the importance of internalizing the anatomical knowledge on display. In this way, a very explicit interpretative framework was placed around the exhibits, one that instructed the audience how, and to what purpose, these bodies were to be viewed. That is, the exhibition was intended to teach its audiences not only what to see, but *how* to see (through the lens of medical discourses). Specifically, by drawing spectators' attention to the various physical disorders that resulted from unwise 'life-style choices' and 'harmful habits', *The Amazing Human Body* encouraged a particular understanding of bodily health as something within our own control, and which we therefore have a personal responsibility to cultivate and protect.

This chapter examines the role of public anatomical exhibitions like *The Amazing Human Body* in the emergence of a specifically modern concept of health, one that is marked by the distinctive intermixing of the medical and the spectacular found in such spaces. Accordingly, the purpose of this chapter is not simply to recover the historical circumstances in which the anatomies of bodies that can be empirically identified as healthy or unhealthy have been exhibited to the public, but rather to track the invention of a particular *idea* of bodily health, once intricately connected to contemporaneous developments in medical and visual technologies. As such, the convergence of the medical and spectacular, of professional knowledge and popular representation that characterizes exhibitions such as *The Amazing Human Body* is an important site of emergence for modern ideas about bodily health. We see this in the way these shows frame their use of anatomical information, which is repeatedly mobilized as a legitimizing discourse through which to make normative medico-moral judgements about the body and its practices (such as smoking, alcohol and food consumption, etc.), in a way that serves to shame or to motivate spectators about their treatment of their own bodies. Although *The Amazing Human Body* encouraged audiences to internalize the medical guidelines it promotes by representing these as an objective and neutral index of the body's condition or well-being, 'health', as represented in *The Amazing Human Body*, denotes not simply a physical condition or set of recommended prescriptives, but rather a cultural space in which particular understandings of the body come to be privileged precisely through their widespread circulation to, and uptake by, a general public.

In this, too, *The Amazing Human Body* is deeply indebted to Von Hagens' *Body Worlds*, which has provided these subsequent exhibitions not only with the anatomical technology on which they depend but also with the justificatory framework that has fuelled *Body Worlds*' own enormous success. Despite being originally advertised as 'event anatomy' and 'anatomy art', since its relocation to the Unites States in 2004, *Body Worlds* has increasingly focused, like *The Amazing Human Body*, on its educational aspects, promoting itself as a public anatomy lesson designed to teach audiences about the importance of understanding and cultivating practices of bodily care, by 'educat[ing] the public about the inner workings of the human body and show[ing] the effects of poor health, good health and lifestyle choices' (exhibition pamphlet).[3] Von Hagens currently enjoys, and actively pursues, institutional acceptance in the United States, where exhibitions are now held exclusively in science and technology museums.[4] Promotional literature repeatedly refers to von Hagens as the 'world's leading anatomist'.[5] Like Castle, von Hagens often appears in publicity photographs attired in the white coat of a medical professional. This contextualization of public anatomical exhibitions as primarily medical in focus serves to provide a strong justificatory framework for the display of human remains, allowing their proprietors to mobilize – with a considerable degree of success – a widespread pre-existing support for public measures to improve general knowledge about bodily health. In Australia, the *Sydney Morning Herald* warmly endorsed the medical value of *The Amazing*

[3] In 2009, *Body Worlds* had exhibitions in Brussels, Heidelberg and London. Exhibitions run by other operators were also staged in other cities across Europe and the United States. (For instance, *Our Body, à corps ouvert* showed in Paris in May 2009, although this show was closed early due to a strong negative public reaction.) The *Body Worlds* exhibition in London is especially notable as it marked von Hagens' first return to London since his notorious public autopsy, held in an East End art gallery in 2002 and screened on Channel 4 – the first public dissection in Great Britain since the establishment of the Anatomy Act in 1832. (For a description of the autopsy and its reception, see Helen MacDonald, *Human Remains: Episodes in Human Dissection* (Melbourne, 2005), pp. 5–7). The *Body Worlds* exhibitions are part of a suite of three interconnected shows together known as 'The Human Saga', and said to be '[i]nspired by the latest advances in neuroscience, cardiology, biology, genetics, gerontology, psychiatry, and physiology' (www.bodyworlds. com/en/prelude/ human_saga.html).

[4] This shift in the tenor and publicity of *Body Worlds* seems motivated primarily by commercial considerations, in response to the fraught legal status of von Hagens' work in the UK subsequent to his public autopsy. As Schulte-Sasse recognizes, in the United States *Body Worlds* has metamorphosed 'from an enticing but dubious form of entertainment into the ideal family-friendly Sunday outing or junior-high field trip' (Linda Schulte-Sasse, 'Advise and Consent: On the Americanization of Body Worlds', *BioSocieties*, 1/4 (2006): pp. 369–84 on p. 371).

[5] This claim is made on publicity flyers for the show, von Hagens' television series now released on DVD, *Anatomy for Beginners*, and on the exhibition website. Available at: www.bodyworlds.com.

Human Body by confirming that 'as well as the general public, the show will attract those in the industry keen for an incredible learning experience, such as medical students, medical researchers, sporting groups and even artists'.[6]

Despite the support for these exhibitions found in some quarters, however, the public display of actual human remains they feature has also – and unsurprisingly – been a source of considerable controversy, especially given their commercial, profit-motivated nature. Both *Body Worlds* and *The Amazing Human Body* have often provoked intense public reaction, becoming targets of vandalism, theft and protests that have sometimes taken a theatrical turn. In London, Martin Wynness draped a blanket over the plastinate of a pregnant woman, which also showed her seventh-month foetus, after strewing the floor around the display with red paint. Wynness explained to the *Guardian* newspaper: 'A womb and a baby is such a private place. It's between the mother and the child. It's sacred in a way, not even from a religious point of view. Just as a parent and a human, I feel it's a sacred place that doesn't deserve to be looked at. I was looking at a kind of freak show in there … It was horrendous'.[7] Several months later, in December 2002, Amanda Wilson streaked nude through the same London show, as a feminist protest to *Body Worlds*' gendering of anatomy, in which standard, or 'normal', anatomy is depicted as exclusively male. (*Body Worlds* now includes a number of female plastinates in active poses that do not focus on the reproductive system, in direct response to Wilson's actions.)

However, by far the single most contentious issue surrounding *Body Worlds* and other exhibitions of this kind is the provenance of the bodies they put on display. Critics of *Body Worlds*, argues Helen MacDonald, question:

> how [von Hagens] obtains so many bodies. They note that the plants at which they are processed are located in remote places thought to lack ethical credentials where human remains are concerned. One is in China, where von Hagens now lives. Another, a medical institute in Novosibirsk, Russia, ships him suspiciously large numbers of bodies, from people who were mentally ill, destitute, or had been imprisoned.[8]

The swirl of rumour and controversy surrounding *Body Worlds*' acquisition of human bodies that MacDonald describes is best understood, she shows, when contextualized as part of a longer history of anatomical study.

---

6 Doble, 'What Lies Beneath', p. 15.

7 Anthony Browne, '*Body Worlds* Visitor Throws Paint in Protest', *Guardian* (24 March 2002): p. 9.

8 MacDonald, *Human Remains*, pp. 5–6. It is precisely for this reason that *Body Worlds* foregrounds the process – and possibility – of body donation, claiming that all the bodies on display in *Body Worlds* have been voluntarily donated. However, given that the donation agreement requires the estate of the deceased person to meet all shipping costs to Germany, one wonders what percentage of bodies are actually acquired by this means.

Controversy and a sense of public distaste have attended the practice of anatomy and human dissection since its re-emergence as a central part of medical study during the mid-eighteenth century, primarily because, as historians of medicine have widely recognized, dissection was widely believed to defile the physical integrity of the dead body – hence its restriction to the bodies of executed criminals.[9] The practice of anatomy became even more disreputable after the Burke and Hare case, in which Burke was convicted of a series of murders in order to sell victims' bodies to an Edinburgh anatomy school in 1828 inextricably linking anatomists in the public imagination with 'body snatching', or grave-robbers.[10] Given this history of reservations about the practice of professional anatomy, it is not surprising that public anatomical displays as a form of popular entertainment have been considered proportionately even less ethical and much more abhorrent, lacking the counterbalancing justification of scientific research.[11] It is precisely for this reason that critics like Martin Wynness so often compare the display of anatomical exhibits in shows like *Body Worlds* to a Victorian freak show. For the Melbourne *Age*, too, *The Amazing Human Body* was 'little more than a freak show', appealing not to a desire for

---

9 See, for instance Jonathan Sawday's *The Body Emblazoned: Dissection and the Human Body in Renaissance Culture* (New York and London, 1996) or Ruth Richardson's *Death, Dissection, and the Destitute* (London, 2001, 2nd edn). However, as Katherine Park has argued in *Secrets of Women: Gender, Generation, and the Origins of Human Dissection* (New York, 2006) the history of practical anatomy and its public reception is more complex than most histories recognize and begins much earlier. Park's own history largely concentrates on the twelfth and thirteenth centuries, during which time autopsies were undertaken as part of a range of religious and other cultural practices that had little to do with medicine, and were extended to the highest echelons of society (such as aristocratic women who had died in childbirth).

10 Detailed accounts of this history can be found in Brian Bailey's *Burke and Hare: The Year of the Ghouls* (Edinburgh and London, 2002) and Jacques Barzun's volume, edited from the Fenwick Beekman Collection at the New York Academy of Medicine, *Burke and Hare: The Resurrection Men* (New Jersey, 1974). Burke's body was itself donated to the medical school at Edinburgh after execution, and his skeleton is still on display at the University Medical School. A pocket book was also made of his skin and this is on display at the Police Museum on the Royal Mile.

11 Relatively little scholarship has been undertaken on the history of popular anatomical exhibitions and even less on their relationship to the practice of anatomy in popular contexts. The most detailed accounts can be found in Michael Sappol, *A Traffic in Dead Bodies: Anatomy and Embodied Social Identity in Nineteenth-Century America* (Princeton, 2002) and Maritha Rene Burmeister, Popular Anatomical Museums in Nineeteenth-Century England (PhD thesis, 2000), while shorter histories are provided by Alan Bates, 'Dr Kahn's Museum: Obscene Anatomy in Victorian London', *Journal of the Royal Society of Medicine*, 99/12 (2006): pp. 618–24 and Kathryn Hoffman, 'Sleeping Beauties in the Fairground: The Spitzner, Pedley and Chemisé exhibits', *Early Popular Visual Culture*, 4/2 (2006): pp. 139–59.

education about human anatomy but to a prurient taste for the macabre.[12] Von Hagens' often whimsical modelling of his plastinates – turning one into a chest of drawers, fanning the flesh of another into a series of lizard frills – has done little to discourage such comparisons, with such exhibits condemned by many as morbid monstrosities of little anatomical benefit.

Von Hagens, it must be recognized, was initially not averse to capitalizing on this perceived association between *Body Worlds* and the freak show, even exploiting it for publicity purposes by commissioning advertising billboards that promised the spectacle of 'real human bodies!'. Von Hagens clearly recognized this element of the show was part of its popular appeal: 'It is an honour to cause this controversy', he declared in an interview with the *Guardian* in 2002. 'I don't mind if you're sensationalist in your article … More people will come if you are'.[13] Despite this PR bravado, and von Hagens' provocative self-description as the 'Disney of Death',[14] *Body Worlds* is really no closer to the freak show than *The Amazing Human Body* is to the medical textbook: in the first place, freak shows primarily display living models rather than human remains;[15] secondly, they rarely advertise their exhibits as morally improving or instructive;[16] and, finally, freak shows focus on figures of anatomical difference – JoJo the Dog-Faced Boy, the Hottentot Venus, the Elephant Man etc. – whereas anatomical exhibitions predominantly feature displays of 'normal' anatomy. In light of these differences, I would suggest that the reason it is the freak show that is so often invoked by critics challenging these exhibitions' claims to education value or anatomical instruction is because the freak show is now the last popularly remaining vestige of what was once a thriving culture of public displays of anatomy and anatomical difference and the only reference point with which contemporary audiences are likely to be familiar.[17]

---

12 Clay Lucas, 'Melbourne in Line for Corpse Exhibition', *Age* (17 January 2006): p. 8.

13 Stuart Jeffries, 'The Naked and the Dead', *Guardian* (19 March 2002): p. 9.

14 *Anatomy for Beginners* DVD.

15 A number of preserved bodies have been exhibited in freak shows, of course, such as the mummified remains of Julia Pastrana, exhibited during her life as a bearded lady, under names such as 'The Bear Woman' and 'The Nondescript'. 'Pickled punks', or bottled foetuses showing severe congenital deformities, have a long history as popular exhibits in side and freak shows.

16 Although many historians of the freak show argue that its decline as a form of popular entertainment coincides with an increasingly medicalized view of the body, in which such spectacularized displays of anatomical difference come to be increasingly seen as cruel and invasive, I would argue that freak shows have simply absorbed popular medical discourses. Contemporary televised spectacles such as *Medical Incredible* and *Embarrassing Illnesses* are reflective of a new tendency to frame public displays of the freak body as a story of medical treatment or cure.

17 The most detailed histories of the freak show can be found in Rachel Adams, *Sideshow USA: Freaks and the American Cultural Imagination* (Chicago, 2001), Robert Bogdan, *Freak Shows: Presenting Human Oddities for Amusement and Profit* (Chicago and

Although they have now been largely forgotten, public spectacles of anatomy like *Body Worlds* and *The Amazing Human Body* once occupied an important and unique position in popular culture, particularly during the eighteenth and nineteenth centuries, over the course of which they served to transform the public's relationship to, and understanding of, bodily health and care. One of the main reasons this history is now widely overlooked, as Michael Sappol recognizes, is that it has been systematically expunged from official histories of medicine, often assumed to represent an obsolete and marginal tradition, and one further tainted by its later decline into the sleazy forms of the dime museum and freak show.[18] Yet, from the late eighteenth century until the turn of the twentieth, popular exhibitions featuring anatomical displays of human bodies – in the form of skeletal remains, teratology specimens, waxwork models and living exhibits – were enormously popular with a wide range of audiences, marketed variously as teaching facilities for medical professionals, diversionary entertainments for the middle classes, and educational opportunities for the (upper) working classes. Such exhibitions were staged by both commercial operators and professional medical organizations, reflecting an important – and culturally very influential – inter-relationship between the popular and professional spheres, and between spectacular and medical displays of human anatomy. Many of the longest-running and best-known of these sites were commercial enterprises such as Rackstrow's Museum of Anatomy and Curiosities in London (1746–1798), Dr Kahn's Museum of Anatomy in London (1851–1878) and Dr Spitzner's Grand Musée Anatomique, which moved between Paris and Brussels (1863–*c.*1939). The disreputable Dr Jordan, who collaborated with Kahn in the late 1850s, opened a dozen anatomical museums in cities across the United States between the 1860s and 1890s. Others were museums attached to medical colleges but also open to the general public, including The Natural History Museum at the University of Florence, also known as la Specola (founded 1775 and the first public science museum in Europe), the Hunterian Museum in London (originally the private collection of the English surgeon and anatomist, John Hunter, opened as a public institution in 1813), the Mütter Museum of the College of Physicians in Philadelphia (established in 1849), and The National Museum of Health and Medicine in Washington, DC, founded as the Army Medical Museum during the American Civil War in 1862. All of the museums associated with professional organizations remain open today.

London, 1988) and Rosemarie Garland Thomson (ed.), *Freakery: Cultural Spectacles of the Extraordinary Body* (New York, 1996).

[18] For this reason, histories of public anatomical exhibitions are largely to be found within the context of the scholarship on charlatanism and quackery. See, for instance, David Armstrong and Elizabeth Armstrong's *The Great American Medicine Show: Being an Illustrated History of Hucksters, Healers, Health Evangelists, and Heroes from Plymouth Rock to the Present* (New York, 1991) or Brooks McNamara's *Step Right Up*: *An Illustrated History of the American Medicine Show* (Jackson, 1996).

Although the commercial and professional museums listed above were not identical kinds of spaces, neither did they offer neatly distinct kinds of exhibition.[19] Rather, the exhibitory styles they used, and their manner of presenting anatomical displays to a general public, were closely interconnected. This can be seen in the way the curatorial practice of professional medical museums reflects the clear influence of the stylistic conventions established by commercial exhibition spaces (the earliest of which, as the dates above indicate, preceded those of official anatomy museums). An exemplary instance of this is provided by the comparative display of the skeletons of Charles Byrne and Caroline Crachami in the Hunterian Museum, which continues to occupy a prominent position today.[20] Both Byrne and Crachami performed in late eighteenth-century exhibition halls, under the stage names the 'Irish Giant' and the 'Sicilian Dwarf' respectively, and their posthumous display reproduces the commercial convention for exhibiting 'human curiosities' – placed side by side in the same glass cabinet in a way that exaggerates the prodigious height of one body while emphasizing the diminutiveness of the other.

The inter-relationship between spectacular and medical modes of exhibition, and between commercial and professional institutions found in these spaces, is further reflected by the regularity with which entire collections have periodically moved from one context to the other. For instance, the personal collection of John Hunter, originally available for viewing by medical students, practitioners and other interested parties in Hunter's own residence, was bought by the Royal College of Surgeons in London in 1799 and opened as a public museum in 1813.

---

[19] For instance, although commercial and professional museums used many of the same exhibitory techniques and were both open to members of the public (usually with some restrictions), their displays were nonetheless directed to different kinds of audiences, which in turn informed the kinds of material they collected. The Army Medical Museum, for example, was originally designed as a central repository for information about new medical procedures and treatments developed during the Civil War: the museum collected specimens of bones broken by gunshot, accounts of amputation techniques and reconstructive surgeries, and photographic records of case studies, which were eventually published in six vast volumes, *The Medical and Surgical History of the War of the Rebellion*. While the museum was opened to the public within its first few years of operation, then, its central purpose – the dissemination of the knowledge it collated and interpreted – was primarily focused on medical professionals.

[20] The means by which Byrne's and Crachami's bodies were acquired by medical authorities raises a number of important questions about the ethics of official medical museums, and whether these historically differed in any significant way from those of freak shows and other commercial spaces. Byrne was so resistant to the idea of medical dissection and posthumous display that prior to his death he paid two men to sink his body in the Thames, who nonetheless sold his remains to the Royal College of Surgeons. The autopsy of Crachami, who was nine years old at the time of her death, was interrupted by her father, who had not given consent for her dissection and who was (falsely) assured it would be definitively halted (see P. Youngquist, *Monstrosities: Bodies and British Romanticism* (Minneapolis and London, 2003), pp. 5–9).

The Musée d'anatomie, part of the University of Paris's Anatomy Department, was similarly constituted from three private collections – those of Delmas, Rouvière and Ofila. (This museum closed to the public in 2005, although the Musée d'histoire de la medicine, maintained by the Faculty of Medicine at the University of Paris-Descartes, remains open.) Tracing an opposing trajectory, during the late nineteenth and early twentieth centuries, as such collections and the medical knowledge they represented became obsolete, they moved once again from public to private ownership: the Liverpool School of Anatomy's collection, for instance, was sold to Louis Tussaud's museum in Blackpool.[21]

While professional medical sites borrowed their modes of spectacularization from commercial spaces, these latter in turn drew on the authority of established medical institutions in their promotion and publicity as popular entertainments, emphasizing their educational value and importance. In terms almost identical to those used by the *Amazing Human Body* and *Body Worlds* today, eighteenth- and nineteenth-century anatomical exhibitions claimed their central purpose was to instruct audiences in the importance of bodily health and the practices by which it could be cultivated. *The Handbook for Dr Kahn's Museum of Anatomy*, for instance, declares that 'the object of the Museum is to enable every one to become acquainted with the Laws of Health and the detrimental effects of neglecting them'.[22] Similarly, Dr Spitzner's Grand Musée Anatomique provides the following epigraph in its exhibition catalogue:

> Health is the happiness of life.
> Health is joy.
> Health is force.
> Health must be everything for you.
> More than money or property.
> For this keep your body clean. And keep it under constant surveillance.

Like their contemporary counterparts, eighteenth- and nineteenth-century anatomical exhibitions combined their exhortations to study and cultivate one's health with stern warnings about the dire consequences for failing to do so. *The Handbook for Dr Kahn's Museum of Anatomy* couples its urging to attend to one's health with a diagnostic list for various debilitating diseases and disorders whose symptoms extend over three pages, and included such tell-tale conditions as 'dark circles under eyes', 'lethargy' and 'lack of confidence'. By listing such vague complaints as potential indicators of serious and/or fatal illnesses, Kahn (re)produced a view of the body's health as something inherently precarious, and therefore requiring vigilant self-monitoring and constant cultivation. As Kahn's text shows, by the nineteenth century it is no longer enough to avoid disease and

---

[21] This museum still exists, now as part of the Ripley chain, although this earlier material is no longer on public display.

[22] Dr Kahn, *Handbook of Dr Kahn's Museum* (London, 1863), p. 75.

treat disorders – in addition, one must constantly work to protect and improve one's health by undertaking reflexive and medicalized practices of self-care.

In this respect, museums like Kahn's and Spitzner's are significant not simply for what they reveal about the actual medical knowledge of health during the periods in which they operated – for the specific information they provided about what constitutes health and how best to cultivate it – but also for the way they reflect the emergence of a newly medicalized view of the body and its broader cultural consequences. As such, these public exhibitions of anatomy were an important space in which the cultural authority of medicine was actively promoted, repeatedly cited as a privileged source of knowledge about the body. In this way, anatomical museums like Kahn's functioned to confirm the growing status of medicine as '[t]he most prestigious social institution in Western culture'.[23] They did this, in part, by providing a forum in which medical discourses could be circulated amongst a wide and general audience, thereby serving to popularize new medical treatments and technologies. At the same time, however, these sites not only communicate a particular kind of medical knowledge but also promote a very specific way of relating to one's own body: as something that requires constant self-surveillance and self-cultivation. As in *The Amazing Human Body* and *Body Worlds*, medical knowledge in nineteenth-century anatomical exhibitions is represented as something to be internalized, a context through which we are increasingly encouraged to see and experience ourselves and our corporealities.

In this way, 'health', in these contexts, less signifies a medically measurable state or recognizable physical condition than it describes a process, an ongoing relationship we are encouraged to develop with our own bodies and through which we are trained to understand their practices and functions. For this reason, we might best understand the idea of 'health' invoked in and by these spaces not as a stable entity or concept, but rather as a domain of knowledge in the Foucauldian sense – a field of (self-)cultivation and (self-)discipline, a discursive field in which the spectacular and the medical, popular culture and professional practice, converge in their representation and understanding of the body. Recognition of the extent to which ideas about health, and the value attributed to its cultivation, are inflected by wider cultural values and assumptions is especially important given how often such information is treated as somehow objectively true and unmediated, presented to the public with all the neutrality of 'a medical textbook'. As Cressida Heyes has recently argued, even feminist critics of the diet industry often assume a direct correlation between body size and health, and between 'amount eaten and body weight'.[24] The apparent neutrality of health discourses is, moreover, a direct result of the particular modes of representation these use, which function in and through their own (self-)erasure. We see this double-gesture

[23] Sander Gilman, *Creating Beauty to Cure the Soul: Race and Psychology in the Shaping of Aesthetic Surgery* (Durham, 1998), p. 25.

[24] Cressida Heyes, *Self-Transformations: Foucault, Ethics and Normalized Bodies* (Oxford, 2007), p. 69.

in anatomical exhibitions like *The Amazing Human Body* and *Body Worlds*, which simultaneously spectacularize figures of the un/healthy body within a commercial context while promoting their exhibits as sources of unmediated, or 'textbook', medical information. This apparently neutral 'non-style', to which, as Amy Werbel recognizes, medical images often lay claim, has its origins in the changing conventions found in nineteenth-century medical photography, itself representing 'a very special mode of rhetoric, the rhetoric of disinterested objectivity'.[25] As a result, notes Sander Gilman, medical professionals and historians of medicine alike have tended to marginalize the role played by visual images in the production and circulation of medical knowledge, assuming these to serve a purely illustrative purpose, despite the fact that 'the culture of medicine is as heavily involved with visual culture as any other aspect of modern cultural history'.[26] Yet visual technologies and conventions are not simply the modes or means by which medical (or any other kind) of knowledge is disseminated but rather, as the anatomical exhibitions examined above show, actually constitutive of that knowledge. For instance, *Body Worlds*' gendering of anatomy – itself consistent with a longer tradition that extends back to the earliest popular anatomical displays[27] – does not simply disseminate anatomical information but actively produces those objects of knowledge in and through the practice of their display.

The idea of health mobilized in such spaces, as we have seen above, thus functions both as a disciplinary technology – requiring one to regulate one's body and its practices in accordance with cultural norms – and also as a process of self-cultivation and self-improvement, a means by which to better and deepen our knowledge of ourselves. Both of these functions are clearly visible in the promotional rhetoric of the twentieth-century anatomical exhibitions examined at the start of this chapter, as well as in that of the eighteenth- and nineteenth-century museums discussed above: in all of these spaces, health is the name given to the injunction to constantly monitor and improve our bodies, to internalize the information on display and thus to constitute ourselves the willing subjects of health.

---

[25] Amy Werbel, *Thomas Eakins: Art, Medicine, and Sexuality in Nineteenth-Century Philadelphia* (New Haven, 2007), p. 103.

[26] Sander Gilman, *Picturing Health and Illness: Images of Difference* (Baltimore and London, 1995), p. 11.

[27] Specifically, von Hagens' representation of pregnant bodies is continuous with that of the waxwork 'anatomical Venuses' manufactured from the mid-eighteenth century onwards, and which were the most popular exhibit in Rackstrow's, Kahn's and Spitzner's museums. And, as the responses to *Body Worlds* already cited above demonstrates, these exhibits continue to be the central focus of public interest and response. The original Venuses were gynaemorphic waxworks that included extraneous details such as pearl necklaces, open mouths and hair ribbons, which reveal as much about contemporaneous ideas of femininity and maternity as they do about female reproductive anatomy (see Ludmilla Jordanova, *Sexual Visions: Images of Gender in Science and Medicine between the Eighteenth and Twentieth Centuries* (Madison, 1989), p. 50).

The practices of self-cultivation they encourage must therefore be understood both as a medico-moral imperative and as part of a broader emergent culture of self-improvement, whose strictures are so often internalized as self-realizing and highly individuating. Moreover, these functions of health are not contradictory but rather mutually reinforcing: as Foucault has so famously argued, the exercise of power is not only repressive but also productive, in this case constituting our subjectivity through our compulsory interaction with health discourses even as it provides new avenues for self-making that often extend beyond the normative constraints of those discourses.

The public exhibitions of human anatomy, which emerged during the mid-eighteenth century and remain popular today, in this way prove and disprove Foucault's argument in *Discipline and Punish*, that the grand spectacles of punishment as seen in grisly public executions disappear by the early nineteenth century, to be replaced by a new disciplinary technology that functions through the constant surveillance and management of bodies. The culture of public anatomical exhibitions examined in this chapter at once represents an ongoing cultural investment in the function of spectacles as a form of discipline *and* their transformation into new normalizing technologies that encourage an internalized self-surveillance. We see this in anatomical exhibitions' insistence that we 'look inside' the body to see 'what lies underneath' (*Body Worlds* exhibition pamphlet), and in their displays of diseased hearts or smokers' lungs that warn that damaged health is not always evident on the surface of the body but only properly visible from within. By this means, exhibitions like *Body Worlds* and *The Amazing Human Body* exemplify the broader trajectory of medical discourses over the last two and a half centuries, with their progressive privileging of the visual and increasing penetration of the interior spaces of the body. The spectacularization of the *écorché* body within the context of public exhibitions (re)produces an 'anatomical vision' in which the body is seen as something that must be opened up to reveal a truth or knowledge hidden inside it. Just as contemporary visual technologies – endoscopes, ultrasounds, magnetic resonance imaging – have made the interiority of the body increasingly transparent to medical professionals, the flayed and sliced bodies in *The Amazing Human Body* and *Body Worlds* promise us the ability to gaze into the recesses of the body with uninterrupted visibility.

As historians of medicine have recognized, this anatomical vision of the body is one that emerged during the early modern period, co-extensive with the gradual resumption of dissection as a public and professional practice, but also indicative of the wider transformations in systems of knowledge at this time.[28] This shift in ways of seeing, exemplified by this newly medicalized vision of the body, played a pivotal role in the construction of the modern subject as an individuated and autonomous entity, while also serving to make that subject's body fully visible to

[28] Sawday, *The Body Emblazoned*; Barbara Stafford, *Body Criticism: Imaging the Unseen in Enlightenment Art and Medicine* (Cambridge, MA, 1991); Michel Foucault, *Birth of the Clinic: An Archaeology of Medical Perception* (London, 1973).

new systems of power. In this way, we can see that, just as the new bio-political systems emergent during the eighteenth century produced the autonomous subject of modernity, so did the rise of practical anatomy invent the healthy subject who is assumed to be rational about, and individually responsible for, the condition of his or her body – increasingly held to be a consequence of 'lifestyle choices' and personal habits, rather than, for instance, economic or environmental factors (such as public sanitation).

In teaching us to see our bodies as the external expression of a constructed interiority, anatomical exhibitions from the mid-eighteenth century to the present have shaped our relationship to our bodies in ways that remain profoundly influential. In particular, public anatomical exhibitions are an important site at which one of the central messages of modern medicine is reproduced and disseminated to a broad audience: that health is always improvable and the body perfectible. With their influential combination of the spectacular and the medical, anatomical exhibitions thus serve to reinforce the cultural status of medicine while also drawing on its authority to justify their own public displays of human anatomy. Despite their apparent cultural marginality, popular anatomical exhibitions have left behind an enduring legacy in the way we understand our relationships to our own bodies, encouraging us to see work on the body as a form of work on the self. As such, anatomical exhibitions have played, and continue to play, an important role in the history of medicine's popularization while also drawing attention to the centrality of medicine to the history of popular culture. It is at the intersection of these two fields, as this chapter has shown, that modern ideas of health and the healthy subject emerge – a subject that continues to be both the focus of professional advice and popular fascination.

Bibliography

Primary Sources

The Amazing Human Body exhibition flyer (Sydney, 2006).
Body Worlds exhibition flyer (Philadelphia, 2006).
www.bodyworlds.com (accessed 6 April 2009).
www. bodyworlds.com/en/prelude/ human_saga.html (accessed 6 April 2009).

Secondary Sources

Adams, Rachel, *Sideshow USA: Freaks and the American Cultural Imagination* (Chicago: University of Chicago Press, 2001).

Armstrong, David and Elizabeth Metzger Armstrong, *The Great American Medicine Show: Being an Illustrated History of Hucksters, Healers, Health Evangelists, and Heroes from Plymouth Rock to the Prese* (New York: Prentice Hall, 1991).

Bailey, Brian, *Burke and Hare: The Year of the Ghouls* (Edinburgh and London: Mainstream, 2002).
Barzun, Jacques (ed.), *Burke and Hare: The Resurrection Men* (Metuchen, NJ: Scarecrow Press, 1974).
Bates, Alan, 'Dr Kahn's Museum: Obscene Anatomy in Victorian London', *Journal of the Royal Society of Medicine*, 99/12 (2006): pp. 618–24.
Bogdan, Robert, *Freak Show: Presenting Human Oddities for Amusement and Profit* (Chicago and London: University of Chicago Press, 1988).
Browne, Anthony, '*Body Worlds* Visitor Throws Paint in Protest', *Guardian*, 24 March 2002: p. 9.
Burmeister, Maritha Rene, Popular Anatomical Museums in Nineteenth-Century England (PhD thesis, Rutgers University, 2000).
Doble, Claire, 'What Lies Beneath', *Sydney Morning Herald*, 2 February 2006.
Foucault, Michel, *Birth of the Clinic: An Archaeology of Medical Perception*, trans. A.M. Sheridan Smith (London: Tavistock, 1973).
Foucault, Michel, *Discipline and Punish: The Birth of the Prison*, trans. Alan Sheridan (London: Allen Lane, 1977).
Garland Thomson, Rosemarie (ed.), *Freakery: Cultural Spectacles of the Extraordinary Body* (New York: University of New York Press, 1996).
Gilman, Sander, *Picturing Health and Illness: Images of Difference* (Baltimore and London: Johns Hopkins University Press, 1995).
Gilman, Sander, *Creating Beauty to Cure the Soul: Race and Psychology in the Shaping of Aesthetic Surgery* (Durham, NC: Duke University Press, 1998).
Heyes, Cressida, *Self-Transformations: Foucault, Ethics, and Normalized Bodies* (Oxford: Oxford University Press, 2007).
Hoffmann, Kathryn, 'Sleeping Beauties in the Fairground: The Spitzner, Pedley and Chemisé Exhibits', *Early Popular Visual Culture*, 4/2 (2006): pp. 139–59.
Jeffries, Stuart, 'The Naked and the Dead', *Guardian*, 19 March 2002.
Jordanova, Ludmilla, *Sexual Visions: Images of Gender in Science and Medicine Between the Eighteenth and Twentieth Centuries* (Madison: University of Wisconsin Press, 1989).
Kahn, Dr, *Handbook of Dr Kahn's Museum* (London: W. Snell, 1863).
Lucas, Clay, 'Melbourne in Line for Corpse Exhibition', *Age*, 17 January 2006.
MacDonald, Helen, *Human Remains: Episodes in Human Dissection* (Melbourne: University of Melbourne Press, 2005).
McNamara, Brooks, *Step Right Up: An Illustrated History of the American Medicine Show* (Jackson: University of Mississippi Press, 1996).
Park, Katharine, *Secrets of Women: Gender, Generation, and the Origins of Human Dissection* (New York: Zone, 2006).
Richardson, Ruth, *Death, Dissection, and the Destitute* (London: Phoenix, 2001).
Sappol, Michael, *A Traffic of Dead Bodies: Anatomy and Embodied Social Identity in Nineteenth-Century America* (Princeton: Princeton University Press, 2002).
Sawday, Jonathan, *The Body Emblazoned: Dissection and the Human Body in Renaissance Culture* (New York and London: Routledge, 1996).

Schulte-Sasse, Linda, 'Advise and Consent: On the Americanization of Body Worlds', *BioSocieties*, 1/4 (2006): pp. 369–84.

Stafford, Barbara, *Body Criticism: Imaging the Unseen in Enlightenment Art and Medicine* (Cambridge, MA: MIT Press, 1991).

Von Hagens, Gunther, *Anatomy for Beginners*, DVD.

Werbel, Amy, *Thomas Eakins: Art, Medicine, and Sexuality in Nineteenth-Century Philadelphia* (New Haven: Yale University Press, 2007).

Youngquist, P., *Monstrosities: Bodies and British Romanticism* (Minneapolis and London: University of Minnesota Press, 2003).

Epilogue
'Thanks for the Thanksgiving Service'

Leo Brown

In 1992 the University of Queensland inaugurated an annual ceremony to say thank you publicly to those people who had chosen to donate their bodies after death for dissection and study by students learning about human anatomy. The Thanksgiving Service is conducted to give the families of those people an opportunity for acknowledgement of their loved ones' generosity and gives the students an opportunity to meet and thank the families face-to-face. As awareness of the ceremony has increased, the service has also now come to play a valuable secondary role in introducing people in the wider community to the idea that donating their body is something that they might themselves consider. I am the programme coordinator of that ceremony and it is also my role to mediate the donation, reception and ultimate burial or cremation of the donor's body, through working with the donor and/or their families.

The early use of deceased human bodies in Australia involved mainly unclaimed bodies and people who died in institutions. This practice has now changed and all bodies made available for educational reasons are obtained through well-established body donor programmes. The teaching of human anatomy, using deceased human bodies, has been conducted at the University of Queensland since 1927 and has provided unique experiences for thousands of students gaining foundation knowledge of the structure of the human body. The aim of the programme is to render as comforting as possible for the donors and their families the transition from living person, to deceased person, to human body, to the less personal, but both humanly and medically valued, 'cadaver'. The students, as well as many practitioners, regularly comment how privileged they feel to have had access to cadavers for their studies.

The wishes of the person whose body is to be used in this way are paramount and my work has been an education in how to understand the ways in which people of all ages think about – or choose not to think about – their own anticipated deaths or the death of a loved one. Over many years I have spoken to thousands of people about the process and the benefits of donating bodies to 'medical science'. Whilst death is accepted as inevitable in a basic, rational sense, detailed discussion on the topic seems often to be avoided for fear of one being characterized as a morbid person. There is never a good time to raise the subject, as it is a very personal matter and people will talk about it when they consider that the time, place and audience is appropriate. It is a question which tends to evoke hesitant responses: 'Not just now', 'Maybe next week', 'I'm not ready to talk about that topic', 'I'd rather talk about that in private'. This seems to change as people age. I have found that end-of-life arrangements do not feature highly in social conversation topics of the younger generation, whereas older people are more inclined to discuss the subject. It appears that as people move through life and become more settled into their careers, there is a realization that there will come a time when they will die. At this time, there is more of an acceptance of talking about death and after-death arrangements for their body. And whilst parents are often prepared to talk about after-death arrangements, their children can be rather reluctant to discuss the matter. I have found that even though the families of body donors generally are aware of the wishes of their relative and are willing to carry out those instructions, it can sometimes be challenging to abide by the bequest of the deceased. Whilst the death of an older person can be expected, it is still surrounded with sadness and grief for the family and, for that reason, these decisions can be more easily made if there has been open discussion prior to the death of the donor. Every effort is made to assist the relatives in making the decision that best suits the situation, taking into consideration the concerns of all parties involved, both living and deceased. Advance directives from the donor are the most common way for bodies to be made available for the programme.

In the programme itself, the bodies are used mainly for the conduct of practical classes to complement the theoretical study undertaken by students studying human anatomy. These donated bodies also provide opportunities for the skill- and knowledge-development of practising surgeons and other health professionals. One of the major advantages in having cadavers is being able to study the structure of the human body in three dimensions and to identify the anatomical variations found in different cadavers. At the beginning of each year, anatomy students receive a general induction to the anatomy laboratory which includes a session on the topic of using human bodies for learning anatomy. It is emphasized to these students that they are in a very privileged position that enables them to gain great benefit from the special gift of the body of a donor. Students are also encouraged to discuss with staff any concerns that they may have about studying or dissecting a human body. At all times, the cadavers are treated with dignity and respect, and our donors are remembered for their generosity and their special contribution to education. The deceased donors are in our care for two to three years after which time they are cremated and their ashes made available to their families for final commitment and memorialization.

In recognition of these donations, the university conducts a Thanksgiving Service for Body Donors annually, paying tribute to the donors and their families. The initial Thanksgiving Service was conducted at the University of Queensland in 1992 following an initiative by a Senior Lecturer in Anatomy, Dr Walter Wood, who considered that it would be appropriate to demonstrate our gratitude to the families of the donors. The Thanksgiving Service was held in Mayne Hall in April 1992, paying tribute to those donors who died in 1990 and their bodies were cremated in 1992. The first organizing committee was made up of representatives from Chaplaincy, Religious Studies, Anatomy and Music Departments as well as Media and Protocol sections. The multi-faith service provides an opportunity for students to talk directly to the families of the deceased donors, express their gratitude and relate to them the benefits gained from having access to human cadavers for their studies. I've always found that both the families and students gain mutual benefit from this interaction.

Initially the service relied on voluntary labour and donations: anatomy students provided floral tributes for distribution to families; the Brisbane Crematoria Group organized the purchase of a Book of Remembrance and the inscription of the donors' names in it and a coffin manufacturer donated a cabinet for the permanent display of the Book of Remembrance. The service starts with a formal processing of the Book of Remembrance and a single candle, accompanied by academic staff and students. The book and candle are placed in a prominent position on stage, to signal the start of the service. A central element of the service is the lighting of commemorative candles, symbolizing the passage of the knowledge from the deceased donors to the student groups. An Anatomy tutor passes the central candle to other students who in turn light a series of candles representing the various groups who gain benefit from the bodies of the donors being honoured. The deceased donors are then honoured by the public reading of their names followed by a period of silence. Throughout the service, students, staff and faith representatives deliver prayers and readings. These are supported by choral and musical arrangements. The service concludes with the Book of Remembrance being carried out by a recent graduate in formal procession to a designated Reflection Area where the Book is placed on display for all attendees to view the names of the donors. The families are invited to light remembrance candles and sign a Visitors' Book prior to joining staff and students for supper.

The families of body donors are encouraged to arrange an event to mark the occasion of the death and the acceptance of the donor's body into the care of the university. Whilst most donor families have made such arrangements with families and friends, those who have not done so find that the Thanksgiving Service provides them with the opportunity to make their final farewell to the deceased donor. Some staff and students attend regularly and comment that it assists them in maintaining a realization of the importance of recognizing the contribution to education that is made by body donors.

With the success of the first Thanksgiving Service and with the support of the senior management of the university, subsequent services gained additional momentum and improvements have continued annually. We have been fortunate to have a variety of students always willing to take part, either as direct participants, or interacting with families expressing their gratitude for the benefits gained. We estimate that around 40 per cent of all students who use the donated cadavers in their studies choose to attend the service. We have also been able to attract donations to assist with the payment or provision of support for the service and we are indebted to all of these people and organizations who have contributed to the establishment and regular conduct of the service.

The Thanksgiving Service has been recognized as an extremely important community outreach event providing an important linkage between the university and the community. The publicity surrounding the Thanksgiving Service continues to generate awareness of the body donor programme, thereby increasing the registration of donors and ensuring a continuing supply of educational opportunities for future students.

The Thanksgiving Service Organising Committee endeavours to introduce a new element each year which adds variety to the service to ensure that each event has its own special appeal and remembrance factor, especially for those families who come along and say ‘Thanks for The Thanksgiving Service’. An example of this initiative is the inclusion of the distribution of student testimonials. A selection of these testimonials is distributed to the families and friends of donors who attend the Thanksgiving Service. Here is a short letter written by a student to demonstrate his gratitude for the gift that had assisted him in his studies. It’s simply titled ‘Thanks to Donors’:

> In your life, you laughed and wept, loved and lost. You have been a son or a daughter, husband or wife, mother or father. But such things must pass.
>
> So you came to us at the end of your life’s journey, just as your family were suffering their bitterest grief.
>
> Now, each day you are helping a future obstetrician to save the life of a mother and infant in difficult labour. You are helping a future surgeon to heal a father rescued from car wreckage.
>
> Except by our Roll of Honour, those people will never know your name. But they will be forever indebted to your life.
>
> We are enmeshed: you and I, doctor and patient, past and future. You have become so many everyday acts of human kindness. Through your gift, others will live; through others, you live on. Your final gift transcends the death that brought you into our care.
>
> We thank your family for their grace. We thank you for your charity, your selfless choice.
>
> A grateful student.

Even though the focus in this short epilogue has been on matters surrounding death and the use of human bodies, organs and tissues, the lesson I take from my experiences is that it is important to develop our capacity to think and speak about life and death more generally and I encourage people to engage more in open dialogue on these deeply personal issues. This will assist us all in gaining a better understanding of each other, help us to respect other people's point of view and share information and knowledge, as well as being better prepared to meet challenges as they arise.

Index